ESSENTIAL
MUSCULOSKELETAL MRI

Commissioning Editor: Claire Wilson
Development Editor: Carole McMurray
Project Manager: Glenys Norquay
Page Design: Stewart Larking
Cover Design: Charles Gray
Illustration Manager: Bruce Hogarth

ESSENTIAL
MUSCULOSKELETAL MRI
A PRIMER FOR THE CLINICIAN

by

Michelle A Wessely BSc (Chiro) DC DACBR FCCR (Can) FCC (UK/Radiology) Dip MEd

Director of Radiology, Institut Franco-Europeen de Chiropratique (IFEC), Ivry-sur-Seine/Paris and Toulouse, France

Martin F Young BSc (Phys) BSc (Chiro) DC FCC MEWI

Private practice, Yeovil, Somerset, UK

With contributions by

Renée M deVries
Nicholas Green
Julie-Marthe Grenier
Kristin L Hurtgen-Grace
Anita L Manne
Peter J Scordilis
David R Seaman

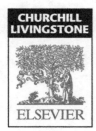

Edinburgh London New York Oxford Philadelphia St Louis Sydney Toronto 2011

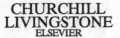

ISBN 9780443067266

British Library Cataloguing in Publication Data
A catalogue record for this book is available from the British Library

Library of Congress Cataloging in Publication Data
A catalog record for this book is available from the Library of Congress

Notices
Knowledge and best practice in this field are constantly changing. As new research and experience broaden our understanding, changes in research methods, professional practices, or medical treatment may become necessary.

Practitioners and researchers must always rely on their own experience and knowledge in evaluating and using any information, methods, compounds, or experiments described herein. In using such information or methods they should be mindful of their own safety and the safety of others, including parties for whom they have a professional responsibility.

With respect to any drug or pharmaceutical products identified, readers are advised to check the most current information provided (i) on procedures featured or (ii) by the manufacturer of each product to be administered, to verify the recommended dose or formula, the method and duration of administration, and contraindications. It is the responsibility of practitioners, relying on their own experience and knowledge of their patients, to make diagnoses, to determine dosages and the best treatment for each individual patient, and to take all appropriate safety precautions.

To the fullest extent of the law, neither the Publisher nor the authors, contributors, or editors, assume any liability for any injury and/or damage to persons or property as a matter of products liability, negligence or otherwise, or from any use or operation of any methods, products, instructions, or ideas contained in the material herein.

your source for books, journals and multimedia in the health sciences
www.elsevierhealth.com

Working together to grow libraries in developing countries
www.elsevier.com | www.bookaid.org | www.sabre.org

ELSEVIER   BOOK AID International   Sabre Foundation

The Publisher's policy is to use paper manufactured from sustainable forests

Printed in China

Contributors

Renée M DeVries DC DACBR
Associate Professor and Dean of the College of
Chiropractic, Northwestern Health Sciences University,
Bloomington, Minnesota, USA

Nicholas Green DC
Chiropractor, Cor Maximus, North Bay, ON, Canada

Julie-Marthe Grenier DC DACBR
Professor, Department of Chiropractic, Université du
Québec à Trois-Rivières, Trois-Rivières, QC, Canada

Kristin L Hurtgen-Grace DC DACBR
Formerly of School of Applied Sciences, University of
Glamorgan, Pontypridd, Wales, UK

Anita L Manne DC DACBR
Professor and Chair of the Department of Diagnostic
Imaging, Northwestern Health Sciences University,
Bloomington, Minnesota, USA

Peter J Scordilis DC CSCS
Clinical Director, Harrison Spine and Rehabilitation,
Director, Scordilis Family Chiropractic, New Jersey, USA

David R Seaman BS MS DC
Assistant Professor, Palmer Chiropractic University,
Florida, USA

Introduction

One of the key components to successful management of a patient is the clinician's ability to communicate with that patient. The more the patient understands about what is wrong with them, what is going to be done about it and what they can expect from their treatment, the more compliant they are, the more positive their attitude and the better their outcome.

Given that a picture can be worth a thousand words, many practitioners' offices are stuffed with anatomical models, charts and diagrams to help them explain the anatomical and physiological detail of a patient's problem. There is, however, one sort of picture that carries a disproportionate weight with patients. Diagnostic imaging has a unique ability to reveal the mysteries hidden beneath the surface. Unlike, say, blood tests, the results are tangible: this is a picture of the person you are addressing, the problem can be seen directly and the patient can easily identify with it.

Most healthcare professionals rub along quite happily with x-rays; even a fairly basic understanding of skeletal anatomy is sufficient to be able to interpret a radiologist's report, and specialists from many disciplines are suitably qualified or experienced to draw their own conclusions from the radiograph. Communicating the findings from plain film examination to the patient is therefore something with which most clinicians feel comfortable.

As soon as specialized imaging is involved, the situation changes dramatically. Each image contains far more information, no longer does one just have to look at bones; suddenly, there is a wealth of detail about the soft tissues and their appearance can vary tremendously from sequence to sequence and plane to plane. There are dozens of images that must be sifted through and dozens of structures that must be evaluated and correlated to the patient's history and examination findings. How much easier then to just read out the radiologist's report ... and how much less effective, both for doctor and patient.

This book is the result of years of work; a collaboration between radiologists who wanted to use the increasing accessibility of digital images to bring radiology back to the consulting room and clinicians who wanted to be able to use magnetic resonance imaging to improve their clinical skills and patient management. It is intended to give anyone involved in treating musculoskeletal conditions the insight to be able to order and interpret magnetic resonance images with confidence and to explain to their patients the details of their findings as easily as they would for physical examination findings or plain film radiographs.

Whether a family doctor, physical therapist, manual physician, orthopaedist or student, the logical development of each chapter should give you the background to understand the nature of what you will see on a magnetic resonance image, the skill to start to understand it and the knowledge to correlate the findings with those from your own examination of the patient ... practice will make perfect, and the accompanying CD-ROM will give you the opportunity to ensure you have grasped the necessary essentials and can apply them.

Instead of a threat, magnetic resonance images should be the clinician's friend; this book should help cement the friendship, regular reference can help make it lifelong.

Martin Young
Michelle A. Wessely

Contents

Magnetic resonance

Principles and application to diagnostic imaging

Martin Young   Michelle A. Wessely   Renée M. DeVries

Introduction

Nuclear magnetic resonance (NMR), the principle on which magnetic resonance (MR) imaging is based, was discovered independently in 1946 by Felix Bloch and Edward Purcell; they were jointly awarded the Nobel Prize for physics in 1952.[1] The first actual image was produced by Paul Lauterbur; although it was grainy and fuzzy, it nevertheless showed the difference between ordinary and 'heavy' water (D_2O). The importance of MR imaging has been such that he too went on to win a Nobel Prize of his own in 2003.[2] The first human image was captured in 1977.[3]

The name 'nuclear magnetic resonance' was altered to 'magnetic resonance imaging' in the 1980s. The official reason given was the public's negative connotation with the word 'nuclear', particularly after the accident at the Three Mile Island power station in 1979. The unofficial explanation was that hospital workers feared that NMR might stand for 'No More Radiographers', whereas MRI could only mean 'More Radiographers Immediately'.[4]

Magnetic resonance imaging uses powerful computer algorithms to generate multiplanar imaging slices through the body.[5] Because it does not utilize ionizing radiation and provides a greater degree of contrast between the different soft tissues of the body than does computed tomography (CT), it is particularly useful in cardiovascular, musculoskeletal, neurological and oncological imaging.[6] The relative lack of attendant safety issues also means that it is a modality that can be used to monitor the course of a condition or the response to treatment by repeat imaging.[6] Although MR imaging is generally safe and

non-invasive, there are circumstances in which it is contraindicated; these are detailed in Box 1.01.[7]

In place of x-rays, MR imaging uses a powerful magnetic field to align the magnetic moments of certain atoms within the body. Radiofrequency fields are then used to alter the alignment of this magnetization, which causes the atomic nuclei to produce a rotating magnetic field, specific to each tissue type, which is detectable by a receptor inside the scanner. This signal can then be manipulated to build sufficient information to construct an image of the body.[4,8]

Magnetic resonance

Subatomic particles, such as protons, neutrons, positrons and electrons, have the property of *spin*, causing the particle to act as a magnetic dipole; that is, having north and south poles.[4,9] If two such particles pair up, the laws of magnetic attraction and repulsion mean that they will point in opposite directions and cancel each other out, so that the resultant particle has no overall magnetism. Certain nuclei, such as ^1H, which consists of a single proton, ^3He, ^{13}C, ^{23}Na and ^{31}P, have an uneven number of protons and neutrons, and therefore have an unpaired particle, giving the nucleus an overall magnetism, known as the **magnetic moment**.[3,4]

This effect is particularly strong in hydrogen, which does not have other particles to 'dilute' the relative strength of its magnetic moment; it is this nucleus, therefore, that is of primary importance in MR imaging.[4,10] Hydrogen has two spin states, sometimes referred to as 'up' and 'down'.[9] When these spins are placed in a strong external magnetic

DOI: 10.1016/B978-0-443-06726-6.00001-9

Box 1.01

MRI contraindications or relative contraindications

- Brain aneurysm clip
- Implanted neural stimulator
- Implanted cardiac pacemaker or defibrillator
- Cochlear implant
- Ocular foreign body (e.g. metal shavings)
- Other implanted medical devices (e.g. Swan Ganz catheter)
- Insulin pump
- Metal shrapnel or bullet
- First trimester pregnancy
- Patients with unstable angina
- Claustrophobia, which affects up to 10% of patients, used to be regarded as a relative contraindication and patients would often need sedation before being able to enter the scanner; however, recent improvement in scanning technology has allowed the advent of the 'open' scanner whereby, instead of entering a narrow tunnel, patients lie between two plates that are open to the sides (see Figure 1.06)
- Extreme obesity
- Certain patients are contraindicated for the administration of MRI contrast agents:
  - lactating women
  - patients with haemoglobinopathies
  - patients with renal disease (decreased glomerular filtration rate)

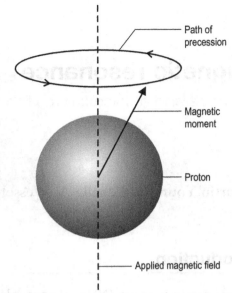

Figure 1.01 • The magnetic moment of the proton precesses about the flux lines of the applied magnetic field.

field, such as that found in an MRI scanner, they precess around an axis along the direction of the field (Figure 1.01).[11] Most protons have low energies and will align with the magnetic field; however, a small number have sufficient energy to have an anti-parallel alignment.[11]

The frequency with which the protons precess (ω_0) is directly proportional to the strength of the magnetic field (B). In a magnetic field of 1 tesla, of the order found in MR scanners, hydrogen atoms will precess at precisely 42.6 MHz, which is in the radio wave band of the electromagnetic spectrum. This value, which varies from nucleus to nucleus as well as with magnetic field strength, is known as the **Larmor frequency**.[4,11]

Energy absorption

Applying a radiofrequency pulse of this value at 90° to the magnetic field causes the hydrogen nuclei, *and only the hydrogen nuclei*, to resonate; other nuclei –

even if they have dipoles – will have their own unique resonance frequency for a given magnetic field. The hydrogen nuclei absorb energy from the pulse, which increases their net energy and, therefore, the number of high-energy anti-parallel protons. If exactly the right amount of energy is applied, this will result in the magnetic fields of the combined hydrogen magnetic moments cancelling each other out; effectively, the **net magnetization vector** of the hydrogen nuclei lies at 90° to the applied field.[4,12]

Phase coherence

The applied radiofrequency pulse also causes the rotating magnetic moments of the hydrogen nuclei to move into phase with each other; this is known as *phase coherence*. It affects all of the nuclei, so the low-energy 'spin up' protons are in phase both with each other and with the high-energy 'spin down' protons. This means that the net magnetization vector now precesses in exactly the same way as the individual protons at the Lamor frequency.[4,12]

The MR signal

The image detector in MR imaging is an electromagnetic coil, which acts as a receiver. It is placed at 90° to the applied magnetic field in what is known as the transverse plane; the direction of the magnetic field is the **longitudinal plane**. Whilst the net magnetization vector lies in the transverse plane, its precession means that it passes across the receiver, inducing a voltage in the coil. This is the **MR signal**. Because the motion of precession is circular, it induces an alternating current in exactly the same way that a spinning magnet induces an alternating current in a power-generating coil.[3,12,13]

When the radiofrequency pulse is removed, the protons begin to lose energy, and the difference between the numbers of spin up and spin down protons increases again until the net magnetization vector lies in the longitudinal plane. As this happens, the MR signal decays: electromotive force is *only* induced by the component of the magnetic field lying perpendicular to it – the longitudinal component of the vector induces no current in the receptor coil. This decrease in the magnitude of the MR signal is called **free induction decay** (free because it happens when the hydrogen nuclei are 'free' of the radiofrequency pulse).[12]

The removal of the radiofrequency pulse also causes the net magnetization vector to stop precessing. This loss of phase coherence is called **transverse (or T2) relaxation** whereas the recovery of longitudinal magnetization is called **longitudinal (or T1) relaxation**.[4]

Contrast

Molecules, unless at the hypothetical limit of absolute zero, are constantly in motion. The greater the motion, the greater the inertia and the more difficult it is for the molecule to release its energy to its surroundings.[4]

Most molecules in the body contain hydrogen; amongst the commonest are fat and water. Water molecules are small and therefore have low inertia; however, they have a high inherent energy, which makes it more difficult for them to absorb more energy efficiently. By contrast, fat molecules consist of long chains of hydrocarbons – a central chain of interlinked carbon atoms with hydrogen attached to the sides. They therefore have high inertia and also possess a low inherent energy, meaning that they readily absorb additional energy.[12]

These characteristics mean that the different tissues in the body have different relaxation times and this is used to produce contrast: areas of high signal (which appears white), medium signal (grey) and low signal (black) which reflect the strength – or, more properly, prolongation – of the MR signal recovered from different locations within the sample.[6]

In addition to relaxation times, contrast is also affected by a number of other factors, including the relative density of the excited hydrogen and the **extrinsic factors** controlled by the radiographer. The two most important of these are the **repetition time (TR)** and the **echo time (TE)**.[14]

Repetition time (TR)

This is the time between the *applications* of the radiofrequency pulses and is measured in milliseconds (ms). The TR affects the length of the relaxation period.[8]

Echo time (TE)

This is the length of time between the start of a radiofrequency pulse and the collection of the MR signal; it is also measured in milliseconds. The TE affects the relaxation times after the *removal* of the radiofrequency pulses and also the peak of the signal induced in the receiver coil.[8] The differentiation of these factors is shown in Figure 1.02.

The precise design of the imaging pulse sequences allows one contrast mechanism to be emphasized while the others are minimized. This ability to choose different contrast mechanisms is what gives MR imaging its tremendous flexibility.[4] In the spine (Figure 1.03), the spinal canal structures have very different appearance on T1-weighting compared to T2-weighting, whilst the vertebral bodies and discs remain almost unchanged. The differences in signal intensities between the two types of images are summarized in Table 1.01.

There are conditions in which it is not possible to generate enough image contrast to adequately show

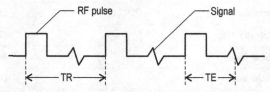

Figure 1.02 • The radiofrequency pulse (RF) is applied at regular intervals. The repetition time (TR) is the time between the applications of the pulse. The echo time (TE) is the time from the application of the pulse to the collection of the magnetic resonance signal.

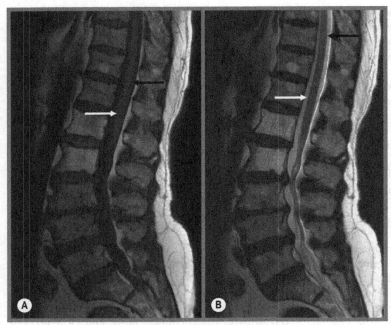

Figure 1.03 • Two midsagittal MR images of the lumbar spine. The image in (**A**) is a T1-weighted image; note how the neurons of grey matter (black arrows), have a medium intensity (grey) signal whilst the cerebrospinal fluid (white arrows) appears dark. These contrasts are reversed in the T2-weighted image (**B**). Of incidental note is the focal higher-intensity signal in the body of the T11 vertebra in both T1-weighted and T2-weighted images; this represents a haemangioma. This finding is also responsible for the lighter appearance of the L1 and L2 vertebral bodies on both images.

Table 1.01 Signal intensities seen in T1-weighted and T2-weighted images

Structure	T1-weighting	T2-weighting
Air	No signal	No signal
Avascular necrosis	Low signal	High signal
Calcification	No/low signal	No/low signal
Cortical bone	No/low signal	No/low signal
Degenerative fatty deposition	High signal	Low signal
Fast-flowing blood	No signal	No signal
Fat	High signal	Low signal
Fluid cysts	Low signal	High signal
Haemangioma	High signal	High signal
Infarction	Low signal	High signal
Infection	Low signal	High signal
Lipoma	High signal	Low signal
Scar tissue	No signal	No signal
Sclerosis	Low signal	High signal
Slow-flowing blood	High signal	High signal
Tendons	No/low signal	No/low signal
Tumours	Low signal	High signal

the anatomy or pathology of clinical interest by adjusting the imaging parameters alone. In such cases, a contrast agent may be administered. This may be as simple as getting the patient to drink a glass of water to assist in imaging the stomach and small bowel; however, most of the contrast agents used in MR imaging are selected for their specific paramagnetic properties.[4]

The most common paramagnetic contrast agent used in musculoskeletal imaging is gadolinium. Gadolinium-enhanced tissues and fluids appear extremely bright on T1-weighted images and this provides high sensitivity for detection of neovascular tissue associated with fibrous tissue, such as that found in tumours, and permits assessment of brain perfusion in cases of cerebrovascular incidents. It also allows assessment of scar tissue following discal surgery. The addition of gadolinium adds a considerable degree of invasiveness and potential toxicity to the imaging procedure and is contraindicated in patients with impaired kidney function (nephrogenic fibrosis).[7]

Proton density weighting

By reducing T1-weighting and T2-weighting effects using a long TR and a short TE respectively, it is possible to create an image that reflects the relative proton density of different tissues. A high signal is produced in areas that have a high proton density and vice versa; this can be used to identify certain pathologies.[3,12]

Pulse sequences

There are a number of ways in which the operator can further manipulate the image. A pulse sequence is defined as a series of radiofrequency pulses, which may be further modified by the application of **gradients**, a change in magnetic flux density along the length of the scanner, and by changing the intervening time periods.[15]

The main purpose of these pulse sequences is to manipulate the TE and TR to produce different *types* of contrast and to rephase the spin of the hydrogen nuclei, which tend to gradually un-phase owing to inhomogeneities in the applied magnetic field causing signal decay.[4,14]

Spin echo (SE)

Spin echo (SE) uses a radiofrequency pulse to rephase in the manner already described; however, in addition to the initial 90° pulse, a second pulse is added at 180°

to rephase any nuclei that have decreased their precessional frequency and reform the net magnetization vector. This regenerates the induced MR signal, which had been decaying, and this regeneration can be measured. The regenerated signal is called an 'echo' and, because a radiofrequency pulse has been used to generate it, it is specifically termed **spin echo**. Spin echo is used to produce T1-weighted (short TR, short TE) and T2-weighted (long TR, long TE) images. By adding an additional 180° pulse (these pulses do not affect TR, which is still defined as the gap between the application of 90° pulses), it is possible to produce two images per pulse. Both will have a long TR; however, the first will have a short TE and produces a proton density weighted image. The second has a long TR and TE and is used to produce a standard T2-weighted image (Figure 1.04). This is known as a **dual echo** sequence.[15]

The main problem with methods of image acquisition is the length of time taken; this can be reduced by **fast** or **turbo spin echo (FSE/TSE)** whereby a chain of 180° rephasing pulses are applied in between the 90° pulses. This can reduce the imaging time by factors of as much as 16; however, there is an inevitable trade-off with image quality and artifacts from

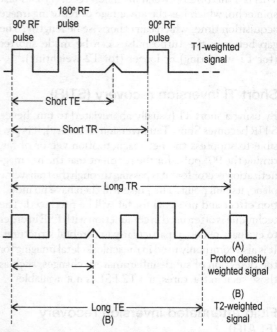

Figure 1.04 • Pulse sequences used to produce T1-weighted, T2-weighted and proton density weighted signals using spin echo and dual echo sequences.

blood flow, which usually is not imaged but can be 'frozen' if the image acquisition is fast enough. This technique depends on altering the gradient between each pulse so that the phase is slightly shifted and can be differentiated by the computer algorithm.[16]

Inversion recovery (IR)

If instead of beginning with a 90° radiofrequency pulse a spin echo sequence begins with a 180° pulse, then the net magnetization vector will be inverted (the TR now becomes the time interval between successive inverting 180° pulses). This pulse is then followed by a second pulse at 90°, which creates a magnetic resonance signal in the induction coils. The time between the two pulses is called the **time from inversion (TI)** and this process is called **inversion recovery**. If this signal is then rephased as before with a rephasing 180° pulse (as distinct from the inverting 180° pulse; this pulse does *not* influence TR), then an echo pulse can be produced.[15,16]

There are three inversion sequences that are in common diagnostic use.

Fast inversion recovery

This is a mixture between inversion recovery and fast spin echo, which has the advantage of reducing image acquisition time, which can otherwise be lengthy. The gap between the turbo pulses can be made shorter (for T1-weighting) or longer (for T2-weighting).[15]

Short TI inversion recovery (STIR)

By using a short TI (usually abbreviated to **tau**, hence STIR becomes Short Tau Inversion Recovery), it is possible to suppress the net magnetization vector of fat, timing the 90° pulse for the moment that the net magnetization vector for fat is passing through the transverse plane, its null point. The pulse will then have no induction effect and no signal for fat will be produced. The technique is often used in conjunction with FSE in order to evaluate oedema, particularly in cerebral structures. It is also commonly used in musculoskeletal imaging for the detection of subtle inflammatory changes, such as those seen in fractures, if a T2 FSE is not available.[4]

Fluid attenuated inversion recovery (FLAIR)

Using exactly the same principles as STIR, by *lengthening* the TI, it is possible to suppress signals from cerebrospinal fluid, which can be a valuable tool in the evaluation of brain tumours.[15]

Clinical aspects of MRI

Although the physics behind NMR and the engineering that allows us to 'see' MR images are complicated, the principles are worth understanding; without them, the clinician can have no real comprehension of what they are seeing on the computer screen or view box – or why. It is therefore worth taking the time to get your head around these terms and their impact on and consequences for the images you are going to learn to interpret; it will also help you to answer the questions that will come from patients about their films and what they mean for them.

Patients will also have questions for you from the moment you decide that imaging is required – why MR imaging and not x-ray? If you cannot readily answer this question, you should revisit your clinical and diagnostic thinking. They will also, as a rule, want to know how much it is going to cost, particularly where the cost of the procedure is not covered by insurance schemes or public health. As a clinician, it is your job to screen the patient for contraindications (Box 1.01); there is nothing guaranteed to infuriate both the imaging centre and patient more than for them to have their time and effort wasted by an inappropriate referral. On occasion, it may be necessary to prescribe tranquillizers (and arrange a chauffeur) for a nervous, claustrophobic patient who cannot gain access to imaging by an open scanner; it may also be necessary to organize a skull x-ray to screen for metal fragments in and around the orbit in those patients who have worked with lathes or sheet metal or who have seen active service in the armed forces.[7]

Most imaging centres will have their own bespoke forms; a typical such form (for the author's own 'local' MR scanner) is shown in Figure 1.05. It is important to give the radiologist as much information as possible so that the appropriate protocols can be used to answer the clinical question that you want answered: the radiologist can't refine your differential diagnosis if you don't have one! Regional protocols are discussed on a chapter by chapter basis; however, as a rule, you can expect to receive back a CD or hard copy films containing T1- and T2-weighted images in at least two planes. These should be correlated with the radiologist's report (a good way to practise) and with your own clinical

Figure 1.05 • A typical referral form for an MR imaging centre. The clinician has room to give a clinical history as well as the patient's demographic details. Contraindications are clearly listed and have to be signed off before sending. (Courtesy of Gloucestershire Magnetic Resonance Imaging Service.)

GLOUCESTERSHIRE MAGNETIC RESONANCE IMAGING SERVICE
Scanner Unit, Linton House Clinic, Thirlestaine Road, Cheltenham, GL53 7AS
Tel: (01242) 535910 Fax: (01242) 535919

Request for MRI Examination CLINICAL SUMMARY			SURNAME	
			FIRST NAMES	
			D.O.B.	SEX M / F	MARITAL STATUS M / S / W
			ADDRESS	
	Patient Weight............			
			POSTCODE	Telephone contact
	Type	Date	Self Pay / Insured	Daytime: Evening:
ATTENTION: Sign below to indicate that you have checked the following contra-indications:			Referred By:	
PATIENT HAS: Pacemaker Monitoring Device	MRI EXAMINATION IS NOT POSSIBLE		ADDRESS FOR REPORT	
PATIENT MAY HAVE: Irritants in the eye (if working with a lathe)	AN ORBITAL X-RAY MAY CLEAR THE PATIENT FOR MRI EXAMINATION		For Office Use Only Protocol	
PATIENT HAS: Vessel Clips or is Pregnant	CONTACT THE MRI UNIT OR A RADIOLOGIST		Appointment Date / Time	Appointment made / letter sent by
Signed.............................. Date..........................			Radiographer	Contrast	Films	Accepted	Rejected

findings and thought processes – remember, the radiologist has not seen the patient, you have.

The patient may also be concerned about the process and what will happen to them, particularly if they have not had a scan before. When they arrive at the centre, they will be asked to complete a consent form and will be rescreened for contra-indications. They will then be asked to change into a gown and to remove all jewellery and eyeglasses. Depending on the region to be imaged, surface coils may be applied to the area; these act as a local receiver that can be placed immediately adjacent to smaller or off-centre structures such as the distal extremities to improve the image quality.

A traditional MR imaging scanner has, from the patient's perspective, the appearance of a long tunnel, around 1.60 m in length. The opening is fairly small; indeed, most centres have an upper limit of 225–280 lb beyond which it is physically impossible to fit the patient in the scanner. In this instance,

the open scanner again provides an alternative (Figure 1.06).

A horizontal table 'feeds' the patient into the scanner, where they will remain for the duration of the scan, usually 25–40 minutes. Communication with the control booth is maintained using speakers or headphones, which can also be used to help reduce the significant banging noises from the radiofrequency pulses turning on and off. Music can help in this regard; patients are often allowed to bring a CD of their choice; this can also help make them feel more comfortable. Instructions usually consist of no more than getting the patient to lie as still as possible while the scan takes place.

Most scanning units are happy to organize visits from referring physicians, and personal knowledge and familiarity with the centre and its personnel can be a significant aid in helping to assuage a patient's concerns or anxieties.

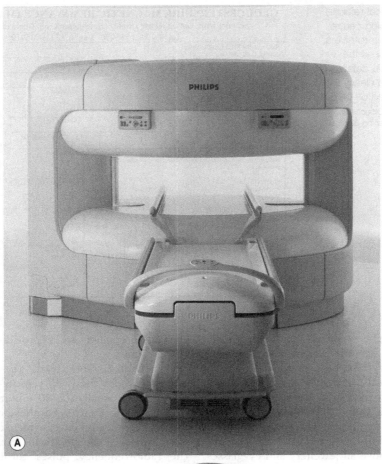

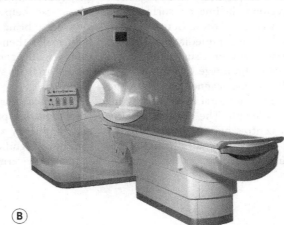

Figure 1.06 • Recent improvements in receptor analysis have allowed the development of open-sided MRI scanners (A), which ameliorate the effects of claustrophobia – a condition that affects up to 10% of people and can preclude the use of a conventional scanner (B).

References

1. *Nobel Lectures*. Amsterdam: Elsevier Publishing; 1964.

2. Lauterbur PC. Image formation by induced local interactions: examples of employing nuclear magnetic resonance. *Nature*. 1973;242: 190–191.

3. Allison W. Imaging with magnetic resonance. In: *Fundamental Physics for Probing and Imaging*. Oxford: Oxford University Press; 2006:207–226.

4. Young MF. Diagnostic imaging. In: *Essential Physics for Musculoskeletal Medicine*. Edinburgh: Elsevier; 2010.

5. Rowe L, Yochum T. Principles of radiological interpretation. In: Yochum T, Rowe L, eds. *Essentials of Skeletal Radiology*. 2nd ed. Baltimore: Williams and Wilkins; 1996:547–585.

6. DeVries RM, Manne A. Cervical MRI. Part I: a basic overview. *Clinical Chiropractic*. 2003;6(4):137–143.

7. Shellock FG. *Safety Information*. 2008 [cited 2009 14th June]. Available from: www.mrisafety.com.

8. Halliday D, Resnick D, Walker J. Magnetic resonance. In: *Fundamentals of Physics*. Hoboken, NJ: John Wiley and Sons; 2005:1015–1016.

9. Garood JR. Nuclear and quantum physics. In: *Physics*. Maidenhead: Intercontinental Book Productions; 1979:276–314.

10. Crooks L, Herfkens R, Kaufman L, et al. Nuclear magnetic resonance imaging. *Prog Nucl Med*. 1981; 7:149–163.

11. Westbrook C. Alignment and precession. In: *MRI at a Glance*. Oxford: Blackwell Science; 2002:16–17.

12. Westbrook C. Resonance and signal generation. In: *MRI at a Glance*. Oxford: Blackwell Science; 2002:18–19.

13. Garood JR. Electromagnetism. In: *Physics*. Maidenhead: Intercontinental Book Productions; 1979:232–275.

14. Westbrook C. Image contrast. In: *MRI at a Glance*. Oxford: Blackwell Science; 2002:20–27.

15. Westbrook C. Pulse sequences. In: *MRI at a Glance*. Oxford: Blackwell Science; 2002:28–47.

16. Helms C, Major N, Anderson MW, et al. *Musculoskeletal MRI*. 2nd ed. Philadelphia: Elsevier Saunders; 2009:1–19.

The cervical spine

2

Renée M. DeVries Anita L. Manne Michelle A. Wessely

Introduction

Cervicalgia, or neck pain, is a common condition that results in work absenteeism and alteration of daily activities for many adults.[1,2] The course of neck pain may be episodic in nature and the condition often fails to resolve completely, resulting in chronic pain. Approximately 20% of patients presenting with musculoskeletal conditions do so with neck pain as their chief complaint[3] and, at any one point in time, over 10% of the adult (>30 years) population complain of cervicalgia; it is more predominant in females than males (3:2).[1]

Radiographs of the cervical spine are often indicated, particularly in those cases that present with acute trauma, or persistent pain[4]; however, the contrast resolution of x-rays does not allow complete evaluation of the soft tissue structures or bone marrow. In cases where there is suspicion of a space-occupying lesion in the central spinal canal or intervertebral foramen, or concern for bone marrow pathology, magnetic resonance (MR) imaging may be indicated. It is important for clinicians to have an understanding of the appearance of normal cervical spine anatomy on MR imaging as well as an appreciation of the more common conditions that may present in an ambulatory care setting.

History and examination

The first step in the evaluation of patients presenting with neck pain is to perform a history and physical examination. The information obtained from these two steps can assist the clinician in narrowing the differential diagnosis and should help guide the diagnostic work-up.

When eliciting a history from a patient with a chief complaint of neck pain, the clinician should obtain a few important pieces of information, starting with the patient's age and past history of similar complaint. It is important to ascertain the duration of pain and whether it was related to a traumatic event. With a history of trauma, the clinician should inquire not only about the mechanism of injury but also about the patient's posture at the time of injury and the direction of the force. The location of the pain, whether diffuse or focal, may also provide an important clue. The presence of radicular symptoms, pain or paraesthesia, and the presence of systemic symptoms such as fever or weight loss are also highly significant.[5]

Physical examination should include vital signs; assessment of cervical range of motion, both active and passive; testing of all major muscle groups; orthopaedic evaluation, wherein foraminal compression tests and assessment of the thoracic outlet are of particular importance; and neurological examination, which should include a check of long tract signs – cervical myelopathy does not affect just the cervical nerve roots![6,7]

Differential diagnosis

Information obtained in the history and physical examination should help the clinician arrive at a differential diagnosis. Focal pain following trauma may raise suspicion of an acute fracture or subluxation/dislocation, whereas diffuse pain following trauma

DOI: 10.1016/B978-0-443-06726-6.00002-0

might be more indicative of soft tissue injury. The presence of radiculopathy might suggest an underlying disc herniation or other pathology in the intervertebral foramen, such as degenerative joint disease. Acute neck pain and fever is a red flag suggesting infection and should prompt immediate follow-up.

Radicular symptoms need to be carefully differentiated from referred or sclerodermal pain and paraesthesia. To this end, in the patient with brachial symptoms, it is important to test the thoracic outlet. Although entrapment by cervical ribs and apical tumours is rare, functional impingement on the cords of the brachial plexus by the anterior and medial scalenes, first rib and pectoralis minor will be a common presentation to the manual physician and can best be differentiated by simple orthopaedic tests such as Adson's, Reverse Adson's, Eden's and Halstead's manoeuvres.[8]

Detailed knowledge of upper limb neurology is also useful in differentiating distal from proximal entrapments: all of the major nerves can suffer functional compression syndromes in the elbow and wrist and a combination of history, neurological testing and compression tests can help refine the differential diagnosis without recourse to nerve conduction studies. MR imaging is often a great help in determining the precise cause – this is dealt with in the chapters dealing with the joints of the upper extremity.[9,10]

A final, and often overlooked, source of pseudo-radicular symptoms is myofascial trigger points, which, of course, are radiographically and electromyographically occult. Although they are often a diagnosis of exclusion – or missed altogether – when sufficiently severe, digital pressure will recreate the patient's symptoms, making the diagnosis easy for the experienced musculoskeletal expert; the deltoid and rotator cuff muscles are particular culprits in this regard and should always be routinely assessed in such cases.[11]

Clinical indications for diagnostic imaging

Although MR imaging is extremely useful in the evaluation of the osseous and soft tissue structures of the cervical spine, plain film radiography is often the initial imaging procedure. Radiographs are indicated with a history of significant trauma, including axial force to the vertex of the cranium; a fall from a height of 1 m or down five stairs; a high-speed (>110 km/h) motor vehicle accident; or a motorized recreation vehicle accident. The presence of paraesthesias and an inability to actively rotate the head to 45° are other criteria that justify the use of radiography.[4]

Standard radiographic views of the cervical spine consist of anterior to posterior (AP) open mouth, AP lower cervical and lateral cervical neutral views. Lateral cervical views taken in flexion and extension posture may be useful to evaluate ligamentous instability; however, it is important to first use the basic routine series to screen the patient for contraindications to these dynamic views. In addition, ligamentous laxity may not become radiographically detectable for several (up to 6) weeks owing to patient limitation and muscular guarding.[12] MR imaging is indicated for evaluation following a high-speed motor vehicle accident, a fall from a height of 3 m, a closed head injury or in the presence of neurologic signs radiating from the cervical spine.[4]

There are many non-traumatic causes of cervical spine problems in which radiographs should be obtained; these are detailed in Box 2.01.[4] If, ultimately, radiographs are inconclusive, advanced imaging may then be required.

Imaging protocol

Though protocols vary slightly between facilities, the standard MR imaging protocol for the cervical spine consists of sagittal T1- and T2-weighted images

---

Box 2.01

Non-traumatic indications for cervical spine radiographs

- Age <20 or >50
- No response to conservative care after 4 weeks
- Significant restriction of activity
- Unrelenting pain at rest
- Neck rigidity
- Dysphagia
- Impaired consciousness
- Long tract signs and symptoms
- Arm or leg pain with neck movement
- Suspected myelopathy
- Sudden onset of acute and unusual pain

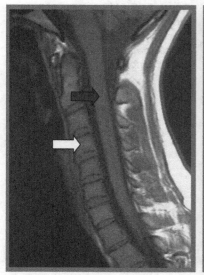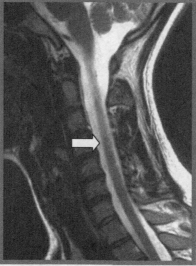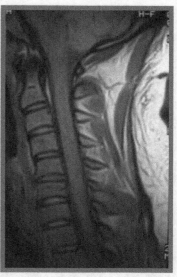

Figure 2.01 • MR imaging of the cervical spine, demonstrating various examples in different patients of the type of sequences that may be performed. All the sequences presented are sagittal slices. The image to the left is an example of a T1-weighted image, wherein the spinal cord and bone marrow are seen as grey signal (note the dark arrow pointing to the spinal cord and the white arrow over the bone marrow within the vertebral body of C4). The image in the centre is an example of a T2-weighted image that is sensitive for fluid, which appears bright – note the bright appearance of the cerebrospinal fluid. The disc signal can then be determined; here, it is of low signal intensity due to multilevel degenerative disc disease. The final image, to the right, illustrates the appearance of a proton density image; here, the signal for fat is intermediate.

(Figure 2.01) along with axial T2-weighted images (Figure 2.02). Additional short TI inversion recovery (STIR) images may be obtained to suppress the signal from fat (a normal marrow constituent) in order to highlight areas with high water content.

Acute fractures, ligamentous injuries, and bony metastasis are all well visualized with STIR imaging (Figure 2.03). Contrast agents, typically chelates of gadolinium, may be utilized in cases where tumour is suspected.[13,14]

Normal anatomy and variants

Vertebral bodies

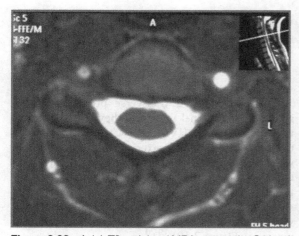

Figure 2.02 • Axial, T2-weighted MR image at the C4 level demonstrating the relationship of the dural sac to the central canal.

The vertebral bodies from C3–C7 are considered *typical* vertebral bodies and they share similar characteristics, in general increasing in size from C3 through C7. C1 and C2 are considered *atypical* as they each have unique characteristics. Their articulation uniquely has no disc; instead, there is an *odontoid process*, or dens, the cephalic extension of the C2 segment, which forms an articulation with the anterior arch of the ring-shaped C1 (Figure 2.04).[15,16] At the base of the dens, a linear area of low signal represents a remnant of the synchondrosis; this is a common

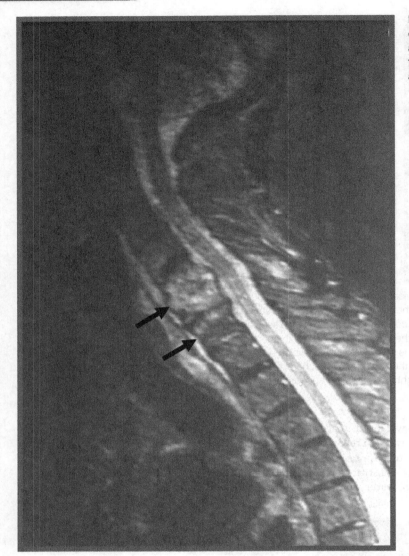

Figure 2.03 • MR imaging of the cervical spine, demonstrating the appearance of a STIR sequence, in this case with pathology seen at C5 and C6 (arrows).

finding and should not be mistaken for fracture (Figures 2.05, 2.06).

The basivertebral veins enter the posterior aspect of the vertebral bodies, midway between the end-plates; although these are most obvious in the lumbar spine, they may be evident on cervical images as well (Figure 2.07). The uncinate processes project superiorly from the lateral aspect of the vertebral bodies from C3 to C7 and, on occasion, from T1, and form the *uncovertebral joints*, or joints of von Luschka, with the inferior bodies of C2 to C6 (Figures 2.08, 2.09).[17,18]

The gutter-shaped transverse processes act as guides for the spinal nerves as they exit the intervertebral foramen (IVF) at each level; they also transmit the vertebral arteries. Arising from the subclavian arteries, the vertebral arteries enter the C6 transverse process and ascend to C1. At C1, the vertebral arteries cross over the posterior arch and meet in the midline to form the basilar artery, which continues superiorly through the foramen magnum (Figure 2.10).[19,20]

The spinal canal dimension is largest at C1, which allows for protection of the upper cervical

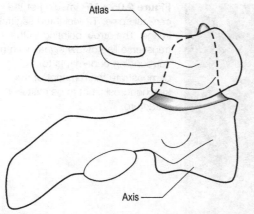

Atlas

Axis

Figure 2.04 • The atlas and axis are considered atypical vertebrae as they have unique features, whereas the remaining, typical, cervical vertebrae all follow the same basic template.

cord. According to *Steele's Rule of Thirds*, one-third of the spinal canal at C1 is occupied by the spinal cord, one-third by the odontoid process, and one-third comprises the subarachnoid space.[21] (More detailed data regarding spinal canal dimensions are given in Table 2.01.[22]) This results in inherent safeguarding of the spinal cord in the event of transverse ligament rupture or odontoid fracture. This explains why some patients with atlantoaxial instability or subluxation may be relatively asymptomatic. The triangular canal decreases in size to C3 and remains approximately uniform in size from C3 to C7.

Facet joints

The articular processes arise from each side of the posterior arch at the junction of the pedicle and lamina. The superior and inferior articular processes from adjacent levels join to form a diarthrodial, plane facet (zygapophyseal) joint (Figures 2.08, 2.11, 2.12). The articular surfaces are lined by cartilage, the thickness of which varies depending on age, sex and the anatomical level; tiny menisci may also be present in each joint,[23] which is surrounded by a synovial-lined, fibroelastic joint capsule.[24] The primary role of the facet joint is not to bear weight, but rather to guide, and limit, movement. Because they are innervated by sensory and autonomic nerve fibres, the facet joints may represent a primary source of pain.[24]

Intervertebral discs

The strongest attachment between vertebral bodies is created by the intervertebral disc, whose main role is to bear weight. In the cervical spine, the lordosis is contributed to by the shape of the intervertebral discs, whose height is greater anteriorly than posteriorly.[24] The three regions of the disc are the annulus fibrosus, the nucleus pulposus, and the vertebral body endplate. The annulus fibrosus is composed of fibrocartilage centrally and collagen fibres peripherally.[25] The cervical annulus fibrosus is crescent-shaped fibrocartilage that becomes increasingly narrow as it extends laterally and posteriorly.[24] The nucleus pulposus lies deep to the annulus and is bound superiorly and inferiorly by the cartilaginous endplates of the adjacent vertebral bodies. The nucleus is formed from glycoproteins and absorbs fluid through the endplates by imbibition, as only the outer region of the annulus fibrosus receives a vascular supply.[24] As can be noted in Figure 2.01, the normal intervertebral disc appears as low signal intensity on T1-weighted images and high signal on T2-weighted images. Though these regions of the disc are anatomically distinct, it is not usually possible to distinguish the interface between the inner annulus and the nucleus pulposus with MR imaging.[25,26]

Spinal ligaments

The role of the spinal ligaments is to connect the vertebral bodies to adjacent segments and to provide smooth motion of the spine. At the same time, these ligaments provide protection for the spinal cord by limiting the amount of intersegmental motion and by acting as shock absorbers during trauma.[24,27] Mechanoreceptor afferent fibres in the interspinous and *supraspinous ligaments* as well as the *ligamentum flavum* allow them to play an additional proprioceptive role.[28] In the cervical spine, the *anterior longitudinal ligament* (ALL) provides anterior stability; this ligament, which extends from the anterior arch of C1 to the first sacral segment, is adherent to the anterior annulus and to the anterior periosteum of the vertebral bodies. Above C1, the anterior longitudinal ligament continues to the anterior margin of the foramen magnum as the *anterior atlanto-occipital membrane* (AAM) (Figures 2.13, 2.14). The function of the anterior longitudinal ligament is to limit extension of the cervical spine.[17]

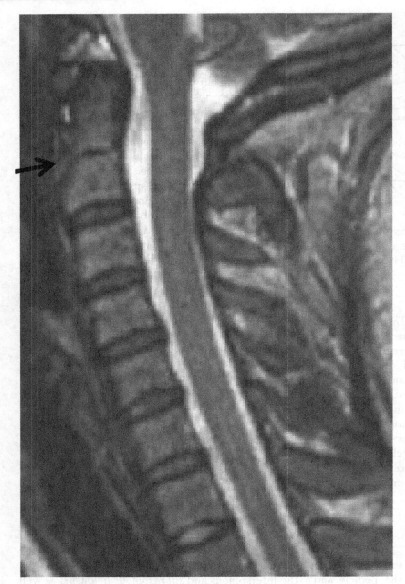

Figure 2.05 • MR imaging of the cervical spine, T2-weighted sagittal image. The arrow pointing to the transverse line of low signal, with no surrounding oedema, is to demonstrate the remnant of the synchondrosis, not to be mistaken for a fracture.

The *posterior longitudinal ligament* (PLL) extends from C2 to the sacrum and acts to limit flexion of the spine. It is tightly adherent to the posterior disc and is indistinguishable from the posterior annulus on MR images.[26] The PLL is narrower than its anterior counterpart and is attached firmly to the vertebral body edges but not to their bodies. Above C2, the PLL continues to the foramen magnum as the *tectorial membrane*, which can be injured in traumatic events such as whiplash, although the long-term effect of such damage is not currently established.[29–31]

Deep to the tectorial membrane, at the junction of the axis (C2) with the atlas (C1), the *transverse ligament* attaches to the posterior aspect of the C1 lateral masses and acts to hold the odontoid process to the anterior arch of C1. The transverse ligament is part of a cruciate ligament whose superior slip attaches to the anterior foramen magnum and inferior slip attaches to the posterior body of C2 (Figure 2.15).[23] Synovial bursae are present between the odontoid process and the anterior arch of C1 and between the odontoid process and the transverse ligament. The odontoid process also attaches to the foramen

Figure 2.06 • MR imaging of the cervical spine, performed in the coronal plane (left, T2-weighted) and sagittal plane (right, T1-weighted), where again the low signal appearance of the synchondrosis of C2 is noted (arrows), a normal appearance.

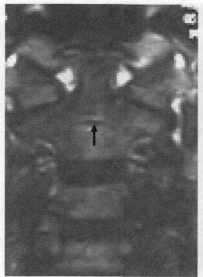 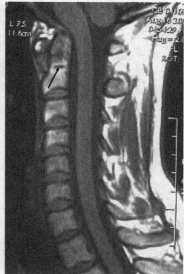

magnum by the apical and alar ligaments. The apical ligament extends from the tip of the dens to the anterior foramen magnum; the alar ligaments run obliquely from the tip of the dens to the occipital condyles and lateral masses of the atlas.[23]

The *ligamentum flavum* connects the laminae at each level, covering the gaps in the posterior wall of the spinal canal and blending with the anterior and medial aspects of the facet joint capsule (Figure 2.16).[24] Extending from the external occipital protuberance to the spinous process of C7 and connecting the spinous processes in the cervical spine is the *ligamentum nuchae*, the cephalic extension of the *supraspinous ligament*.

Spinal cord and spinal nerves

The spinal cord has a characteristic shape in each spinal region; in the cervical spine, it is slightly elliptical in cross-section and demonstrates slight enlargement from C3 to C6.[23] It is best assessed on T2-weighted images, which create contrast between the cord and surrounding cerebrospinal fluid (CSF) (Figures 2.17, 2.18). T2-weighted images are also useful in screening for medullary signal abnormalities (Figure 2.19).

The cervical spine gives rise to eight spinal nerves, each composed of a dorsal sensory root and a ventral motor root. The nerves exit through the IVFs formed by adjacent vertebral bodies and

are named by the *inferior* segment: thus, the first nerve exits between the occiput and C1; the second between C1 and C2 and so on. The eighth cervical nerve exits between C7 and T1; thereafter, the nerves are named for the *superior* segment. The dorsal root is the larger and contains the dorsal root ganglion before joining the ventral root and forming a spinal nerve.[26] In the cervical spine, the dorsal root ganglion lies in the IVF at all levels except C1 and C2 (where there is no IVF), where the dorsal root ganglions lie instead on the respective posterior arch.[26]

The dorsal root of the nerve lies near the superior articular process whilst the ventral root lies adjacent to the uncovertebral joint and posterior to the intervertebral disc.[23] On sagittal images, the nerve roots will be found in the inferior portion of the IVF. The cerebellar tonsils will be also visualized on the sagittal images and their relationship with the skull base should be assessed. The cerebellar tonsils should not project more than 5 mm below the foramen magnum in adults.[32]

Pathological conditions

Intervertebral disc herniation

Cervical disc herniations are a relatively common disorder, affecting 5.5 out of 100,000 people in the United States.[33] Disc herniations are more

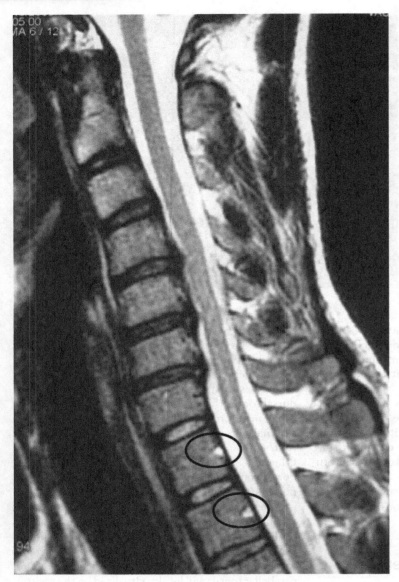

Figure 2.07 • MR imaging of the cervical spine, performed in the sagittal plane, using a T2-weighted sequence. The basivertebral vein entrance, visible in the lower cervical spine, is seen as foci of increased signal intensity along the mid posterior portion of the vertebral bodies of T1 and T2 (ovals). This phenomenon is one that can be found at any level of the spine. (Note also that there is significant disc pathology in the mid cervical spine!) (This case is reproduced courtesy of Sylviane de Vergie DC.)

common in adult populations, with males affected more often than females. The C6/7 and C5/6 levels are most commonly involved.[32,33]

On MR images, the disc should normally lie in line with the edge of adjacent vertebral bodies. A *disc bulge* is defined as extension of disc material beyond the adjacent vertebral body edges, involving over 50% of the circumference of the disc.[34] A *disc herniation* is extension of disc material that involves less than 50% of the circumference of the disc. If the herniation is broader at its base than at any point distal to its base, it is considered a *disc protrusion*.

A *disc extrusion* is a herniation that is broader at a point distal to its base at the parent disc. A disc herniation that migrates superiorly or inferiorly along the posterior body would also be considered an extrusion. A *free fragment* is the term that is used to describe a disc herniation that has separated from the parent disc.

Patients with cervical disc herniations will most commonly present with neck pain and dermatomal paraesthesia. Shoulder pain, arm pain and weakness are other common presenting complaints. Orthopaedic and neurologic testing should elicit findings

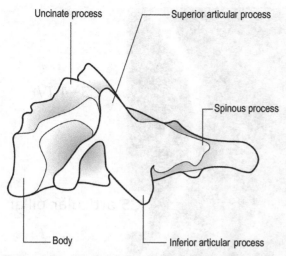

Figure 2.08 • The articular processes of the cervical spine arise from each side of the posterior arch at the junction of the pedicle and lamina. The superior and inferior articular processes from adjacent levels join to form the facet (zygapophyseal) joint.

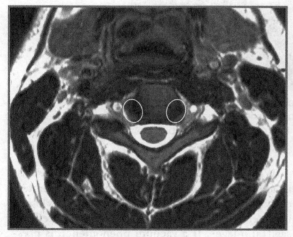

Figure 2.09 • MR imaging of the cervical spine, axial T2-weighted imaging demonstrating the low-signal normal osseous uncovertebral structures seen on either side of the posterolateral aspect of the vertebral body (ovals). Note the relationship between the uncovertebral joints and the foramen.

consistent with nerve root compromise and will likely guide the clinician to the level of involvement. Radiographs of the cervical spine will not reveal the herniation, though they will often still be indicated from the history and examination.

MR imaging is, however, the procedure of choice for evaluating a suspected disc herniation

(Figures 2.20, 2.21). In addition to assessing the intervertebral discs, MR imaging allows for evaluation of the spinal cord to rule out other causes of neurologic compromise, such as cord tumour or syrinx (see Chapter 3).

Myelomalacia of the cord, secondary to compromise, is also evident on MR images and will appear as high signal intensity on the T2-weighted sequences at the site of compression on both sagittal and axial slices. On T1-weighted imaging, the same zone will be seen as thinner and lower in signal compared to normal. The cause of the myelomalacia can be noted directly using dynamic MR imaging where, particularly on extension, buckling of the ligamentum flavum, the joint capsule and degenerative changes can be seen to indent or contact the dural sac and contents directly (Figure 2.22).

On MR imaging, the disc herniation will appear as a lesion, most commonly in the ventral aspect of the spinal canal. It is important to determine whether the herniation is contacting, displacing, or compressing the dural sac, as the nature of the neural compromise will inform treatment; the relationship of the herniation to the dural sac and contents is best evaluated on axial images. It is also necessary to evaluate the disc lesion with respect to the take-off sites of the ventral nerve root and its passage through the intervertebral foramen, either of which may result in discoradicular conflict. On T1-weighted images, the disc herniation will most often have signal characteristics that are isointense to the disc and the herniation will appear continuous with the disc. T2-weighted signals will vary depending upon the relative hydration of the disc. Typically, herniations do not enhance following the administration of contrast, though peripheral granulation tissue surrounding the herniation will show enhancement. This principle has important ramifications in patients with recurrent pain after surgery: scarring versus recurrent disc herniation is a common diagnostic dilemma as the signal intensity may be heterogeneous corresponding to a mixture of discal and haemorrhagic components. Gadolinium may also help in the detection of annular tears.[35]

Degenerative disease

Degenerative disc and joint disease in the cervical spine is a common condition with a multifactorial aetiology. Factors such as repetitive stress, familial predisposition, cigarette smoking, obesity, and diet

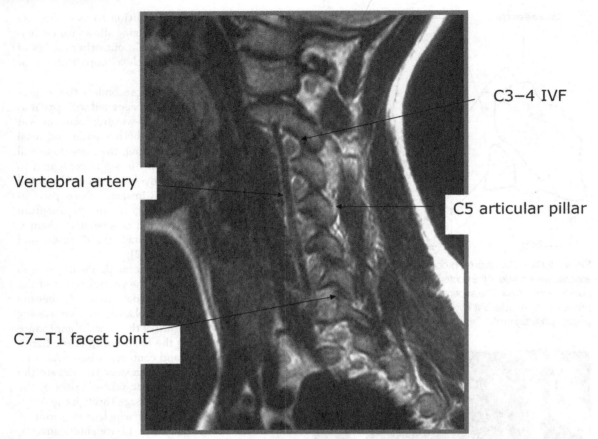

C3–4 IVF

Vertebral artery

C5 articular pillar

C7–T1 facet joint

Figure 2.10 • MR imaging of the cervical spine, sagittal T2-weighted images demonstrating a focal longitudinal region of low signal intensity representing the vertebral artery. The vertebral arteries ascend through the transverse processes of C6 to C1 where they cross over the posterior arch and meet in the midline to form the basilar artery.

Table 2.01 Spinal canal dimensions			
Level	Spinal canal width (mm)	Spinal canal area (mm²)	Spinal cord area (mm²)
C1	15.6	264.6	72.9
C3	13.0	190.9	74.8
C6	12.9	186.2	73.9

can all contribute to degenerative joint disease.[32,36] In the cervical spine, degenerative changes can occur at the intervertebral disc and adjacent vertebral body endplates, the facet joints, and the uncovertebral joints. Degenerative changes in each of these locations can contribute to central canal or IVF stenosis, resulting in symptoms of central or peripheral neurologic compromise.

Well-established degenerative disc disease is easily identifiable on radiographs. On MRI, degenerative disc disease appears on T1-weighted images as loss of intervertebral disc height best appreciated on sagittal images. If a vacuum phenomenon is present, it will appear as signal void or low signal within the disc, though several disorders can give this MR imaging appearance, including calcification and blood products, depending on their age. On T2-weighted images, disc degeneration will show as a loss of signal intensity, representing the altered biochemical content and decreased hydration within the disc.

In addition to demonstrating the changes within the degenerative intervertebral disc, MR imaging is sensitive to physiological changes in the adjacent vertebral body endplates. Modic described three distinct types of endplate changes in the lumbar

Figure 2.11 • MR imaging of the cervical spine, parasagittal T1-weighted sequence demonstrating the alignment of the articular pillars, described as 'tiles on a roof'. The articular processes of the cervical spine arise from each side of the posterior arch at the junction of the pedicle and lamina. The superior and inferior articular processes from adjacent levels join to form the facet (zygapophyseal) joint.

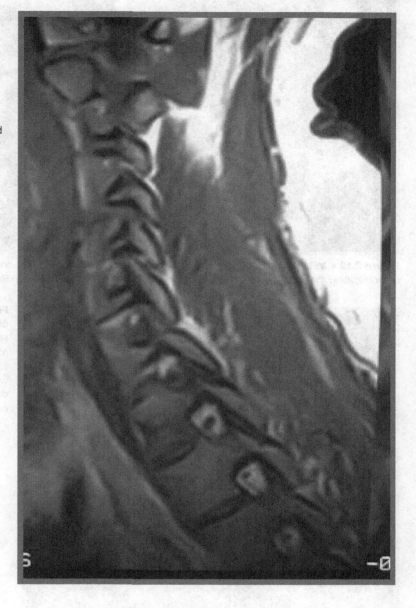

spine: these may also be applied to the cervical spine, although less evidence has been produced to discuss this (Table 2.02).[37] The earliest change in the subchondral endplates is the replacement of normal marrow with fibrovascular marrow. This type 1 endplate change appears on T1-weighted images as hypointense to surrounding marrow. On T2-weighting, type 1 Modic changes appear hyperintense to marrow.

In Modic type 2 endplate changes, fibrovascular marrow is replaced by fatty marrow and appears hyperintense to marrow on T1-weighted images and isointense on T2-weighting. The final stage, Modic type 3, is represented by bony sclerosis which is hypointense to marrow on both T1- and T2-weighted MR images.

The type 3 changes can also be visualized on radiographs as subchondral sclerosis. In addition to endplate changes, the altered biomechanics produced by diminished disc height may result in anterior or posterior osteophytic formation from the vertebral body margins. The combination of decreased disc

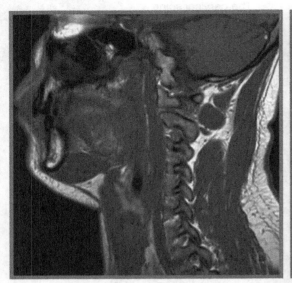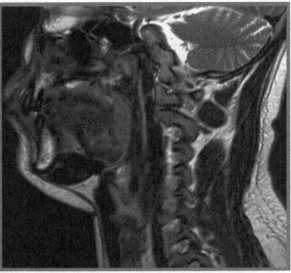

Figure 2.12 • MR imaging of the cervical spine, parasagittal T1-weighted (left) and T2-weighted (right) images demonstrating the appearance of the articular pillars in the same patient using different sequences.

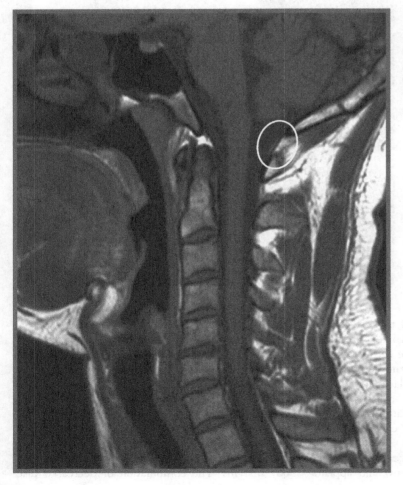

Figure 2.13 • MR imaging of the cervical spine, sagittal T1-weighted image demonstrating the posterior atlanto-occipital membrane (oval), important to evaluate in cases of whiplash, where it may be disrupted or discontinuous. In this patient, it is normal, intact.

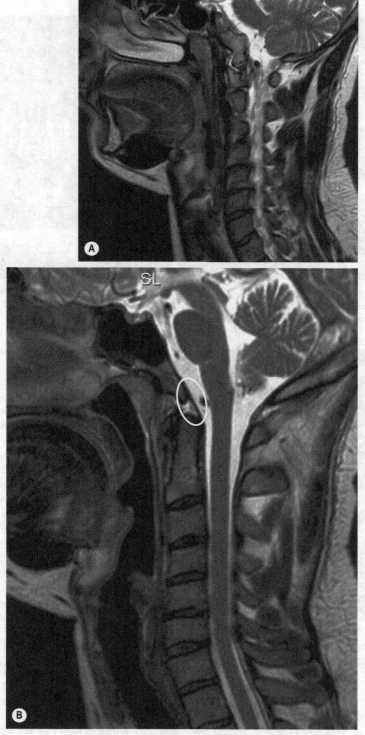

Figure 2.14 • MR imaging of the cervical spine, parasagittal, T2-weighted imaging demonstrating, with difficulty, a small longitudinal low signal intensity extending superiorly from the C2 (A). The same protocol (B) demonstrates a thin oblique signal extending from the posterior longitudinal ligament, representing the anterior atlanto-occipital membrane (oval), which here, as normal, appears as a continuous band. Trauma may cause disruption of this band.

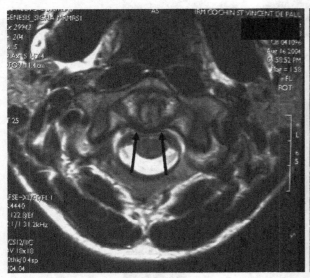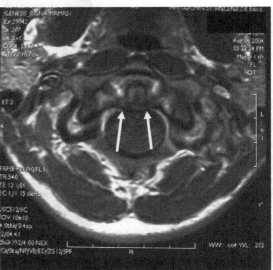

Figure 2.15 • MR imaging of the cervical spine in a female patient with a history of rheumatoid arthritis. The MR imaging was performed in the axial plane, on the left using T2 and on the right using proton density to evaluate the status of the transverse ligament (arrows), which was reported as normal.

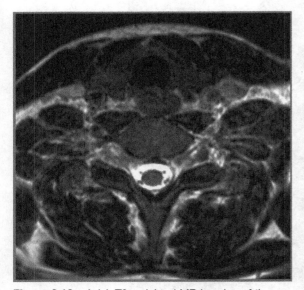

Figure 2.16 • Axial, T2-weighted MR imaging of the cervical spine demonstrating low signal tissue seen to hug the medial aspect of both lamina. This represents the ligamentum flavum in its normal appearance.

height and spondylophytes (osteophytes) may produce central canal stenosis. This will appear on T2-weighted images as a loss of CSF signal around the cord at the level of the intervertebral disc. T2-weighted images are also useful to evaluate for high signal within the cord, which would indicate myelomalacia.[32]

In addition to intervertebral disc degeneration, the facet joints also commonly undergo degenerative changes. These changes are seen on radiographs as diminished joint space and osteophytes originating from the superior and inferior articular surfaces. Overgrowth of the articular surfaces leads to anterolisthesis of the vertebral body, a degenerative type of spondylolisthesis. The facet osteophytes can project into the IVF, where they may impinge on the dorsal root ganglion. Patients may present with symptoms of neck pain and paraesthesia in the upper extremity and may exhibit diminished reflexes, hypoaesthesia, or decreased muscle strength. MR imaging is particularly useful in evaluating the relationship of facet osteophytes to the spinal nerves, and to assess the ligamentum flavum for thickening, which may occur in response to degeneration and can cause neural impingement.

Inflammatory arthropathies

Inflammatory arthropathies share a common pathological feature of degradation of the synovial lining of affected joints. The synovial lining is replaced by vascular granulation tissue, called *pannus*, which progressively fills the joint. The pannus erodes adjacent articular cartilage, bone, and ligaments. Once

Figure 2.17 • MR imaging of the cervical spine, axial T2-weighted image demonstrating the detail that MR imaging achieves, here noting the difference between the different tracts within the spinal cord.

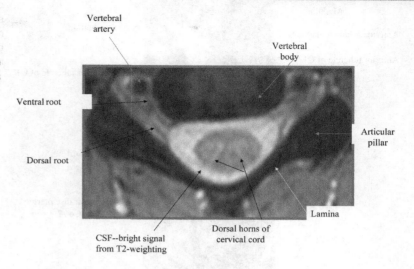

Vertebral artery

Vertebral body

Ventral root

Articular pillar

Dorsal root

Lamina

CSF--bright signal from T2-weighting

Dorsal horns of cervical cord

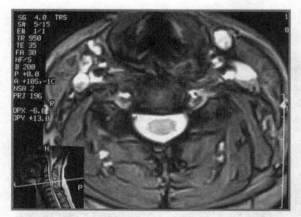

Figure 2.18 • MR imaging of the cervical spine, axial gradient-echo image. Note the high signal (bright) CSF in the central canal, suggestive of a T2-weighted image. The TR and TE numbers are low, similar to T1 images, but the flip angle is less than 90 degrees, making this a gradient-echo sequence.

the joint is filled with pannus, it becomes fibrous, and the joint may eventually fuse.[38]

Ankylosing spondylitis, rheumatoid arthritis and psoriatic arthritis are inflammatory spondyloarthropathies that can affect the cervical spine. Ankylosing spondylitis affects the discovertebral and facet joints, eventually producing ankylosis. Rheumatoid arthritis and psoriatic arthritis are less likely to produce ankylosis of the disc and facet joints, but both can affect the atlantoaxial joint. There are three synovial bursae at the atlantoaxial joint, one between the anterior

tubercle of C1 and the odontoid process, the second between the odontoid process and the transverse ligament, and the third at the apex of the odontoid process. Pannus infiltration into any of these bursae may erode the osseous or ligamentous structures (or both), producing instability. Radiographs of the cervical spine in flexion may reveal widening of the atlantodental interspace and perhaps erosion of the odontoid process and anterior tubercle.

MR imaging is useful to assess the relationship of C1 and C2 to the spinal cord and also allows visualization of the pannus, which may in itself be a cause of cord compression. On MR imaging, the pannus appears as low signal intensity on T1-weighted images. On T2-weighted images, pannus has a heterogeneous appearance, with areas of high and low signal intensity.[25] The use of gadolinium contrast causes the pannus to enhance.[38]

Hydroxyapatite crystal deposition disease (HADD)

HADD, more colloquially known as calcific tendonitis, of the longus colli tendon may present as a sudden onset of neck pain and stiffness in an adult. The aetiology of HADD is not clear, but trauma, repetitive injury, and ischaemia have all been implicated as predisposing factors.[39,40] HADD occurs most frequently around the shoulder, but may also affect the cervical spine, where longus colli is most commonly affected; this muscle extends from C1 through T3 and acts as a principal flexor of the cervical spine.[41]

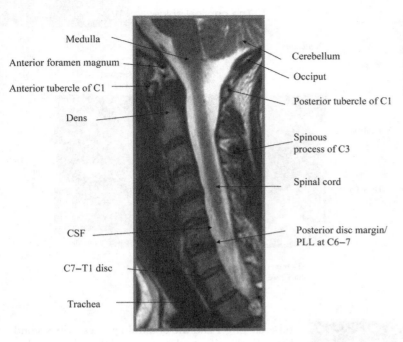

Medulla

Anterior foramen magnum

Anterior tubercle of C1

Dens

CSF

C7–T1 disc

Trachea

Cerebellum

Occiput

Posterior tubercle of C1

Spinous process of C3

Spinal cord

Posterior disc margin/ PLL at C6–7

Figure 2.19 • MR imaging of the cervical spine, sagittal T2-weighted sequence demonstrating some of the many various anatomic structures, both bone and soft tissue, that can be identified.

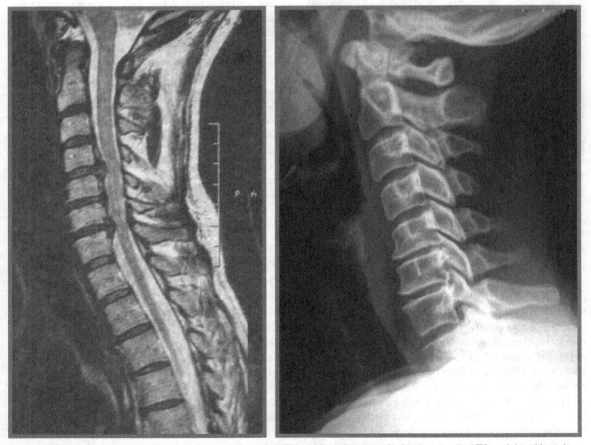

Figure 2.20 • Imaging of the cervical spine: on the left, MR imaging of the cervical spine, sagittal T2-weighted imaging, and on the right, a lateral radiograph of the same patient taken within a week of each other. Note the focal disc lesions present in the cervical spine at C3 through to C7, visible on the MR image only.

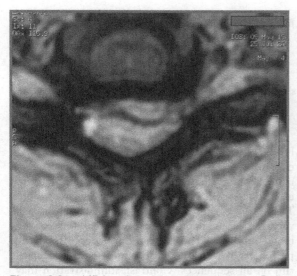

Deposition of hydroxyapatite crystals in the longus colli tendon following trauma results in non-specific neck pain and possibly difficulty swallowing. Though painful, this condition is self-limiting, often resolving in 1 to 2 weeks. Radiographs of the cervical spine will demonstrate a radiopacity in the retropharyngeal interspace, which is homogenous in density.[42] Though MR imaging is not necessary to make the diagnosis, this condition may appear on scans obtained to evaluate the cause of the patient's pain. Advanced imaging is especially useful when trying to exclude the presence of a retropharyngeal abscess or disc space infection. In addition, MR imaging may demonstrate the adjacent bone marrow oedema that may accompany the HADD of the longus colli, although this phenomenon has been more commonly described affecting the extremities.

On MR imaging, the calcific deposits will appear as low signal on both T1- and T2-weighted images. Adjacent prevertebral soft tissue swelling will appear as high signal intensity on T2-weighting. The presence of normal intervertebral discs and vertebral body marrow helps to rule out infection.[39]

Figure 2.21 • MR imaging of the cervical spine at C4/5. This axial T2-weighted image demonstrates a large focal disc lesion, a sizeable disc extrusion occupying the central, predominantly left paracentral and left foraminal zones. This is the same patient as in Figure 2.20.

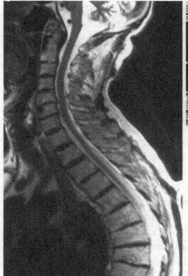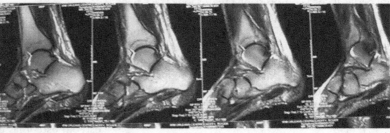

Figure 2.22 • MR imaging of the cervicothoracic spine, sagittal T2-weighted in a patient with neck pain and with a history of repeatedly falling over owing to a sensation of unsteadiness on the feet. Due to the unsteadiness, MR imaging of the ankle (sagittal T1-weighted) had also been previously performed to determine the cause. On MR imaging of the cervical spine, narrowing of the central canal at C5–C6 is due to a degenerative disc lesion in the ventral central canal and hypertrophy of the ligamentum flavum in the dorsal aspect of the central canal. These findings would likely be exaggerated on dynamic MR imaging, particularly from posteriorly, due to buckling of the ligamentum flavum.

Table 2.02 The appearance of Modic endplate changes on MR imaging

Modic endplate changes	T1 signal	T2 signal	Histopathologic correlation
Type 1	Decreased	Increased	Vascular fibrous (fibrovascular) tissue
Type 2	Increased	Isointense or slightly increased	Fatty subchondral marrow replacement
Type 3	Decreased	Decreased	Bony sclerosis

Calcification of intervertebral discs is a common radiographic finding, typically associated with degenerative disc disease. This is more common in the thoracic and lumbar spine and is typically asymptomatic.[35] Disc calcification in children and adolescents behaves differently from that in adults. In young patients, disc calcification is typically associated with neck pain, possibly torticollis in particular.[43] It is more common in the cervical and upper thoracic spine, and it is considered as self-limiting in nature.

Cervical spine neoplasms

Symptoms of neck pain with radiculopathy, although relatively easy to correlate with specific spinal levels, can result from any space-occupying lesion within the spinal canal. More generalized myelopathy from central cervical cord compression creates long tract signs that can be far harder to localize. Both benign and malignant neoplasms can present with a similar symptomatic picture. Benign tumours of the spine include aneurysmal bone cyst, osteoid osteomas, and osteoblastomas. Malignant lesions that affect the cervical spine include metastatic disease, multiple myeloma, and chordoma. The most common benign tumour of the spine is haemangioma; however, these vascular bone tumours rarely cause symptoms.

Aneurysmal bone cyst

Aneurysmal bone cysts are expansile lesions, containing thin-walled, blood-filled cavities. They are, in essence, intra-articular arteriovenous malformations that may occur in any bone, though 30% occur in the spine, where they have a particular affinity for the cervical spine, generally affecting the posterior elements. Patients are typically between the age of 10 and 30 years, with a peak incidence in the second decade; the gender prevalence is unclear.[44-46] Symptoms are related to the expansile nature of the lesion and patients may present with neurological signs. Radiographs typically reveal a 'soap-bubble', expansile

lesion of the posterior elements, similar to other expansile lesions; however, the MRI features of aneurysmal bone cysts are unique. The lobulated posterior arch lesions will often exhibit fluid levels on both T1- and T2-weighted images. The signal intensity will vary, depending upon the stage of breakdown of the blood products. The haemosiderin deposits at the periphery of the lesion will appear as a low signal rim on all sequences. Contrast administration may show enhancement at the periphery of the lesion. MR imaging is also very useful for determining the extent of cord compromise.

Osteoid osteoma and osteoblastoma

Differing only in size, osteoid osteomas and osteoblastomas are pathologically related benign tumours of bone. These lesions should be considered in the differential diagnosis of young patients who present with a painful scoliosis. Osteoid osteomas measure less than 1.5 cm in diameter and may incite extensive reactive sclerosis in the surrounding bone.[47] Osteoid osteomas occur most often in patients 10 to 20 years of age, with osteoblastomas occurring in a slightly older population. In addition to affecting the long bones, such as the femur, approximately 10% of osteoid osteomas occur in the spine.[48]

The classic presentation of a patient with an osteoid osteoma is focal pain, worse at night, which is relieved by salicylates. Given time, these lesions usually spontaneously regress, but they are treated easily with radiofrequency ablation.

On MR imaging, osteoid osteomas can be difficult to see, as the nidus is small and can lie between sequential slices. The tumour nidus is isointense to muscle on T1-weighted images and remains low signal on T2-weighted images. The surrounding oedema appears hyperintense to bone on T2-weighted images and both the nidus and the surrounding oedema will enhance with contrast.[47]

Osteoblastomas are giant osteoid osteomas and are given this designation if the lesion measures over

1.5 cm in size. They occur in patients under 30 years of age, with a peak incidence slightly greater than that of osteoid osteomas.[47,48] Approximately one-third occur in the spine and one-third of those affect the cervical spine. Like osteoid osteomas, these lesions involve the posterior elements, though they may extend into the vertebral body. Because of their expansile nature, these lesions are more likely to produce neurologic symptoms than are osteoid osteomas.[48] The symptomatic picture of night pain, relieved by salicylates, is also similar to osteoid osteomas although typically less intense.

The radiographic appearance of osteoblastomas is similar to aneurysmal bone cysts, in that they appear as a 'soap bubble', locally expansile lesion of the posterior arch. As such, they are considered aggressive but benign tumours. MR imaging will reveal a low-signal lesion on T1-weighted images that becomes mixed-signal or high-signal on T2-weighted images. Surrounding oedema will appear as low signal on T1-weighted images and high signal on T2-weighted images.

Metastatic disease

Osseous metastasis is the most common malignancy of bone. Up to 40% of patients with non-osseous primary malignancies will develop metastasis to their viscera or bones. When metastatic disease involves the skeletal system, the vertebral column is most often affected. The thoracic spine is most often involved, followed by the lumbar and then cervical spine. Prostate, lung, and breast carcinoma represent the source of most spinal metastases. The most common mechanism of extension to the axial skeleton is through haematogenous spread; tumour cells seed to the vertebral bodies via Batson's vertebral plexus.[32]

Patients with metastatic disease to their spine will typically present with unrelenting back pain without substantial objective findings. Radiographs may appear normal or reveal osteoblastic or lytic changes in the vertebral bodies. On MR images, lesions will appear as low signal on T1-weighted images and high signal on T2-weighted images. Contrast-enhanced images should be obtained using fat suppression techniques to avoid masking the inconsistently enhancing lesions.[32] The differential diagnosis for multiple lesions in cancellous bone includes marrow disorders such as multiple myeloma, lymphoma, and leukaemia.

Disc space infection

Infection of the disc space is a serious, potentially life-threatening, condition that requires early detection and prompt treatment for the most favourable outcome. Approximately 2–4% of osteomyelitis affects the spine, with the cervical spine least commonly involved.[49–51] The three mechanisms of spread are implantation through surgery or trauma, direct spread from an adjacent focus of infection, or haematogenous spread. Bloodborne pathogens arrive in the vertebral body through Batson's venous plexus (retrograde flow) or the vertebral body arterioles.[52]

The infection starts in the anterior aspect of the vertebral body and spreads through the disc to the adjacent level. Patients with disc space infection are likely to present with back pain of insidious onset. The pain will appear non-mechanical, constant, and unaffected by rest.[50] Additional constitutional symptoms such as fever, chills and weight loss may be present but are not necessary for the diagnosis. Laboratory evaluation may reveal elevated white blood cells, erythrocyte sedimentation rate, and C-reactive protein. Radiographic findings of early disc space infection are subtle and may consist only of disc space narrowing and subtle endplate irregularity.[49] MR imaging is the imaging procedure of choice for the evaluation of suspected infection and clinical suspicion should prompt an immediate referral (Figure 2.23). Findings will include decreased marrow signal on T1-weighting and increased signal on T2-weighting in adjacent vertebral bodies and the intervening disc.[49] MR imaging may also demonstrate endplate destruction in more advanced cases of infection. Administration of contrast will demonstrate enhancement of infected tissues.[49] One of the biggest mimickers of disc space infection, and one that causes anxiety amongst clinicians on MR imaging, is the findings seen with Modic degenerative endplate changes.[50] With Modic type 1 changes, there is increased marrow signal on T2-weighted images secondary to replacement of normal bone marrow by fibrovascular tissue. The presence of increased T2 signal within the disc in disc space infection is an important diagnostic clue that helps to distinguish between infection and degenerative disc disease, which produces a reduction in the disc signal on T2-weighted images.

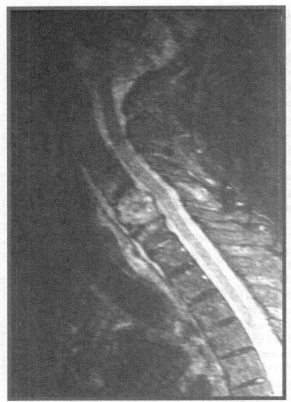

Figure 2.23 • MR imaging of the cervical spine, sagittal STIR sequence demonstrating heterogeneous increased signal at C5–C6 with bright signal in the disc space extending even to involve part of the inferior portion of C4. Extension is also occurring posteriorly in this case of osteomyelitis/disc space infection. (This case is reproduced courtesy of Francois-Xavier Fournier.)

Cervical spine trauma

Neck pain following cervical trauma is a common presenting complaint in primary care. A thorough history and physical examination, including neurological assessment, is crucial in arriving at a diagnosis and in guiding appropriate treatment or follow-up. Injury patterns vary depending upon the mechanism of injury and understanding the direction of force is helpful in narrowing the differential diagnosis (Table 2.03).[53]

The initial imaging work-up following cervical spine trauma typically consists of a three-view radiographic series. Often, flexion and extension views are also obtained, though in the acute setting the usefulness of these images to detect instability may be limited if the patient has a decreased ability to perform

Table 2.03 Mechanisms of cervical spine injury

Axial compression	Jefferson's fracture
	Burst fracture
Flexion	Ligamentous instability
	Odontoid fracture
	Transverse ligament rupture
	Vertebral body compression fracture
	Bilateral facet dislocation
	Hyperflexion teardrop fracture
Flexion-rotation	Unilateral facet dislocation
	Rotary facet joint subluxation
Extension	Ligamentous instability
	Hangman's fracture (spondylolysis of C2)
	Posterior arch fracture (articular pillar, lamina, spinous process)
	Odontoid fracture
	Hyperextension teardrop fracture?

range of motion.[54] In the evaluation of static or flexion/extension radiographs, the presence of more than 3.5 mm of motion at one level, compared to adjacent levels, constitutes instability and warrants a referral for neurosurgical evaluation.[12]

In an acute, post-traumatic situation, CT may be obtained to assess the spine for fracture. CT gives greater detail than MR imaging regarding the amount of cortical offset and is better in detecting displacement of small fragments. MR imaging is superior, however, for evaluating soft tissue injuries and for evaluating the spinal cord, intervertebral discs, and ligamentous structures.[55] MR imaging is also highly sensitive for detecting fractures, and, in a patient with neurologic impairment following trauma, MR imaging is the imaging procedure of choice.

Cervical injuries are often occult on plain film and clinical suspicion should drive imaging decisions. On MR imaging, the oedema produced by fracture or ligamentous injury will appear as low signal on T1-weighted images and high signal on T2-weighted images. Injuries to the spinal cord can occur in the absence of fracture or dislocation and will also be best evaluated on MR imaging. During extension injuries, the ligamentum flavum buckles into the canal, reducing its cross-sectional diameter. In the presence of pre-existing degenerative disease, a physiologically narrow canal or momentary subluxation at the time of injury, the cord may be contused.[53] The cord contusion will appear as a high signal focus within the cord on T2-weighted images. The advent of seated MR imaging allows patients to be imaged in a weight-bearing posture and in a position that recreates their pain. Patients can also be imaged in flexion and extension positions to evaluate stability. Upright imaging may reveal disc herniations and antero- or retro-listheses not present on recumbent studies; this may help inform prognosis and guide treatment decisions.[56]

References

1. Cote P, Cassidy DJ, Carroll LJ, Kristman V. The annual incidence and course of neck pain in the general population: a population-based cohort study. *Pain*. 2004;112: 267–273.

2. Makela M, Heliovaara M, Sievers K, et al. Prevalence, determinants, and consequences of chronic neck pain in Finland. *Am J Epidemiol*. 1991;134(11):1356–1367.

3. Christensen MG, Kollasch MW. *Job Analysis of Chiropractic 2005: A Project Report, Survey Analysis, and Summary of the Practice of Chiropractic within the United States*. Greeley, CO: National Board of Chiropractic Examiners; 2005.

4. Bussieres AE, Taylor JAM, Peterson C. Diagnostic imaging practice guidelines for musculoskeletal complaints in adults—an evidence-based approach—Part 3: Spinal disorders. *J Manipulative Physiol Ther*. 2008;31(1):33–88.

5. Berkow R. Neck, shoulder and upper limb pain. In: *Merck Manual of Diagnosis and Therapy*. 16th ed West Point, PA: Merck & Co; 1992:1362.

6. Bates B. The musculoskeletal system. In: Bates B, ed. *A Guide to Physical Examination*. 3rd ed. Philadelphia: JB Lippincott; 1983:324–370.

7. Lindsay K, Bone I, Callander R. *Localised neurological disease and its management. Neurology and Neurosurgery Illustrated*. Edinburgh: Elsevier; 1991.

8. Demirbag D, Unlu E, Ozdemir F, et al. The relationship between magnetic resonance imaging findings and postural maneuver and physical examination tests in patients with thoracic outlet syndrome: results of a double-blind, controlled study.

Arch Phys Med Rehabil. 2007;88(7):844–851.

9. Wessely M, Grenier JM. Elbow MRI. Part 2: The imaging of common disorders affecting the elbow region. *Clinical Chiropractic*. 2007;10(1): 43–49.

10. Wessely M, Grenier J-M. MR imaging of the wrist and hand—a review of the normal imaging appearance with an illustration of common disorders affecting the wrist and hand. *Clinical Chiropractic*. 2007;10(3):156–164.

11. Travell J, Simons D. *Myofascial Pain and Dysfunction*. Baltimore: Williams and Wilkins; 1992.

12. White A, Johnson R, Panjabi M, Southwick W. Biomechanical analysis of clinical stability in the cervical spine. *Clin Orthop Rel Res*. 1975;109:85–96.

13. Helms C. Trauma. In: *Fundamentals of Skeletal Radiology*. Philadelphia: Elsevier Saunders; 2005:78–112.

14. Helms C, Major N, Anderson MW, et al. Basic principles of musculoskeletal MRI. In: *Musculoskeletal MRI*. 2nd ed. Philadelphia PA: Elsevier Saunders; 2009:1–19.

15. Moore K. The back. In: *Clinically Oriented Anatomy*. 2nd ed. Baltimore: Williams and Wilkins; 1985:565–625.

16. Green J, Silver P. The vertebral column and the back. In: *An Introduction to Human Anatomy*. Oxford: Oxford University Press; 1981:52–68.

17. Standring S, ed. *Gray's Anatomy – The back (Section 45)*. Edinburgh: Elsevier; 2009.

18. Rowe L, Yochum T. Radiograpic positioning and normal anatomy. In: Yochum T, Rowe L, eds. *Essentials of Skeletal Radiology*. Baltimore: Williams and Wilkins; 1987:1–93.

19. Standring S, ed. *Gray's Anatomy – Neuroanatomy: vascular supply of

the brain (Section 17)*. Edinburgh: Elsevier; 2009.

20. Green J, Silver P. The blood supply to the head and neck. In: *An Introduction to Human Anatomy*. Oxford: Oxford University Press; 1981:253–267.

21. Steel HH. Anatomical and mechanical considerations of the atlanto-axial articulations. *J Bone Joint Surg Am*. 1968;50: 1481–1482.

22. Ulbrich E, Schraner C, Busato A, et al. Cervical spinal canal dimensions. In: *16th Annual Congress of the European Society of Musculoskeletal Radiology*. Italy: Genoa; June 11–13, 2009.

23. Clark C. *The Cervical Spine*. 3rd ed. Philadelphia: Lippincott-Raven; 1998.

24. Cramer GD, Darby SA. *Basic and Clinical Anatomy of the Spine, Spinal Cord, and ANS*. 2nd ed. St. Louis: Mosby; 2005.

25. Kaplan P, Helms CA, Dussault R, et al. *Musculoskeletal MRI*. Philadelphia: WB Saunders; 2001.

26. White M. Cervical spine: MR imaging techniques and anatomy. *Magn Reson Imaging Clin N Am*. 2000;8(3):453–469.

27. Teo E, Ng H. Evaluation of the role of ligaments, facets and disc nucleus in lower cervical spine under compression and sagittal moments using finite element method. *Med Eng Phys*. 2001;23:155–164.

28. Swinkels A, Dolan P. Spinal position sense is independent of the magnitude of movement. *Spine*. 2000;25(1):98–105.

29. Kaale BR, Krakenes J, Albrektsen G, Wester K. Head position and impact direction in whiplash injuries: associations with MRI-verified lesions of ligaments and membranes in the upper cervical spine. *J Neurotrauma*. 2005;22(11): 1294–1302.

30. Kaale BR, Krakenes J, Albrektsen G, Wester K. Whiplash-associated disorders impairment rating: neck disability index score according to severity of MRI findings of ligaments and membranes in the upper cervical spine. *J Neurotrauma.* 2005;22(4):466–475.

31. Kaale BR, Krakenes J, Albrektsen G, Wester K. Clinical assessment techniques for detecting ligament and membrane injuries in the upper cervical spine region—a comparison with MRI results. *Man Ther.* 2008;13(5):397–403.

32. Ross JS, Brant-Zawadzki M, Chen MZ. *Diagnostic Imaging: Spine.* Salt Lake City: Amirsys; 2007.

33. Braga-Baiak A, Shah A, Pietrobon R, et al. Intra- and inter-observer reliability of MRI examination of intervertebral disc abnormalities in patients with cervical myelopathy. *Eur J Radiol.* 2008;65:91–98.

34. Fardon DF, Milette PC. Nomenclature and classification of lumbar disc pathology. *Spine.* 2001;26(5):E93–E113.

35. Boutin R, Steinbach L, Finnesey K. MR imaging of degenerative diseases in the cervical spine. *Magn Reson Imaging Clin N Am.* 2000;8(3): 471–490.

36. Sangha O. Epidemiology of rheumatic diseases. *Rheumatology.* 2000;39(suppl 2):3–12.

37. Modic M, Steinberg P, Ross J, et al. Degenerative disk disease: assessment of changes in vertebral body marrow with MR imaging. *Radiology.* 1988;166: 193–199.

38. Imhof H, Nobauer-Huhmann I-M, Gahleitner A, et al. Pathophysiology and imaging in inflammatory and blastomatous synovial diseases. *Skeletal Radiol.* 2002;31:313–333.

39. Feydy A, Liote F, Carlier R, et al. Cervical spine and crystal-associated diseases: imaging findings. *Eur Radiol.* 2006;16:459–468.

40. Hayes C, Conway W. Calcium hydroxyapatite deposition disease. *Radiographics.* 1990;10:1031–1048.

41. Chung T, Rebello R, Gooden E. Retropharyngeal calcific tendonitis: case report and review of the literature. *Emerg Radiol.* 2005; 11:375–380.

42. Hviid C, Salomonsen M, Gelineck J, et al. Retropharyngeal tendinitis may be more common than we think: a report on 45 cases seen in Danish chiropractic clinics. *J Manipulative Physiol Ther.* 2009;32(4):315–320.

43. Donmez H, Mavili E, Ikizceli T, Koc RK. Pediatric intervertebral disc calcification. *Diagn Interv Radiol.* 2008;14(4):225–227.

44. Zehetgruber H, Bittner B, Guber D, et al. Prevalence of aneurysmal and solitary bone cysts in young patients. *Clin Orthop Rel Res.* 2005;439: 136–143.

45. Leithner A, Windhager R, Lang S, et al. Aneurysmal bone cyst: a population based epidemiologic study and literature review. *Clin Orthop Rel Res.* 1999;363:176–179.

46. Pennekamp W, Peters S, Schinkel C, et al. Aneurysmal bone cyst of the cervical spine (2008:7b). *Eur Radiol.* 2008;18(10):2356–2360.

47. Ozaki T, Liljenqvist U, Hillmann A, et al. Osteoid osteoma and osteoblastoma of the spine: experiences with 22 patients. *Clin Orthop Rel Res.* 2002;397:394–402.

48. Pettine K, Klassen R. Osteoid-osteoma and osteoblastoma of the spine. *J Bone Joint Surg Am.* 1986;68:354–361.

49. Maiuri FI, Iaconetta G, Gallicchio B, et al. Spondylodiscitis: clinical and magnetic resonance diagnosis. *Spine.* 1997;22(15): 1741–1746.

50. Hong SH, Choi J-Y, Lee JW, et al. MRI imaging assessment of the spine: infection or an imitation. *Radiographics.* 2009;29(2):599–611.

51. Tins BJ, Cassar-Pullicino VN, Lalam RK. Magnetic resonance imaging of spinal infection. *Top Magn Reson Imaging.* 2007;18(3): 213–222.

52. Dagirmanjiian A, Schils J, McHenry M. MR imaging of spinal infections. *Magn Reson Imaging Clin N Am.* 1999;7:525–538.

53. Cusick JF, Yoganandan N. Biomechanics of the cervical spine 4: major injuries. *Clin Biomech.* 2002;17:1–20.

54. Insko EK, Gracias VH, Gupta R, et al. Utility of flexion and extension radiographs of the cervical spine in the acute evaluation of blunt trauma. *J Trauma.* 2002;53(3): 426–429.

55. Wenger M, Adam P, Alareon F, Markwalder T-M. Traumatic cervical instability associated with cord oedema and temporary quadriparesis. *Spinal Cord.* 2003;41:521–526.

56. Perez AF, Isidro MG, Ayerbe E, et al. Evaluation of intervertebral disc herniation and hypermobile intersegmental instability in symptomatic adult patients undergoing recumbent and upright MRI of the cervical or lumbosacral spines. *Eur J Radiol.* 2007;62(3):444–448.

The thoracic spine

3

Michelle A. Wessely   Renée M. DeVries

Introduction

Perhaps more than any other area, pain in the thoracic spine and its associated rib articulations requires differentiation from referred visceral pain and pathology, which can easily mimic musculoskeletal problems.[1] However, the thoracic spine is one of the most difficult areas to image with plain film radiography. On an x-ray, the thoracic cage is superimposed over the vertebral bodies; the discrepancy in tissue density between the osseous thoracic spine and the lung parenchyma creates a confluence of densities that precludes the acquisition of high-quality radiographic images.[2] This is particularly true for the lower thoracic spine, owing to the superimposition of the diaphragm, and the upper regions of the thoracic spine, owing to the soft tissues of the shoulder.

Cross-sectional imaging of the spine, spinal cord and surrounding anatomical structures has therefore contributed substantially to the detection and characterization of disorders affecting the thoracic spine; however, magnetic resonance (MR) imaging of this area is not without its own complications, which mainly arise from motion artifacts. Image quality can be affected by the pulsation of the heart, the respiratory cycle, and the vertical pulsatile movement of the blood and the cerebrospinal fluid through the thoracic region (Figure 3.01).[3] It is therefore important to recognize that the method of imaging the thoracic spine has been designed to reduce the effect of motion artifacts by utilizing techniques such as peripheral gating or saturation pulses.[4,5]

MR imaging of the spine has distinct advantages over computed tomography (CT), in particular the lack of ionizing radiation and spectacular resolution of the soft tissues, which offers a greater appreciation of the anatomic structures that may be contributing to the clinical syndrome; however, CT is the modality of choice to assess for certain conditions, especially osseous lesions, for example fractures.

Although MR imaging of the thoracic spine can be performed to assess a variety of disorders presenting to the manual physician, it is less commonly performed than that for the lumbar or cervical spine. Parts of the thoracic spine are, however, included both on cervical studies, where the upper three or four thoracic segments are routinely included, and on lumbar studies, when the lower three or four thoracic segments are often included.

Often, evidence of lower thoracic spine pathology, such as disc lesions or osseous trauma, is detected when the imaging has been performed to ostensibly evaluate a lumbar pathology. Knowledge of the thoracic spine and the disorders that can affect it is therefore important, not only for those dedicated MR imaging studies for the thoracic spine, but also when the thoracic spine is incidentally included on a study of the lumbar or cervical region.

MR imaging of the thoracic spine is often performed to determine the presence of a disc lesion. Although such lesions tend to be less common and also smaller in volume than those in other spinal areas, because the dimension of the thoracic spinal canal is relatively smaller, the risk of neurological compression is correspondingly higher.[6,7]

MR imaging has superior imaging quality of epidural and bone marrow involvement compared to other general imaging modalities, providing a means for the

© 2011, Elsevier Ltd.
DOI: 10.1016/B978-0-443-06726-6.00003-2

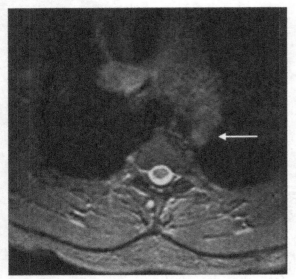

Figure 3.01 • MR imaging of the thoracic spine in the axial plane demonstrating a T2-weighted sequence. Note the blurred appearance of the great vessels and heart (white arrow indicating the proximal portion of the descending thoracic aorta) anterior to the spine due to the cardiac rhythm. Optimal imaging techniques allow for the subtraction of such artifacts, which may otherwise interfere with the interpretation of the imaging study.

differentiation of normal haematopoietic marrow from infiltrative processes such as metastatic disease. MR imaging, by virtue of the differing signal intensities, allows for the diagnosis and evaluation of disorders affecting the epidural fat, spinal cord, subarachnoid and intramedullary regions.[8]

By contrast, CT provides beautiful detail of bony structures but is somewhat limited in its depiction of canal lesions. MR imaging also allows the depiction of the soft tissue structures around the spine, including paraspinal soft tissue and neural structures; this is useful in conditions such as paraspinal abscess formation and neural tumours.[9,10]

History, examination, diagnosis and indications for imaging

Examination of the thoracic spine is considerably more difficult than that of the cervical and lumbar areas. There is a dearth of orthopaedic tests of diagnostic significance; the dermatomes overlap to the point whereby a single root lesion remains occult; there are no reliable myotomal indicators and no deep tendon

reflexes, although the umbilical reflexes can sometimes indicate a radicular lesion and long tract signs can also be an important indicator of central cord pathology.[6,11]

This makes the history even more important: apart from a thorough review of the cardiovascular and respiratory systems, the thoracic spine also contains the sympathetic trunk and so a generalized screen of the patient's systemic health is also essential.[12,13]

Observation of the patient can provide important clues. Scoliosis is a condition that commonly affects the thoracic spine, and which is easily seen.[14] Hyperkyphosis can also be associated with Scheuermann's disease (juvenile discogenic disease), ankylosing spondylitis and compression fractures, most commonly secondarily to osteoporosis; the age and sex of the patient is therefore important in indicating the differential diagnosis (Figure 3.02).[15]

Palpation can also be suggestive of conditions such as thoracic facet injury, costovertebral syndrome and costochondritis (Tietze's syndrome), all common causes of thoracic pain; however, because of the difficulty involved in definitive testing, diagnostic imaging is all the more important.[16,17]

Protocol

MR imaging of the thoracic spine requires the patient to lie supine during the examination; usually the patient enters the magnet headfirst. The complete MR examination lasts approximately 30–45 minutes, depending on the sequences required. It is, however, possible for patients to move between the various sequences, each of which commonly lasts for around 2 to 3 minutes. A spinal coil is placed under the patient to increase the quality of the image and a triangular foam pad is frequently placed under the knees, which may affect the normal spinal curvature. A positioning light is centred over the sternum in the midline.[4,5]

The field of view in MR images of the thoracic spine is approximately 16 cm in the sagittal plane and 14 cm in the axial plane. Slice thickness is usually 3–4 mm.[4,5] The initial sequence is the **coronal localizer (scout view)**; this is taken to verify the patient positioning and ordinarily includes C2 in order to correctly identify the thoracic levels. Imaging slices may be acquired either from the left to right field borders or from right to left of the vertebral bodies and it is important to verify this by noting the order of the slice numbers on the localizer view.

MR imaging of the thoracic spine commonly consists of T1-weighted and fast spin echo (FSE) T2-weighted

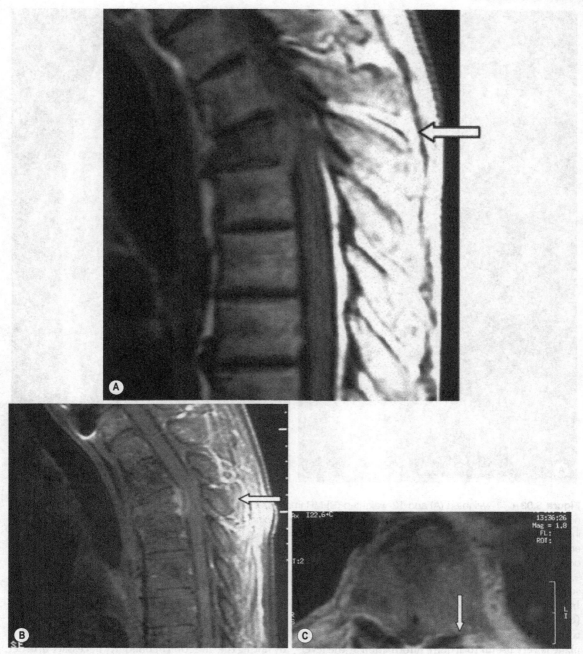

Figure 3.02 • Pathologic compression fracture. (A) T1-weighted sagittal MR imaging of the thoracic spine shows decreased marrow signal and decreased vertebral body height both anteriorly and posteriorly in the upper/mid-thoracic spine. Notice the soft tissue extension into the central spinal canal (at the level of the arrow). (B) A contrast-enhanced, T1-weighted sagittal MR image of the thoracic spine shows increased signal of the soft tissue mass (at the level of the arrow). (C) T1-weighted axial MR imaging of the thoracic spine shows compression of the thoracic cord from the soft tissue mass (arrow).

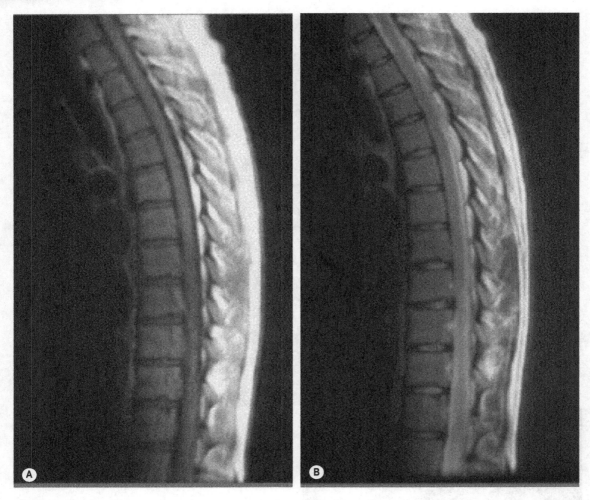

Figure 3.03 • T1-weighted (A) and T2-weighted (B) MR images of the thoracic spine in the sagittal plane: note the normal thin appearance to the disc heights at each level. The spinal cord and vertebral body are of increased signal intensity, especially when compared with the surrounding cerebrospinal fluid. In addition, the lower thoracic spine endplates demonstrate irregularity and focal indentation due to the presence of Schmorl's nodes, likely Scheuermann's disease residuals.

sequences in the sagittal plane (Figures 3.03, 3.04). In the axial/axial oblique plane, T2-weighted FSE (or intermediate weighted axial FSE) images parallel to the disc are acquired (Figure 3.01). The oblique plane is very useful to acquire information at the level of the intervertebral disc and in cases of scoliosis; the coronal/frontal plane may also be included, again particularly in scoliotic patients (Figure 3.05).

Patients with a significant scoliosis may present a challenge during MR imaging owing to the deviation of the spine from the midline in the parasagittal views. It is, therefore, important to inform the MR imaging centre of the clinical suspicion of a scoliosis in order

for the MR radiographer to make allowance for this when performing the imaging. The initial scout view will give the staff a depiction of the scoliosis and allow them to plan their sequences around it by noting the direction of obliquity necessary in order to obtain the most uniform sagittal images.

Contrast may be used in patients with suspicion of infection, intradural, non-traumatic cord lesions and to evaluate postoperative changes. Prior to contrast being given, the patient should be screened for contraindications such as renal disease; nephrogenic fibrosis can be a complication of the use of gadolinium-based contrast agents.

Figure 3.04 • A T2-weighted sequence of the thoracic spine in the sagittal plane: a common appearance of the normal thoracic intervertebral discs is that of apparent decreased signal intensity compared with that of the cervical and lumbar spine due to the relative smaller size of the disc in the thoracic spine. Each disc level should be evaluated to ensure that the consecutive slices demonstrate evidence of fluid signal, though it may be a small amount that is visible. This should not be confused with disc degeneration which appears as low signal intensity on the fluid-sensitive sequences on all consecutive slices. Use of fat suppression in the T2-weighted sequences has been added.

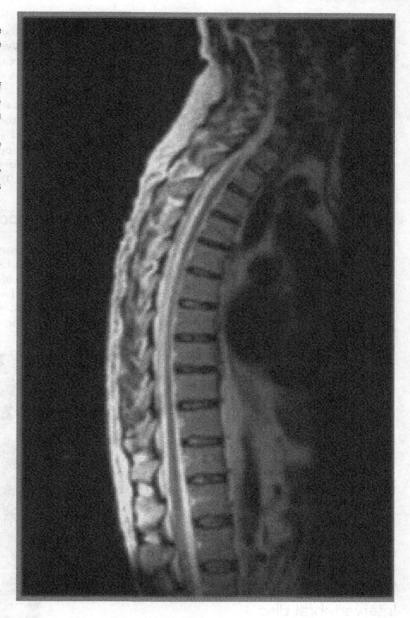

Specific protocols may be used in particular clinical circumstances. Most MR imaging thoracic spine protocols for metastases include T1- and T2-weighted sagittal and axial images with repetition of the T1-weighted images following the addition of gadolinium.[18] Alternative imaging sequences may include short tau inversion recovery (STIR) and fat suppression. The use of STIR is especially useful in increasing the sensitivity of lesion detection in the posterior elements of the vertebrae.[19]

Out-of-phase gradient echo (GRE) imaging is used to provide better lesion detection; the reason for this is that bone marrow metastases are characterized by the alteration of the fat:water ratio in the marrow, increasing the water content. T1-weighted imaging reveals this increased water content as *hypo*intensity; STIR will demonstrate this as *hyper*intensity. However, there are occasions when changes are more subtle and out-of-phase gradient echo sequences improve lesion conspicuity in all situations in which the difference in

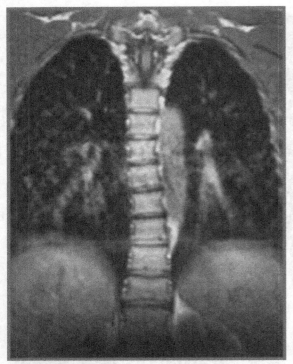

Figure 3.05 • A T1-weighted MR image of the thoracic spine in the coronal plane in a patient with a minimal C-shape, left thoracolumbar convexity. Notice also the possibility of visualizing the liver and spleen.

the fat:non-fat marrow ratio in the abnormal area is reduced when compared to the adjacent normal marrow.

Normal anatomy and variants

In the sagittal and axial planes, there are several important anatomical structures that require evaluation, including the intervertebral disc, vertebral body, spinal cord, intervertebral foramen, and the mediastinal and posterior soft tissues.

Intervertebral disc

The thoracic intervertebral disc is important to evaluate owing to the relatively smaller spinal canal diameter in this area of the spine, which predisposes to a higher risk of neurological involvement in thoracic disc herniations.[7] The hydrated nucleus of the normal intervertebral disc should be appreciated, together with its relationship to the cerebrospinal fluid of the anterior subarachnoid space. In degenerative disc disease, a reduction in hydration is demonstrated as hypointensity in the disc on T2-weighted sequences.[20]

Symptomatic thoracic disc lesions, such as extrusions, are uncommon, and present a particular diagnostic challenge to the clinician.[21] Sagittal, T2-weighted FSE sequences are excellent for displaying indentation of the ventral thecal sac and effacement of the spinal cord by a thoracic disc extrusion. Axial images help delineate lateralization of the disc lesion and evaluate impingement of the traversing nerve roots.

Because of the relatively smaller size of thoracic discs, they may appear hypointense on T2-weighted sequences compared to discs in other areas of the spine (Figures 3.03B, 3.04).

Vertebral body

The individual osseous components of the vertebral bodies are evaluated well using MR imaging; this is particularly true of the bone marrow. Cortical bone should appear as low signal intensity owing to the lack of mobile protons, especially on T1-weighted images (Figure 3.06). There should be no evidence of change

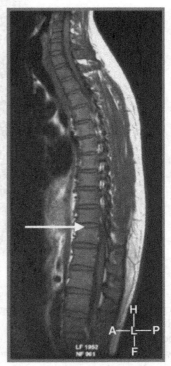

Figure 3.06 • T1-weighted MR imaging of the thoracic spine in the sagittal plane. The cortical bone of the osseous structures should appear as low signal intensity (white arrow), especially on T1-weighted images, owing to the lack of mobile protons.

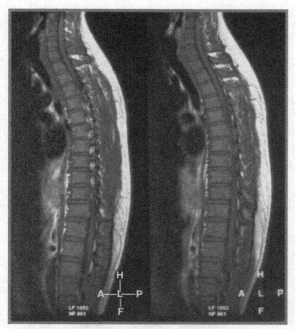

Figure 3.07 • T1-weighted MR imaging of the thoracic spine in the sagittal plane, demonstrating consecutive slices. The vertebral bodies have a homogeneous signal intensity on T1-weighted sequences, which is intermediate or higher signal intensity relative to the adjacent disc owing to the fat content in the normal adult patient.

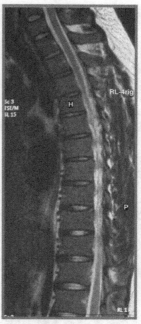

Figure 3.08 • A T2-weighted image of the thoracic spine in the sagittal plane, demonstrating the normal appearance of the vertebral body; that of a homogeneous low signal intensity when compared to the intervertebral discs and cerebrospinal fluid. There is a minimal convexity noted by the sagittal aspect of the spinal cord superiorly and conus inferiorly and a lack of visualization of the mid-thoracic region of the spinal cord.

in the contour of the vertebral bodies, which should have a homogeneous signal intensity on T1-weighted sequences (Figure 3.07).[22] Because of the higher fat content of the marrow, the vertebral body will be of intermediate or higher signal intensity relative to the adjacent disc.

The normal appearance of the vertebral body on T2-weighted sequences is that of homogeneous low signal intensity when compared with that of the intervertebral discs and cerebrospinal fluid (Figure 3.08).

A variation of the normal MR imaging appearance of bone marrow may include the presence of small foci of high signal (relative to the surrounding bone marrow) on T1-weighted imaging, which reduces on the T2-weighted sequences. This most likely represents an intraosseous lipomatous deposit, a normal variation.[4,5]

Another common phenomenon is high signal intensity in the bone marrow on both T1-weighted and T2-weighted sequences, representative of an intraosseous haemangioma. This condition does not usually have clinical consequences for the patient and is almost invariably an incidental finding. In less

than 1% of patients, haemangiomas may become symptomatic – particularly if they begin to expand, and the expansion is posterior. Such expansion is determined by evaluating the posterior wall of the vertebral body for evidence of slight posterior bulging of the cortical margin; this may suggest the presence of expansion before there is frank clinical evidence.[23,24]

By contrast, if high signal intensity is evident in the bone marrow on T2-weighted sequences and *decreased* signal intensity on T1-weighted sequences, this should be a cause for concern, since this pattern is suggestive of an infiltrative process such as metastatic disease, and should be followed with more specific sequences such as STIR or out-of-phase GRE MR imaging, and T1-weighted images with the addition of gadolinium.[4]

Spinal cord

The spinal cord should appear as intermediate (grey) signal intensity on all pulse sequences (Figure 3.09),

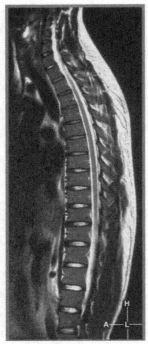

Figure 3.09 • A T2-weighted image of the thoracic spine in the sagittal plane. The spinal cord should be evaluated for shape, size, symmetry and internal signal intensity. If there is suspicion of a disorder such as multiple sclerosis, contrast should be ordered to determine evidence of active plaques.

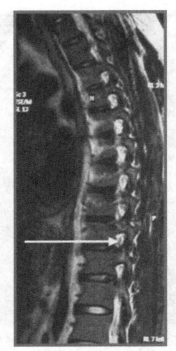

Figure 3.10 • A T2-weighted image of the thoracic spine in the sagittal plane with the slice representing a parasagittal slice demonstrating the intervertebral foramen and its contents (white arrow).

although on T2-weighted sequences it may be possible to distinguish the white and grey matter of the spinal cord. The spinal cord should be evaluated for shape, size, symmetry and internal organization to exclude the presence of disorders such as spinal cord impingement or syrinx formation.

The anterior, lateral and posterior columns (white matter) are demonstrated as hypointense signal intensity on the T2-weighted sequences. The cerebrospinal fluid is visible on MR imaging, visualized well on T2-weighted sequences as hyperintense signal and on T1-weighted sequences as hypointense signal, compared to the bone marrow signal intensity.[5]

Intervertebral foramen

MR imaging allows for definition of the size and morphology of the intervertebral foramen as well as its contents. The thoracic foramina are best visualized on the axial and sagittal sequences (Figure 3.10).

Identification of the exiting nerve roots surrounded by their perineural fat may be possible. Disorders that can involve the IVF in the thoracic spine include nerve root tumours, such as neurinomas, or abnormalities affecting the nerve root sleeve such as meningocoele or diverticulum formation (Figure 3.11).[25]

Pathological conditions

Thoracic disc lesions

The articulations with the ribcage make the thoracic spine the least mobile of the spinal regions; injuries to the thoracic spine and intervertebral discs are, therefore, less common than to the adjacent cervical and lumbar regions. There are, however, some factors that may predispose individual patients to disc lesions in the thoracic spine. Owing to the thoracic

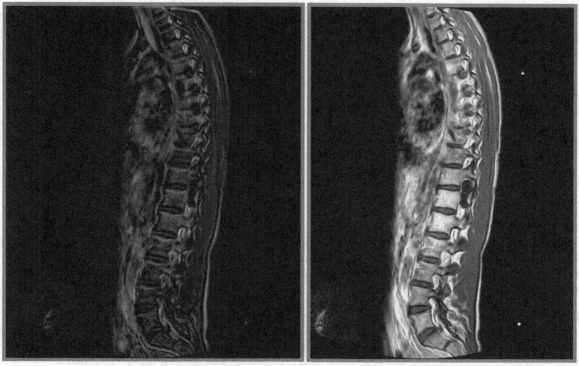

Figure 3.11 • T2-weighted (left) and T1-weighted (right) imaging of the thoracolumbar spine demonstrating a large area of low signal at T11/12 in the region of the intervertebral foramen. This represents a **diverticulum** or **root sleeve cyst**.

kyphosis, the spinal cord lies anteriorly in the spinal canal, approximating to the posterior longitudinal ligament and providing a greater propensity for ventral cord compression.[26] The thoracic spinal canal is also smaller than its cervical and lumbar counterparts and, although the spinal cord too is less massive, the size relative to the canal is still greater than in other areas of the spine. The clinical consequences of this are that although thoracic disc lesions may be less common, there is a higher chance of them being symptomatic, as the neural structures are more prone to compressive or irritative pathology.[13]

Though not a common entity, thoracic disc lesions are, nevertheless, considerably less rare than once thought. Due to the paucity of associated clinical findings, thoracic disc lesions were difficult to diagnose before the advent of MR imaging and they were once thought to represent fewer than 5% of all disc lesions.[21] The incidence of symptomatic thoracic disc lesions is still thought to be low (although this is difficult to ascertain and there is often no way to accurately determine whether a patient's symptoms relate to discal pathology by clinical

examination alone), whilst the presence of asymptomatic thoracic disc lesions may be as high as 37%[21]; certainly, clinicians should not readily correlate disc bulges identified by MR with their patient's pain syndromes unless there is compelling clinical evidence to the contrary, such as a history of significant trauma causing spinal compressive impaction or indications of a space-occupying lesion such as a positive Valsalva's sign/manoeuvre. Disc lesions in the lower thoracic spine are more likely to produce symptoms; however, thoracic disc lesions can also spontaneously reduce in size and will often spontaneously resolve.[27]

The mechanism of discal injury in the thoracic spine is somewhat different to that affecting the cervical and lumbar spine, principally due to the differing anatomy and biomechanical demands in this area. The thoracic region, with the thoracic cavity and rib attachments, is afforded a greater degree of functional rigidity and, to some degree, protection from the shearing forces that can progressively damage the annular fibres; however, there does appear to be some correlation with torsional movement such as that found in a golfer's swing. The predominant mode of disc injury in the thoracic spine, however, involves vertical compressive forces, usually related to trauma such as 'spearing' injuries.[26]

When present at all, the symptoms of thoracic disc lesions are varied and often vague, increasing the difficulty of an accurate and timely diagnosis. In addition to the local thoracic spine, the pain may be referred to the abdomen or chest, providing further confusion as to the origin of the pain. Upper thoracic lesions may present with symptoms similar to thoracic outlet compression syndrome type complaints, neck pain, and sensory or motor changes. Horner's syndrome has also been reported.[28]

In the lower thoracic spine, it becomes even more difficult to correlate symptomatology with a specific spinal level (Box 3.01).[29] Additionally, sympathetic trunk compression can cause visceral symptoms that may be easily confused with cardiac and abdominal disorders or with postherpetic neuralgia.[30]

The reason for this plethora of neurologically diverse symptomatology relates to the increased chance of thoracic spinal cord compression discussed above and the fact that the lumbar and sacral nerves are, of course, traversing the thoracic canal; this can give rise to a *thoracic spinal myelopathy*.[31] Since the spinal cord/conus medullaris terminates at L1–L2 in most adult patients, the segments of the spinal cord do not match vertebral body levels below T4.[32] Lesions of the thoracolumbar region are described as *epiconus syndrome*, involving the L4–S2 cord segments at the T12 vertebral body level, and *conus syndrome*, involving cord segments S3–S5 at the T12/L1 intervertebral disc level. These syndromes can mimic cauda equina syndrome (Figures 3.12, 3.13).[29]

Box 3.01

Symptoms associated with a lower thoracic disc lesion*

- Midline back pain
- Increased patellar tendon reflex
- Sensory disturbance of the entire lower extremity
- Bowel and bladder dysfunction
- Foot drop
- Diminished Achilles' reflex

*From DeVries & Wessely[10]

The presence of myelopathy is an indication for surgical intervention. Given the anatomy of the thoracic region, surgical intervention is complex and is considered controversial for pain relief alone.[10] Owing to the high incidence of asymptomatic thoracic disc lesions, their identification should be carefully correlated with the patient's clinical history (Figures 3.14, 3.15). The classification of a thoracic disc lesion should be related to its anatomical level, just as in the cervical and lumbar spine; however, as we have seen, this can be clinically challenging, if not impossible, even with the aid of MR imaging, which may correlate poorly to clinical or, indeed, represent incidental findings.

Thoracic disc lesions can be categorized into five types, related to the position of the disc lesion.

Central disc lesions, which are detected particularly well on axial slices, will be purely posterior and may cause the patient to develop myelopathic symptoms related to the frank compression of the spinal cord, leading the patient to develop signs of an upper motor neuron lesion, including weakness, hyperreflexia and increased muscle tone.

Centrolateral thoracic disc lesions, best determined on the axial images, can cause the development of weakness unilaterally and pain or sensory alterations on the contralateral side of the patient.

Lateral thoracic disc lesions, again detected on the axial slices, may present with symptoms of local radiculopathy due to nerve root irritation/ compression.

Intradural thoracic disc lesions are very rare and will be best appreciated on the axial and sagittal images. Most commonly, intradural thoracic disc lesions are located in the middle third of the thoracic spine and the most prominent neurological deficit that the patient will present with is that of a spastic paraparesis. The pathogenesis of this somewhat unusual phenomenon may be based on the ventral dura having regions of relative weakness located along it (like the blebs noted in the pleura in patients who are predisposed to pneumothorax).

Intraosseous disc lesions are more commonly termed *Schmorl's nodes*. This lesion is frequently encountered in clinical practice, where it is easily identifiable on plain film x-ray (Figures 3.16–3.18); it is usually asymptomatic. Whilst the routine radiograph will demonstrate the focal indentation along the superior or inferior endplate of one or multiple levels of the thoracic spine (though these may also

Figure 3.12 • MR imaging of the thoracic spine, performed using a T2-weighted sequence in the sagittal plane, to demonstrate a large focal disc extrusion T12–L1 with an associated reduced fluid signal from the disc. The axial slice is necessary to discern if there is true dural sac contact and displacement.

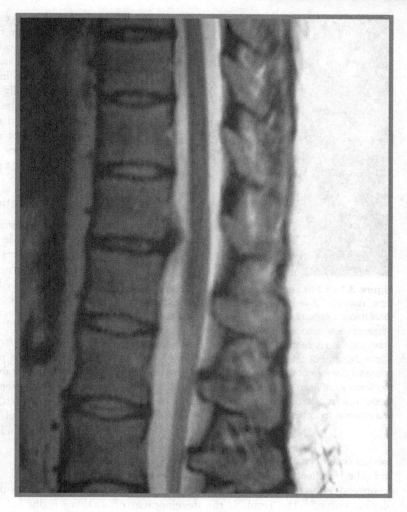

be encountered in the lumbar spine too), special imaging may also detect these lesions. Often, degenerative disc disease is noted to be associated with the intraosseous disc lesion. Although MR imaging is not the imaging modality of choice for the diagnosis of these lesions, routine radiography being sufficient to make the diagnosis, it is useful to determine the imaging appearance on MR imaging that may have been performed to determine the origin of the patient's complaint.

Scheuermann's disease

Multiple intraosseous disc lesions may be associated with *Scheuermann's disease* (also occasionally termed *juvenile kyphosis* or, when seen in the lumbar spine, *juvenile discogenic disease*), a condition affecting the development of the endplates during teenage skeletal growth and characterized by hyperkyphosis, anterior vertebral body wedging, endplate irregularities and the development of Schmorl's nodes. It may be asymptomatic and is found commonly on thoracic spine radiographs. When symptomatic, Scheuermann's disease typically produces an 'aching' type of pain. In addition to the changes seen on plain film, MR imaging may show the presence of associated intervertebral disc lesions (Figure 3.19).

The condition appears to arise from a combination of genetic factors, rendering the vertebral endplates

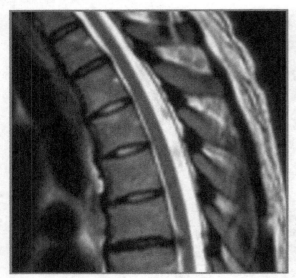

Figure 3.13 • MR imaging of the thoracic spine, sagittal slice, using a T2-weighted sequence, demonstrating a focal mid-thoracic disc lesion, likely extrusion and possibly sequestration associated with degenerative disc disease changes. Also note that there is a second, less voluminous upper thoracic disc lesion with a focal alteration of the posterior contour of the disc accompanying a reduction in the fluid signal from the disc. It is important to correlate these findings with the axial slices and also with the clinical examination to determine the clinical correlation.

weaker than normal because of a fragile blood supply, and the application of trauma, usually vertical compressive forces along the normal thoracic physiological curve.[33] The result is the development of multiple, intraosseous herniations together with irregularity of the endplates, a cuneiform aspect to the shape of the vertebral bodies with anterior wedging, and an apparent increase in the sagittal dimension of the vertebral body. The latter finding is due to the disproportionate growth in the sagittal dimension relative to the vertical height following an interruption of the normal growth pattern of the endplates. Degenerative disc disease is often associated, with a decrease in the disc height and osteophyte formation.

Annular tears

As well as identifying the location of the thoracic disc lesion and its anatomical relationship with surrounding structures, it is also useful to determine whether there is evidence of any tear in the annulus. Annular tears or fissures, often termed HIZ (high intensity zones, owing to their MR appearance seen in Figure 3.20), may, in the thoracic spine, be associated with pain in the local area, and can therefore be a diagnostically useful finding. A thoracic annular tear or fissure is best identified on the axial or sagittal slices, and noted on the T2-weighted sequence as a small region of increased signal intensity, usually in the outer one-third of the annulus along the posterolateral margin.

Disc calcification

Additional findings in disc lesions in the thoracic spine may include calcification. In general, calcification of disc lesions is relatively uncommon, although children have a higher likelihood of disc calcification than do adults. Although usually asymptomatic, it can be associated with torticollis in the cervical and upper thoracic spine; however, this tends to be self-limiting.[34–36] Whilst disc calcification is a relatively unusual phenomenon in the adult population, it may be more prevalent in the thoracic spine.[37] Although detectable on routine radiographs, if MR imaging of the thoracic spine is the only modality that has been provided, it is useful to recognize calcification as a region of low signal intensity at the level of the disc both on T1- and T2-weighted sequences.

Conclusion

MR imaging provides a relatively simple way in which a thoracic disc lesion can be confirmed; however, cost may be a limiting factor. MR imaging of the thoracic spine for the detection of disc lesions comes in to its own when it is necessary to quantify the lesion and its relationship with surrounding anatomic structures. Although both the sagittal and axial images can be used to determine the presence of a thoracic disc lesion, it is the latter that is the more useful for determining the effect of the lesion on the surrounding structures, particularly the epidural fat and the spinal cord. Evidence of cord displacement and/or effacement either posteriorly or laterally are factors that are useful in determining the severity of the disc lesion. It is also important to evaluate the intracordal signal, particularly in those cases of chronic or long-standing compressive lesions where myelomalacia may develop; this is best done on T2-weighted sequences.

Figure 3.14 • Thoracic disc herniation: a T2-weighted sagittal MR image of the thoracic spine demonstrates a focal posterior disc lesion in the mid-thoracic area (curved arrow).

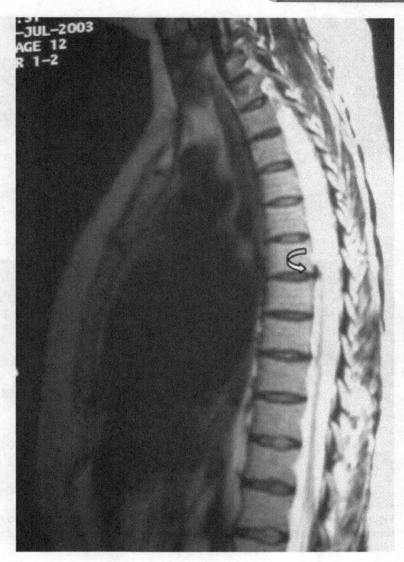

Tumours

Whilst a number of osseous and cord tumours can arise in the thoracic spine, this section will focus on those that are most frequent and have the greatest clinical relevance.

Vertebral body haemangioma

Haemangiomas are benign, primary, vascular neoplasms that may be regarded as an abnormality in the development of bone; they are considered the

most common benign neoplasm of the spine. Most lesions are asymptomatic and are considered incidental findings when seen on plain film radiography; however, occasionally, they may expand into the spinal canal, producing central canal stenosis.[38,39]

Haemangiomas are vascular malformation anomalies that predominate in the spine (they may also be located in soft tissues) and most frequently occur in the thoracic region. On biopsy, haemangiomas are full of thin-walled vascular channels lined with flattened endothelial cells, interspersed with adipose tissue. These, together with sinuses, lie between

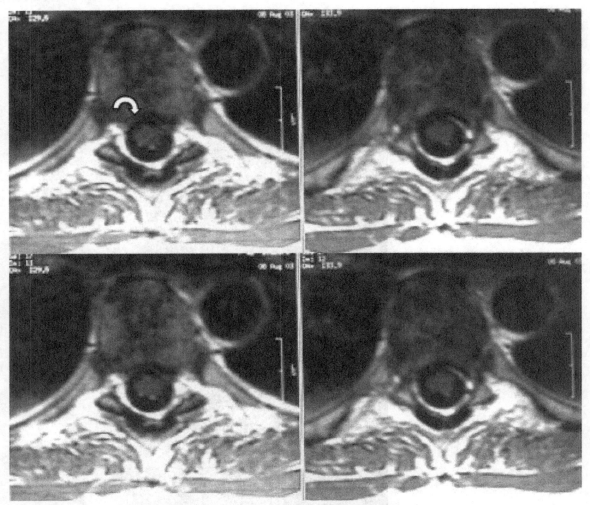

Figure 3.15 • Thoracic disc herniation: a contrast-enhanced axial T1-weighted MR image of the thoracic spine demonstrates a central/right paracentral disc lesion (curved arrow) with contact with the ventral dural sac resulting in minimal cord displacement in the left posterolateral direction.

vertically oriented trabeculae, giving the bone its classical striated appearance on radiographs, known as a 'corduroy cloth' vertebra.[40]

These, however, are not the only lesions that can give rise to this appearance. The classical radiographic appearance is due to local bone resorption by the vascular channels lying between the vertically oriented traberculae; therefore, other conditions such as lymphoma, metastatic disease, focal fatty fibrous deposits and multiple myeloma may also produce this appearance. It is thus very important to correlate the clinical history, physical examination, and appropriately ordered laboratory tests with imaging findings to determine the most probable cause of the imaging appearance.

MR imaging can detect very small haemangiomas not evident on plain film radiography. The location of these small haemangiomas is characteristic: on the sagittal, T2-weighted images there will often be a small linear region of high signal intensity along the posterior vertebral body; this represents the entrance of the basivertebral vein. Where this vein terminates anteriorly, a focal region of circular increase in signal intensity is often noted, which is often of the

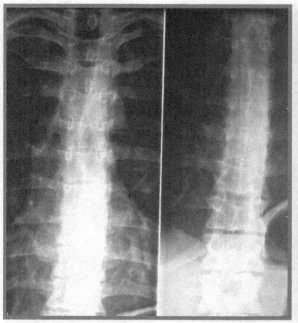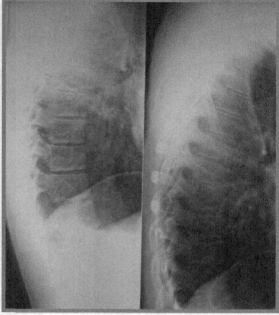

Figure 3.16 • Anteroposterior and lateral radiographs demonstrating, particularly on the lateral view, the irregularities along the endplates in the thoracic spine due to Scheuermann's disease residuals. Note also the unnecessary dose of radiation to this patient, which could have been reduced had a filter been placed in front of the x-ray beam to begin with!

same form and signal intensity on the T1-weighted image; this region represents a small haemangioma (Figures 3.21–3.23).

This increased signal intensity on both T1- and T2-weighted sequences differentiates haemangiomas from most other tumours, which often show decreased signal intensity on T1-weighted sequences owing to their water content. However, if the haemangioma is predominantly vascular – thus with a correspondingly lower level of adipose – a less intense signal is noted on the T1-weighted sequence (the increased signal intensity of haemangiomas on T1-weighted sequences is thought to be due to the fatty components of these lesions, whereas the increased signal intensity on T2-weighted sequences is due to the water content of the tumour).[38,40]

In most cases, haemangiomas affect the vertebral body rather than the posterior arch. They may be of differing sizes, located in the centre of the vertebral body only or occupying the totality of the vertebral body in question. Having determined the presence of any osseous haemangioma, it is important to ascertain whether there is evidence of bony expansion, particularly posteriorly. Normally, there is a slight concavity in the posterior wall (this is not to be confused with posterior scalloping, which is a clinically significant accentuation of this normal concavity). If there is loss of this concavity or any appearance of a bulge (deformation posterior of the posterior wall), this is suggestive of posterior expansion of the haemangioma, which may provoke not only local pain but also the development of neurological symptoms and signs, dependent on the level involved.[4,24] Highly vascular/low adipose haemangiomas (the ones with lower signal intensity on T1-weighted images) are also suggestive of lesions that are more likely to be associated with focal pain.

Symptoms from haemangiomas are most commonly produced from pathological fractures, haematomas, extension of the lesion into the epidural space, or from bony expansion.[38,40,41] Symptomatic lesions are more likely to involve the entire vertebral body and appear more irregular and less well defined.[40] Previously, treatment for symptomatic haemangiomas has included radiotherapy, embolization, and surgical excision. Vertebroplasty, the injection of methylmethacrylate (bone cement) into the vertebral body, has been used and can produce both symptomatic relief and bone

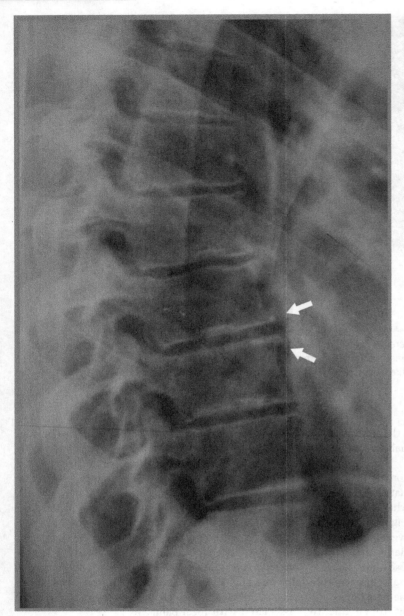

Figure 3.17 • Lateral thoracic spine radiograph demonstrating the irregularity of the endplates with small Schmorl's nodes noted and resultant degenerative disc disease, with evidence of spondylophyte formation anteriorly (black arrows).

strengthening. Injection of the lesion with ethanol represents another method of treatment, the ethanol acting as a sclerosing agent that shrinks the tumour.[42]

Metastasis

Aggressive tumour processes may also affect the thoracic spine; by far the most commonly encountered is metastatic disease. Metastasis tends to affect the older population (over the age of 50 years), although if there is a history of a child-hood tumour – for example a Wilms' tumour – the patient may develop metastatic disease at a younger age.[43,44] Osseous metastatic deposits tend to affect the axial skeleton in the older patient, since the red marrow located in this region acts as the

Figure 3.18 • The multiple Schmorl's nodes of Scheuermann's disease are commonly seen on thoracic radiographs. Note the irregular endplates and the increase in the physiologic thoracic curve, kyphosis, in this young adult male patient. (Image courtesy of Marco Colombo)

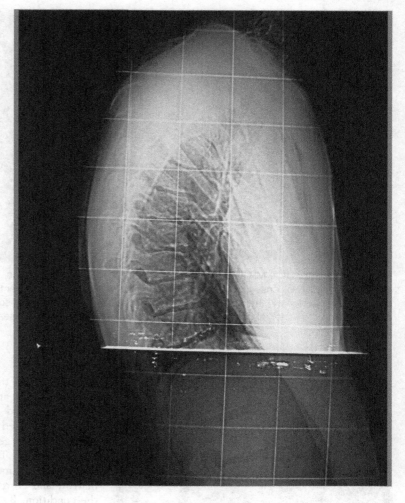

nutrient bed. In an adult, red marrow is located primarily in the axial skeleton and the proximal halves of the femurs and humeri. Where there is a clinical suspicion of metastatic disease, then, depending on local protocols, imaging may comprise routine radiography, bone scanning and then cross-sectional imaging.[2]

MR imaging is particularly valuable in the assessment of metastatic disease as well as the response to treatment; however, with the development of newer techniques, future evaluation may include the use of positron emission tomography (PET) as part of the routine assessment of the patient.[45,46]

In order to recognize the presence of metastatic disease in the thoracic spine, it is essential to be thoroughly familiar with normal radiographic anatomical appearance. As we saw earlier in the chapter, the bony marrow in the thoracic spine should be of a relatively high signal on the T1-weighted images and, moreover, should be homogeneous in appearance. On the fluid-sensitive, T2-weighted sequences, the vertebral marrow should be of a lower signal intensity compared with that on the T1-weighted sequence, and again should be homogeneous (Figures 3.07, 3.08). There are, however, a number of factors that can affect the normal appearance of the marrow, including age, general health status, smoking, and anaemia.[47,48]

If there is metastatic disease in the thoracic spine, a focal area of increased signal intensity will initially be seen on T2-weighted sequences, usually in the vertebral body although the posterior arch can also be

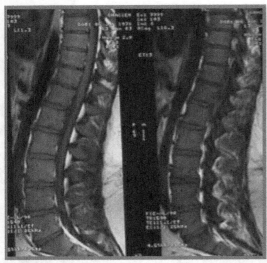 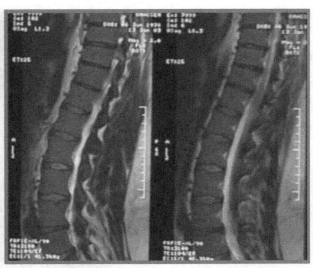

Figure 3.19 • Alternative MR imaging of the lumbar spine, in the sagittal plane, T1-weighted (two consecutive slices) and T2-weighted (two consecutive slices), where it can be noted that in the lower thoracic spine T8 through to T12 there is a reduced fluid signal in the discs, and that the endplates are irregular with a somewhat cuneiform or wedge-shaped appearance to the vertebral bodies due to the residuals of Scheuermann's disease with resultant degenerative disc disease.

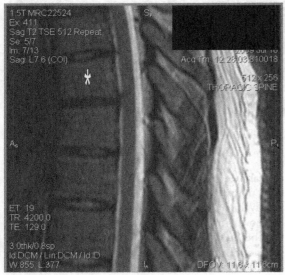

Figure 3.20 • A high intensity zone (HIZ) represents an annular tear or fissure, seen on a T2-weighted image as a small area of increased signal intensity, usually in the outer third of the annulus along the posterolateral margin. In this patient, sagittal T2-weighted MR imaging of the thoracic spine demonstrates that there is a reduction in the signal intensity of the disc in general between the vertebra (*) and the level below, as well as a focus of high signal noted in the posterior aspect of this disc, a HIZ.

affected. Over time, depending on the patient's treatment, the area of increased signal intensity may enlarge and be noted at multiple levels. On the T1-weighted sequences, the corresponding region will, in general, have low signal intensity (Figure 3.24). This represents the commonest appearance of metastatic disease affecting the bony marrow and corresponds to the osteolytic form of the condition. By contrast, osteoblastic lesions will cause a decrease in signal intensity on both the T1- and T2-weighted sequences.[4,24]

Once the radiographic probability of metastatic disease in the vertebral body has been confirmed, it is important to determine whether the posterior arch is also affected; often an indicator of the spread and extent of invasion. It is also important to assess for the common complications of metastasis: pathological fractures and extension of the tumour into the spinal canal.

Vertebral body fracture

Pathologic fractures can be difficult to appreciate on routine, plain film radiography, particularly in the thoracic spine; therefore, MR imaging may be particularly useful in this area. It can, at times, be

Figure 3.21 • T2-weighted sagittal imaging of the thoracic spine. Notice the high signal intensity in the posterior half of the vertebral body in the mid-thoracic spine, a characteristic of a vertebral body haemangioma, although it is important to view the T1 image to determine that this is likely a haemangioma. No evidence of bony expansion is noted.

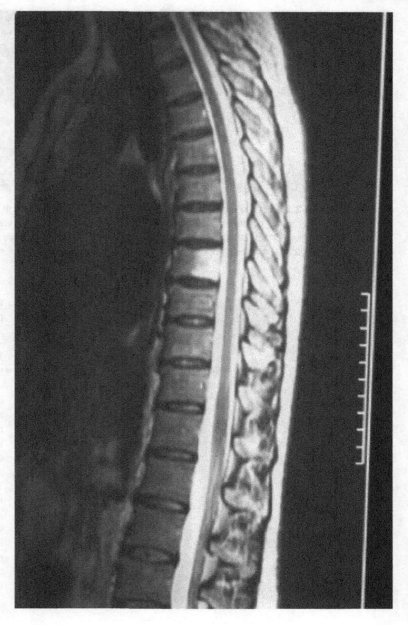

extremely hard to differentiate between a simple compression fracture and a pathologic fracture; however, there are some general rules that can help guide both the radiologist and the clinician.

Simple compression fractures, be they due to the generalized demineralization related to senile osteoporosis or to trauma, will tend to have a preservation of the posterior vertebral body height and a reduction of the anterior height. By contrast, a pathological fracture commonly causes a global reduction in vertebral body height, both posteriorly and anteriorly (see Figure 3.11).[2] Osteoporotic compression fractures are by far the commonest form of spinal fracture, affecting at least one million women every year in the USA alone, and they are particularly prevalent in the thoracic spine.[49]

In the case of a simple compression fracture, the majority of the increased signal intensity on the

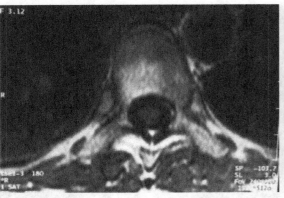 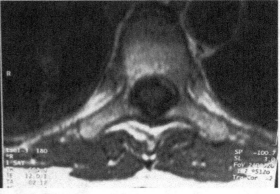

Figures 3.22 and 3.23 • In the same patient a T1-weighted axial image through the mid-thoracic spine demonstrates high signal intensity in the posterior half of predominantly the right side of the vertebral body due to the presence of a haemangioma; these classically appear as high signal on both T1- and T2-weighted images. There is again no evidence of posterior expansion, a rare but possible finding associated with a haemangioma.

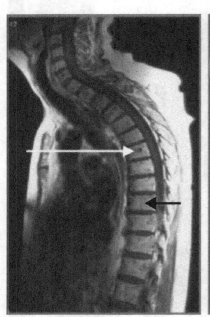 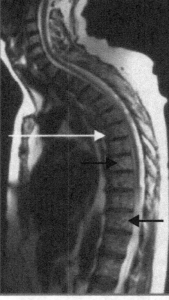

Figure 3.24 • A 71-year-old lady presented with progressively worsening, diffuse spinal pain that occasionally awoke her from sleep. A bone scan was ordered and, following these results, MR imaging was obtained: the T1-weighted image is on the left and the T2-weighted image on the right. Notice the markedly abnormal bone marrow throughout all the visualized spine, well demonstrated as a decreased signal intensity of the bone marrow on the T1-weighted image of T6 marked by the arrow on the left image, and the increased signal intensity at the same level on the T2-weighted image. Biopsy was performed and confirmed metastatic disease to the spine from a previously undetected primary adenocarcinoma of the breast.

T2-weighted sequence will be located immediately underneath and parallel to the superior endplate. This is known as the *zone of condensation*, and is produced by the overlapping, compressed trabeculae. On the T1-weighted sequence, this appears as a region of grey, or as a slightly decreased signal (corresponding to oedema) with a hypointense signal just underneath the superior endplate (corresponding to the fracture).[4]

In a pathologic fracture, there may be diffuse or patchy alteration in signal intensity that may involve a significant portion of the vertebral body. This will manifest as a focus of increased signal on the T2-weighted sequence and decreased signal on the T1-weighted sequence. Furthermore, with a simple compression fracture, no additional deformation of the vertebral body will be noted posteriorly, whereas with the pathologic fracture, posterior deformation may be apparent with perhaps evidence of a soft tissue mass extending into the spinal canal (Figure 3.25).

Figure 3.25 • The thoracic spine is the commonest area for compression fractures. Simple compression fractures will tend to maintain their posterior body height (**A**); by contrast, a pathological fracture will tend to cause a global reduction in vertebral body height (**B**). Notice the multiple foci of increased signal intensity within the vertebral bodies, associated with the anterior wedging of the anterior vertebral bodies, due to multiple compression fractures sustained during a snowmobile accident. (This case is courtesy of Tim Mick DC, DACBR, CDI/Minnesota.)

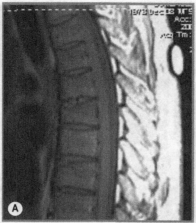
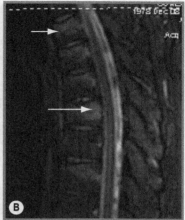

Another sign of an acute fracture is the *step defect*, the buckling of the anterior vertebral body margin that represents a break in the anterior cortex, again from the compressive injury. Both the step defect and the zone of condensation disappear with the remodelling that occurs during fracture healing, and the absence of these signs is helpful in determining if a fracture is healed, or old. In highly osteoporotic patients, the bone density is so diminished on plain films that the step defect and zone of condensation cannot be detected, even with recent fractures. MR imaging is useful in cases such as these. An acute compression fracture will show decreased signal intensity in the bone marrow on T1-weighted sequences and increased signal on T2-weighted sequences with respect to the adjacent, normal segments.

These generalized rules may not, however, be enough to differentiate a simple vertebral compression fracture from a pathological fracture. In some cases, special MR imaging sequences may be needed to determine the underlying cause of the altered marrow signal. The sequences that may be of particular use are *in-phase* and *opposed phase* whereby the differing precession of hydrogen atoms in water and fat can be used to differentiate a compression fracture with normal marrow from pathological fracture in which there will most probably be altered marrow physiology.

What this means is that on the normal spin echo sequence, the previous cited imaging findings will be noted with each type of fracture. However, when the opposed phase imaging is performed, in a simple compression fracture, given that the marrow surrounding the fracture site is by definition normal, suppression of the signal will be noted. In a patient with a pathological fracture, because the surrounding marrow is usually to some degree abnormal, altered signal intensity will be noted.

MR imaging is particularly useful in fracture assessment, evaluating the amount of vertebral body collapse and, therefore, differentiating the possible treatment options. One technique for alleviating the pain associated with thoracic body fractures, as well as helping prevent further alteration to the patient's thoracic kyphosis, is vertebroplasty: injection of stabilizing cement into the damaged bone. Before this technique is employed, it is helpful to know the degree of vertebral collapse and whether there are any complications, such as in a *'burst' fracture* where bony fragments may be located in the spinal canal.

Syrinx

A syrinx is a cyst-like expansion of the spinal cord. The term 'syringomyelia' is used for cysts that are lined with glial cells, whilst the term 'hydromyelia' implies that the cyst is lined with ependymal cells. The former usually represents an acquired cavity, whilst the latter is typically of congenital origin.[50] Patients with a syrinx may present with symptoms of back pain, headaches and paresis and have altered reflexes.[33] The clinical signs may also consist of a loss of pain and temperature sensations owing to interruption of the spinothalamic tracts; muscular weakness due to involvement of the anterior horn cells; and hyperreflexia due to involvement of the upper motor neurons.[6]

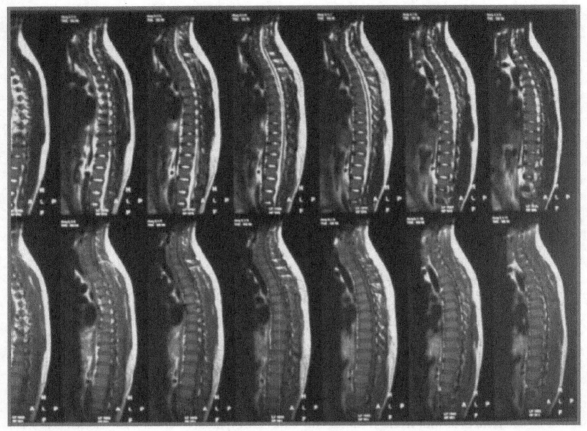

Figure 3.26 • MR imaging of the thoracic spine performed in the sagittal plane – the top imaging panel is the T2-weighted imaging and the lower imaging panel is the T1-weighted imaging. Always use the scout views when provided (not in this case) to determine the orientation, i.e. left to right or, conversely, right to left.

There appears to be an association between syringomyelia and atypical scoliosis patterns.[33,51,52] In particular, the presence of a left-sided scoliosis and hyperkyphosis have been associated with cord syrinx, and also with Arnold-Chiari type I malformations. Syringohydromyelia may be associated with additional abnormalities of the nervous and osseous systems, including Arnold-Chiari malformation, Klippel–Feil syndrome or occipitalization of the atlas. Cord syrinxes can also occur following spinal trauma or can arise as a postsurgical complication.[51]

The syrinx is usually imaged in both the sagittal and axial planes (imaging of the coronal plane is not commonly performed unless scoliosis is suspected). The author's preference is to use the sagittal T2-weighted sequence to initially determine the extent of the syrinx in the longitudinal dimension; the sagittal plane will also give an idea of the loculations associated with the syrinx. The axial slices are then useful to determine the extent of spinal cord displacement and direction of expansion (see Figure 3.26).

The MR imaging appearance of syringomyelia is that of low signal on T1-weighted sequences and high signal on T2-weighted sequences, consistent with the imaging characteristics of CSF (Figure 3.27). Following the initial identification of the syrinx, it is important to determine if there are other important associated findings, for example the presence of Arnold-Chiari malformation (see Chapter II) whereby the cerebellar tonsils will be noted to be engaged, ectopic or frankly displaced inferiorly. When symptomatic, a syrinx may be treated with surgical shunting to reduce the collection of CSF; however, syrinxes may recur and, if symptomatic, may need to be re-drained.

Figure 3.27 • Syrinx. (A) A T2-weighted sagittal MR image of the cervicothoracic spine with a large cyst-like cavity in the cervicothoracic cord, extending from C2 into the mid-thoracic spine. The syrinx is of high signal intensity on this T2-weighted image, consistent with CSF. (B) A T1-weighted image showing the fluid-filled syrinx as low signal intensity (white arrow). The cerebellar tonsils extend below the foramen magnum and are slightly peg shaped, representing an Arnold-Chiari type I malformation, a common concomitant of congenital/developmental/type 1 syringomyelia.

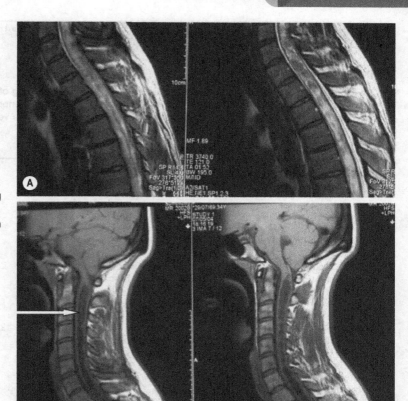

Clinical pearls

- MR imaging of the thoracic spine presents a variety of artifacts that may interfere with the quality of the final image, including the cardiac and respiratory cycles and the continuous cerebrospinal fluid flow. Techniques have been developed to negate the effects of these motion artifacts.
- Identify the T2-weighted sequence first and locate abnormal regions of increased signal intensity. Following this, use the T1-weighted image to identify the nature of the altered signal intensity.
- MR imaging of the thoracic spine is performed with the patient supine and therefore interpretation of the thoracic curvature should be guarded.
- If a scoliosis is detected on physical examination or plain film x-ray, it is important to inform the MR imaging unit to optimize the imaging sequences used.
- Bone marrow in an adult patient is usually hyperintense (relative to the intervertebral disc) on T1-weighted

sequences and hypointense (relative to the intervertebral disc) on T2-weighted sequences (see Figure 3.12).
- Suspicion of an infiltrative process should be considered if the bone marrow is hyperintense on T2-weighted sequences and hypointense on T1-weighted sequences (Figure 3.28).
- The soft tissue structures surrounding the thoracic spine should be evaluated, including the thoracic aorta, inferior vena cava, diaphragm and paraspinal musculature.
- Because thoracic disc herniations can compress the spinal cord or nerve roots, consider the diagnosis of thoracic disc lesions in patients who present with a clinical appearance of a lumbar disc lesion but who have a normal lumbar MR image.
- Consider MR imaging to evaluate for extraosseous extension of the lesion if a patient with a haemangioma presents with neurological symptoms.

Continued

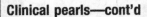

Clinical pearls—cont'd

- Atypical scoliosis has been associated with cord syrinx and Arnold-Chiari type I malformations. Findings that are considered atypical for scoliosis include: male gender, left-sided convexity, pain, and neurological symptoms.

- On MR imaging of a compression fracture, the extension of abnormal marrow signal into the posterior elements of the vertebral body suggests underlying pathology.

References

1. Gatterman MI, ed. *Chiropractic Management of Spine Related Disorders*. Baltimore: Williams and Wilkins; 1990.

2. Rowe L, Yochum T. Principles of radiological interpretation. In: Yochum T, Rowe L, eds. *Essentials of Skeletal Radiology*. 2nd ed. Baltimore: Williams and Wilkins; 1996:547–585.

3. Henry-Feugeas MC, Idy-Peretti I, Baledent O, et al. Origin of subarachnoid cerebrospinal fluid pulsations: a phase-contrast MR analysis. *Magn Reson Imaging*. 2000;18(4):387–395.

4. Helms C, Major N, Anderson MW, et al. Spine. In: *Musculoskeletal MRI*. 2nd ed. Philadelphia: Elsevier Saunders; 2009:273–323.

5. Wessely M. Magnetic resonance imaging of the thoracic spine: Part 1: normal imaging. *Clinical Chiropractic*. 2008;7(4):187–195.

6. Lindsay K, Bone I, Callander R. Localised neurological disease and its management. In: *Neurology and Neurosurgery Illustrated*. Edinburgh: Elsevier; 1991:213–466.

7. Standring S, ed. *Gray's Anatomy – The back (Section 45)*. Edinburgh: Elsevier; 2009.

8. Wade A. Imaging with magnetic resonance. In: *Fundamental Physics for Probing and Imaging*. Oxford: Oxford University Press; 2006:207–232.

9. Wade A. Medical imaging and therapy with ionising radiation. In: *Fundamental Physics for Probing and Imaging*. Oxford: Oxford University Press; 2006:233–266.

10. DeVries RM, Wessely M. Magnetic resonance imaging of the thoracic spine: Part 2: common disorders. *Clinical Chiropractic*. 2008;8(1):33–40.

11. Bannister R. Disorders of the nerve roots and peripheral nerves. In: *Brain and Bannister's Clinical Neurology*. 7th ed. Oxford: Oxford University Press; 1992:420–458.

12. Green J, Silver P. The vertebral column and the back. In: *An Introduction to Human Anatomy*. Oxford: Oxford University Press; 1981:52–68.

13. Moore K. The back. In: *Clinically Oriented Anatomy*. 2nd ed. Baltimore: Williams and Wilkins; 1985:565–625.

14. Wong HK, Hui JH, Rajan U, Chia HP. Idiopathic scoliosis in Singapore schoolchildren: a prevalence study 15 years into the screening program. *Spine*. 2005;30(10):1188–1196.

15. Bates B. The musculoskeletal system. In: Bates B, ed. *A Guide to Physical Examination*. 3rd ed. Philadelphia: JB Lippincott; 1983:324–370.

16. Beers M, Berkow R. Musculoskeletal abnormalities. In: *The Merck Manual*. 17th ed. West Point, PA: Merck & Co; 1999:2198–2241.

17. Berkow R. Neck, shoulder and upper limb pain. In: *The Merck Manual*. 16th ed. West Point, PA: Merck & Co; 1992:1362.

18. Kim HJ, Ryu KN, Choi WS, et al. Spinal involvement of hematopoietic malignancies and metastasis: differentiation using MR imaging. *Clin Imaging*. 1999;23(2):125–133.

19. Ghanem N, Altehoefer C, Hogerle S, et al. Comparative diagnostic value and therapeutic relevance of magnetic resonance imaging and bone marrow scintigraphy in patients with metastatic solid tumors of the axial skeleton. *Eur J Radiol*. 2002;43(3):256–261.

20. Arana E, Marti-Bonmati L, Molla E, Costa S. Upper thoracic-spine disc degeneration in patients with cervical pain. *Skeletal Radiol*. 2004;33(1):29–33.

21. Wood KB, Garvey TA, Gundry C, Heithoff KB. Magnetic resonance imaging of the thoracic spine. Evaluation of asymptomatic individuals. *J Bone Joint Surg Am*. 1995;77(11):1631–1638.

22. Goh S, Price RI, Song S, et al. Magnetic resonance-based vertebral morphometry of the thoracic spine: age, gender and level-specific influences. *Clin Biomech (Bristol, Avon)*. 2000;15(6): 417–425.

23. Stoller D. *Magnetic Resonance Imaging in Orthopaedics and Sports Medicine*. 2nd ed. Philadelphia: Lippincott Williams and Wilkins; 1996.

24. Berquist T. *MRI of the Musculoskeletal System*. 4th ed. Philadelphia: Lippincott Williams and Wilkins; 2000.

25. Lecouvet F, Cosnard G. Thoraco-lumbar disc disease with nerve root impingement and differential diagnosis. *J Radiol*. 2002;83(9 Pt 2): 1181–1189.

26. Eustace S, Johnston C, O'Neill P, O'Byrne J. *Sports Injuries: Examination, Imaging and Management*. Edinburgh: Elsevier Churchill Livingstone; 2007.

27. Wood KB, Blair JM, Aepple DM, et al. The natural history of asymptomatic thoracic disc herniations. *Spine*. 1997;22(5):525–529; discussion 9–30.

28. Caner H, Kilincoglu BF, Benli S, et al. Magnetic resonance image findings and surgical considerations in T1–2 disc herniation. *Can J Neurol Sci*. 2003;30(2):152–154.

29. Tokuhashi Y, Matsuzaki H, Uematsu Y, Oda H. Symptoms of thoracolumbar junction disc herniation. *Spine*. 2001;26(22): E512–E518.

30. Wilke A, Wolf U, Lageard P, Griss P. Thoracic disc herniation: a diagnostic challenge. *Man Ther*. 2000;(3): 181–184.

31. Dimar 2nd JR, Bratcher KR, Glassman SD, et al. Identification and surgical treatment of primary thoracic spinal stenosis. *Am J Orthop*. 2008;37(11):564–568.

32. Clemente CD. *Anatomy: A Regional Atlas of the Human Body*. Baltimore: Urban and Schwarzenberg; 1983.

33. Whitaker C, Schoenecker PL, Lenke LG. Hyperkyphosis as an indicator of syringomyelia in idiopathic scoliosis: a case report. *Spine*. 2003;28(1):E16–E20.

34. Beluffi G, Fiori P, Sileo C. Intervertebral disc calcifications in children. *Radiol Med*. 2009;114(2): 331–341.

35. Dhammi IK, Arora A, Monga J. Calcified thoracic intervertebral disc at two levels as a cause of mid-back pain in a child: a case report. *J Orthop Sci*. 2002;7(5):587–589.

36. Bagatur AE, Zorer G, Centel T. Natural history of paediatric intervertebral disc calcification. *Arch Orthop Trauma Surg*. 2001;121(10): 601–603.

37. Bazzi J, Dimar JR, Glassman SD. Acute calcific discitis in adults. *Am J Orthop*. 2002;31(3):141–145.

38. Ross JS, Masaryk TJ, Modic MT, et al. Vertebral hemangiomas: MR imaging. *Radiology*. 1987;165(1): 165–169.

39. Yochum TR, Lile RL, Schultz GD, et al. Acquired spinal stenosis secondary to an expanding thoracic vertebral hemangioma. *Spine*. 1993;18(2): 299–305.

40. Friedman DP. Symptomatic vertebral hemangiomas: MR findings. *Am J Roentgenol*. 1996;167(2):359–364.

41. Doppman JL, Oldfield EH, Heiss JD. Symptomatic vertebral hemangiomas: treatment by means of direct intralesional injection of ethanol. *Radiology*. 2000;214(2): 341–348.

42. Bas T, Aparisi F, Bas JL. Efficacy and safety of ethanol injections in 18 cases of vertebral hemangioma: a mean follow-up of 2 years. *Spine*. 2001;26(14):1577–1582.

43. Sikorski CW, Pytel P, Rubin CM, Yamini B. Intradural spinal Wilm's tumor metastasis: case report. *Neurosurgery*. 2006;59(4): E942–E943; discussion E3.

44. Klein SL, Sanford RA, Muhlbauer MS. Pediatric spinal epidural metastases. *J Neurosurg*. 1991;74(1):70–75.

45. Young MF. Diagnostic imaging. In: *Essential Physics for Musculoskeletal Medicine*. Edinburgh: Elsevier; 2010.

46. Allison W. Imaging with magnetic resonance. In: *Fundamental Physics for Probing and Imaging*. Oxford: Oxford University Press; 2006: 207–226.

47. Tall MA, Thompson AK, Vertinsky T, Palka PS. MR imaging of the spinal bone marrow. *Magn Reson Imaging Clin N Am*. 2007; 15(2):175–198, vi.

48. Vande Berg BC, Malghem J, Lecouvet FE, Maldague B. Magnetic resonance imaging of normal bone marrow. *Eur Radiol*. 1998;8(8): 1327–1334.

49. Kaplan P, Helms C, Dussault R, Anderson M. *Musculoskeletal MRI*. Philadelphia: WB Saunders; 2001.

50. Resnick D. *Diagnosis of Bone and Joint Disorders*. 3rd ed. Philadelphia: WB Saunders; 1995.

51. Spiegel DA, Flynn JM, Stasikelis PJ, et al. Scoliotic curve patterns in patients with Chiari I malformation and/or syringomyelia. *Spine*. 2003;28(18):2139–2146.

52. Ouellet JA, LaPlaza J, Erickson MA, et al. Sagittal plane deformity in the thoracic spine: a clue to the presence of syringomyelia as a cause of scoliosis. *Spine*. 2003;28(18): 2147–2151.

The lumbar spine

Michelle A. Wessely   Julie-Marthe Grenier
Peter J. Scordilis   David R. Seaman   Martin Young

Introduction

Low back pain is one of the most common presenting complaints to any primary healthcare physician. With the wide variety of structures capable of generating pain and the common inclusion of pathological conditions in the differential diagnosis, it is important for the clinician to be able to reach specific and accurate conclusions as to the precise nature of their patient's complaint.[1] This involves a detailed clinical history, physical examination and appropriate diagnostic imaging.[2,3] Magnetic resonance (MR) imaging plays a crucial role in determining the cause of the clinical picture when used in the appropriate clinical context.[4]

MR imaging is an invaluable tool for the clinician assessing the lumbar spine. Although previously radiographs were always the mainstay for imaging diagnosis of disorders arising from the low back (and, in some countries, this still holds true), it is now generally accepted that cross-sectional imaging, in particular MR imaging, is the perfect tool to assess the potential pain-generating structures of this region.[5,6] MR imaging now has the added benefit of being able to be performed in different positions; therefore, if the patient experiences pain only in a particular position, this posture can be recreated within the MR scanner, in order to better identify the origin of the symptoms. This determination is clearly an important factor in the subsequent management of the patient. Positional and upright MR imaging are not widely available at the time of writing, but the benefits are such that the utilization is likely to increase in the near future.[7–9]

MR imaging's role in assessment of the lumbar spine is well established. In most clinical situations, it is preferred over computed tomography (CT) and myelography, although the former can still be used in conjunction with MR imaging to more fully assess the multiple components of severe trauma.[10] MR imaging has been shown to be superior to both these modalities in the evaluation of degenerative disc conditions, infections, spinal neoplasms and other intrinsic cord diseases; it allows visualization of both components of the intervertebral disc and direct imaging of the bone marrow.[11–15] Computed tomography may show an advantage over MRI for the evaluation of postoperative stenosis due to arthrosis, particularly in the case of an instrumented spine, where the artifact produced by the implant affects MR images to a greater extent than CT; however, CT does not allow for distinction between postsurgical fibrosis and scarring and a recurrent disc lesion, even with the use of intrathecal contrast agents (Figure 4.01), a particularly challenging and important clinical determination to make because of the differing management options available.[10,16]

This chapter is designed to give an overview of the basics of MR imaging for the lumbar spine, the indications for imaging and relevant procedures to the ordering clinician. Familiarity with these topics will allow for appropriate patient examination and optimization of this diagnostic tool and help achieve a comprehensive assessment of the patient's clinical requirements.

History and examination

Low back pain is one of the most common complaints presenting to the offices of any primary care

DOI: 10.1016/B978-0-443-06726-6.00004-4

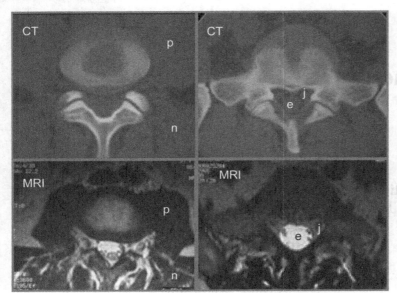

Figure 4.01 • Comparison of structures visualized on a non-contrast computed tomography CT (bone window) axial image [upper images] and MR axial T2-weighted image [lower images] at the lumbosacral junction. The contents of the central canal (filum terminale) are well visualized on the T2-weighted images as well as the relationship between the neural structures and the surrounding borders, which may be involved in neural compromise. MR imaging also allows for closer evaluation of the paraspinal soft tissue including the musculature. The key to the legend is detailed in Box 4.01.

physician – and one of the most poorly understood and badly managed. Part of the problem is that the condition is frequently treated as a disease in itself rather than a symptom that can emanate from dozens of different causes. Family doctors frequently fail to differentiate these causes beyond a basic elimination of 'red flag' pathologies; their argument is that such differentiation is not necessary as any musculoskeletal problem will be treated in the same way: non-steroidal anti-inflammatories and analgesia. There is also a belief that back pain is a self-limiting condition that will spontaneously resolve within 6 weeks.[17,18]

Unfortunately, the evidence shows that this treatment regimen does little other than to moderately alleviate symptoms in the short term and, rather than self-resolve, many patients simply stop attending their family practice owing to the lack of effective treatment; this, however, is interpreted as evidence of resolution by the treating physician. Current guidelines emphasize early return to normal activities, acupuncture and spinal manipulative therapy, preferably followed by individually tailored prescriptive exercise.[19,20]

An accurate and concise differential diagnosis is important not only to inform management protocols but also to determine what, if any, diagnostic imaging may be required. Orthopaedic textbooks are replete with tests for low back pain, usually eponymic, and usually of unproved or dubious reliability and sensitivity.

The diagnostic dilemma is further compounded by the prevalence of comorbid conditions: sacroiliac syndrome is frequently linked with lumbosacral facet dysfunction and with myofascial syndromes arising from the muscles of the gluteal area; many discal lesions arise following years of low-grade back pain,

Box 4.01

Key to legend for figures

a: spinal cord
b: epidural fat
c: intervertebral disc
d: spinous process
e: cerebrospinal fluid
f: dura
g: filum terminale
h: ligamentum flavum
i: articular facet and joint space
j: nerve root
k: lamina
m: intervertebral foramen
n: paraspinal musculature
o: pedicle
p: psoas
q: epidural vein
r: pars interarticularis
s: aorta

again often linked to lumbosacral dysfunction; any acute back pain will cause muscle guarding and spasm that can, in their own right, contribute to and perpetuate the condition.

So, what is the clinician to do? As with any presentation, the key is a thorough history and examination; with experience, this will become honed both with practice and with the rejection of tests that prove regularly unhelpful or invariably duplicate the findings from other tests; remember, many orthopaedic tests are aggravational ... too much aggravation and the patient may never return! The detail of this clinical encounter will depend on the discipline of the clinician; the specificity of diagnosis required prior to spinal manipulation is likely to differ from that needed in general family practice.

Differential diagnosis

Of the many causes of low back pain, sacroiliac joint syndrome and facet joint syndrome are perhaps the most commonly presenting conditions, contributing to approximately 50% of cases. The accurate diagnosis of these entities, which are best identified by orthopaedic testing and by response to conservative care, either manipulation or injection, is complicated by comorbidity: 30% of low back patients have more than one anatomical source of pain.[21] MR imaging is, however, considered the gold standard for several other common low back disorders, including disc lesions and central canal stenosis.[22,23]

The common differential diagnoses for the lumbar spine are detailed in Table 4.01.[24,25]

Table 4.01 Differential diagnosis for low back pain

Condition	Example	Historical correlation	Physical correlation
Trauma	• Fracture • Ligamentous sprain	Obvious, significant precipitating trauma	Diagnostic imaging usually indicated prior to examination
Mechanical	• Lumbosacral dysfunction • Scoliosis • Pregnancy	Chronic, often intermittent history with activity-related exacerbation	Positive orthopaedic testing
Degenerative	• Degenerative disc disease • Degenerative joint disease	Older population often with history of trauma or significant back pain	Restricted range of motion; positive imaging findings
Infections	• Osteomyelitis • Tuberculosis • Spinal abscess • Basilar pneumonia	History of infection; severe nocturnal spinal pain	Signs of systemic illness including pyrexia
Metabolic	• Osteoporosis • Osteomalacia	Familial history	Diagnostic imaging findings
Vascular	• Abdominal aortic aneurysm • Spinal infarction	Often occult	Vascular or neurological findings
Neoplastic	• Multiple myeloma • Hodgkin's disease • Metastasis	Systemic symptoms from primary or secondary deposits; severe nocturnal spinal pain	Evidence of weight loss

Continued

Condition	Example	Historical correlation	Physical correlation
Gastrointestinal	• Inflammatory bowel disease • Pancreatitis • Cholelithiasis	Altered bowel habit	Localized abdominal tenderness
Renal	• Calculus • Pyelonephritis • Hydronephrosis	Altered urinary function	Palpatory tenderness
Haematological	• Sickle cell crisis • Haemolysis	Familial history plus symptoms of anaemia	Signs of anaemia
Gynaecological	• Fibroids • Endometriosis • Uterine prolapse • Ovarian cyst	Dysmenorrhoea	Lower abdominal tenderness
Inflammatory	• Ankylosing spondylitis • Psoriatic arthritis • Reiter's syndrome	Morning stiffness History of condition Iritis, foot pain and non-specific urethritis	Reduced sacroiliac joint movement/lumbar extension Subungual psoriasis Haematological markers
Psychogenic	• Malingering • Hysteria • Anxiety	Abnormal illness behaviour	Positive 'functional' tests (e.g. Bench test)

Table 4.01 Differential diagnosis for low back pain—cont'd

Clinical indications for diagnostic imaging

The symptoms and presentations associated with back pain that are indications for spine imaging are detailed in Box 4.02.[21,26] It is important that the clinician orders MR imaging only with valid clinical suspicion and appropriate history and examination findings because, without these, the results of the study may be misleading; in the early years of MR imaging, there were frequent examples of inappropriate back surgery, with its attendant risks and complications, on disc bulges that were not only asymptomatic but simply failed to correlate to the radicular level of the patient's complaint.

Box 4.02

Indications for MR imaging of the lumbar spine

• Unresolved non-complicated low back pain following one month of conservative care
• Neurological symptoms including, but not limited to:
   • Paraesthesias
   • Radicular pain
   • Changes to deep tendon reflexes
   • Pathological reflexes
   • Muscle weakness
   • Upper or lower motor neuron lesion symptoms
• Bowel or bladder dysfunction related to a trauma or the onset of pain (This condition should be referred to the emergency room but will typically necessitate an MR imaging evaluation)
• Muscular atrophy
• Fever associated with the onset of pain
• Unexplained weight loss
• Swollen lymph nodes
• Night pain or pain that does not resolve with rest
• Inconclusive radiographic findings
• Age over 50 years

After determining the indications for MR imaging, it is important to clearly communicate them to the facility or attending radiologist; although few, the risks and contraindications need to be evaluated on a case-by-case basis. Additionally, depending on the clinical question or differential diagnoses, intravenous contrast use may be recommended and the need for this has to be assessed by the imaging team. Findings from any plain film imaging *or the absence thereof* should also be included in the referral details.

Contraindications

Whilst MR imaging is generally considered safe, the procedure does have a few cautions and contraindications. The following situations are common but do not comprise an inclusive list and should merely serve as a guide for patient screening and consideration. Before undergoing an MR imaging examination, the facility performing the procedure should screen the patient, but it is important that referring doctors are familiar with common contraindications and cautions to better inform the patient and avoid referring inappropriately.[27]

Caution needs to be taken when referring patients experiencing claustrophobia, anxiety or panic attacks for MR imaging examination. It is important that the process is thoroughly explained to the patient in order to decrease stress and anxiety prior to the procedure. Also, there are several options offered to these patients to minimize the discomfort. Sedatives, open tube architecture, headphones and prisms that allow the patient to see outside the unit all may help to calm these individuals and allow the acquisition of higher-quality images. The first trimester of pregnancy also requires caution with regard to MR imaging.[27] The necessity for the imaging procedure should be made on an individual clinical basis if:

- the information cannot be obtained by non-ionizing means
- the emergent data could affect the care of the patient and/or fetus
- the referring physician feels the test is necessary and cannot be postponed.

It is important that the patient is aware of the benefits and risks of the examination and any alternatives if applicable.[27]

Absolute contraindications to MR imaging generally involve implants or foreign bodies. The most important concern is whether or not the object is

Box 4.03

Common foreign bodies and implants that constitute a contraindication to MR imaging

- Aneurysm clips[1,5]
- Intraocular bodies
- Subcutaneous or other various foreign bodies
- Shrapnel
- Certain prosthetic heart valves[1]
- Neurostimulators
- Cochlear implants[1,5]
- Most cardiac defibrillators or pacemakers[1,5]
- Electronic drug infusion pumps[1]

ferromagnetic; objects with ferromagnetic properties need to be assessed for size, shape and anatomical location. The magnetic field strength of the unit also needs to be considered. Common foreign bodies that represent contraindications to MR imaging are detailed in Box 4.03.

Most surgical clips or orthopaedic devices will not contraindicate MR imaging. Electrically, magnetically or mechanically activated devices that cannot be removed during an examination represent another category of contraindications to MR examination and are also included in Box 4.03.

Contrast

Gadolinium is the most frequently used contrast agent in MR imaging. It is a paramagnetic ion that is attached to a chelating agent in the form of gadolinium diethylenetriaminepentaacetic acid (Gd-DTPA), which decreases the toxicity of the gadolinium, restricts its activity and alters its pharmacokinetics. The contrast agent is intravenously administered.

Total incidence of adverse reactions for all types of MR contrast ranges from 2% to 4%. Gadolinium is safer than the iodinated contrast utilized in plain film and CT imaging, with fewer side effects.[28–30] When side effects do occur, the most common reactions are nausea, emesis, hives, headaches and local injection site symptoms.[29,31] Adverse events following gadolinium injection are more common in patients who have had previous reactions to MR imaging or iodinated contrast; therefore, it is necessary to inquire about past reactions and take these into account before requesting studies with contrast. MR contrast agents have been shown to cross the placenta and are therefore not routinely given to pregnant patients, who should only receive contrast medium if the potential benefits outweigh the risk to the fetus; this should be determined by the attending radiologist.[27]

The traditional recommendation for breastfeeding is a 24-hour suspension following gadolinium injection; however, it has now been shown that less than 0.04% of the administered dose is absorbed by the nursing infant (100 times less than the permitted intravenous dose for infants) and the length of the suspension needs to be reviewed based on the potential risks against the stress that may be placed on a nursing infant due to the suspension.[32]

An additional, though rare, reaction to gadolinium contrast has also now been recognized: nephrogenic fibrosis. This tends to occur in those patients with kidney failure or where a patient has a dramatically lowered glomerular filtration rate; therefore, if gadolinium is to be used, the patient's renal status must be assessed. Where clinical suspicion exists, the glomerular filtration rate must be evaluated prior to the imaging study, and, if lowered, gadolinium cannot be used – nephrogenic fibrosis is an irreversible condition that is both debilitating and extremely severe.[29,33]

Techniques and protocols

The most common sequences used for imaging the lumbar spine are T1-weighted and T2-weighted; fat suppression techniques are added on occasion. T2-weighted sequences will highlight fluid and, to some extent, fatty tissues as well (Figure 4.02). Sequence combinations are determined by the clinical question being addressed; in most centres, routine orders include T1-weighted and T2-weighted sagittal and continuous axial images from L1 to S1. Slice

thickness usually varies from 3 to 4 mm with a 0.5–1.0 mm gap.[10,34]

When evaluating degenerative disc conditions or patients with radiculopathy, contiguous axial slices through the plane of the disc are obtained in addition to the regular continuous axial images (Figure 4.03). Axial, T1-weighted slices will nicely demonstrate the outline of the intraspinal fat against disc material, bone and nerves. On the T2-weighted sequences, the cerebrospinal fluid (CSF) will act as a contrast agent (the *myelographic effect*) and allow for good distinction between the disc and adjacent structures (Figure 4.04).

Axial slices of the lumbar spine are very useful in determining the morphology of the disc, particularly posteriorly and posterolaterally. They can also be used to accurately assess the dimensions of the central canal, subarticular recesses and foramen, providing information regarding their patency, which is important to determine not only from the clinical explanation of the patient's complaint but also for the interventional clinician, where injections are being considered.

Also in this plane, the clinician can get a good feel for the volume and state of the paraspinal and psoas muscles, both of which have been identified among the multifactorial contributors to low back pain. Individual nerve roots can also be followed to their point of exit, establishing evidence of impingement by surrounding structures. As the nerve exits, the sagittal images become more useful for evaluating the intervertebral foramen and determining whether there is evidence of impingement, most commonly from degenerative facet hypertrophy or a far lateral, extraforaminal disc lesion.

The sagittal sequences are also useful in assessing the status of both discal and ligamentous structures.

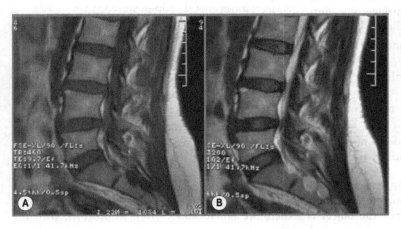

Figure 4.02 • Sagittal, T1-weighted (A) and T2-weighted (B) MR imaging of the lumbar spine demonstrating a Tarlov (perineural) cyst at the level of the second sacral segment. Bright structures on T1-weighted images have a high fat content; fluid produces the brightest signal on T2-weighted sequences.

Figure 4.03 • MR imaging of the lumbar spine, T2-weighted sagittal planning scans (**A** and **B**) and corresponding axial images (**C** and **D**) through the disc obtained on a 25-year-old patient with radicular symptoms. Note on the plan scans (**A** and **B**) that the slices are at the level of the disc only in (**A**), whilst in (**B**) they are continuous through both the intervertebral discs and vertebral bodies. It is important to evaluate the whole of the spine since it is possible to miss diagnoses using (**A**) alone, for example in cases of sequestered discs and vertebral metastatic deposits that might be located between the slice levels.

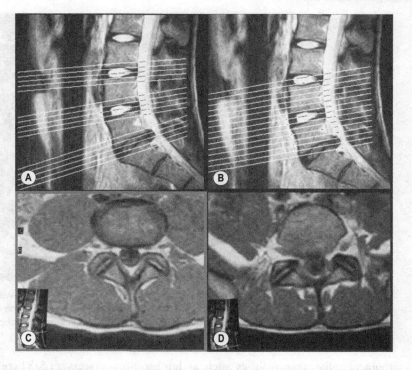

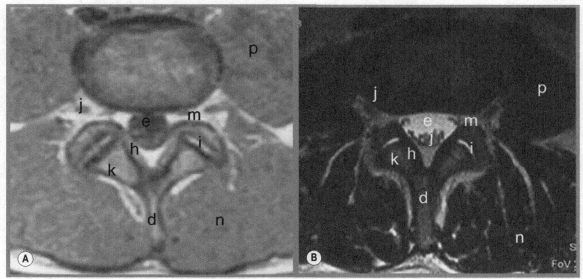

Figure 4.04 • MR imaging of the lumbar spine in the axial plane using T1-weighted (**A**) and T2-weighted (**B**) sequences. The key to the identification of structures is given in Box 4.01; note the different structures that appear with different signal on each type of imaging sequence.

Parasagittal slices depict the intervertebral foramen and the position of the dorsal root ganglion (Figures 4.05, 4.06). Locating levels on a sagittal slice can be difficult; rudimentary disc spaces and transitional lumbosacral segments are fairly common,

making a precise count effectively impossible in certain circumstances. Although identification of the twelfth rib can help to suggest the levels distally, even this is prone to error since transitional lumbosacral anomalies are commonly associated with

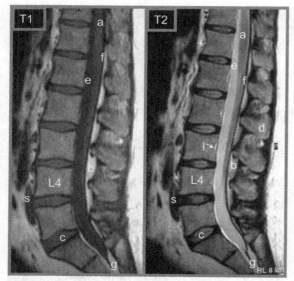

Figure 4.05 • MR imaging of the lumbar spine showing T1- and T2-weighted, mid-sagittal slices, demonstrating the osseous and soft tissue anatomy visible. The key to the identification of structures is given in Box 4.01.

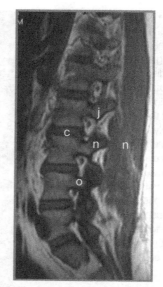

Figure 4.06 • T1-weighted parasagittal MR imaging of the lumbar spine at the level of the pedicles. The key to the identification of structures is given in Box 4.01.

thoracolumbar abnormalities such as lumbar ribs; or hypoplasticity or agenesis of the twelfth rib.[35] Correlation with plain film radiography can be helpful in this regard, along with identification of the conus medullaris and right renal artery, both usually located at the level of L1 or L2. On the axial images, assessment of the orientation of the lumbosacral facet can be used to clarify the findings. Lumbar facets are oriented in the sagittal plane from L1 to L5. The articular

facets at L5/S1 are often in the coronal plane. In cases where a count is still uncertain but necessary, a single cervicothoracic sagittal scout can be obtained.[30]

Coronal images are not routinely used in evaluation of the lumbar spine except as 'scouts' and in scoliotic patients. Severe curvatures can prevent full visualization of all intraspinal structures in all three planes; the scout can allow data to be acquired in an oblique plane, making interpretation simpler (Figure 4.07).

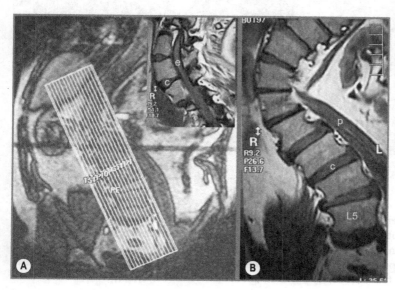

Figure 4.07 • MR imaging of the lumbar spine in a patient with a severe scoliosis. By taking a coronal plan scan (A), it was possible to modify the T1-weighted sagittal images to compensate for the curve, avoid volume averaging and to prevent the area of anatomical and clinical interest falling outside the plane of imaging (B and **insert**). The key to the identification of structures is given in Box 4.01.

Contrast media in lumbar spine imaging are routinely used in three situations, details of which are given below.

Following disc operations, gadolinium is used to differentiate between postsurgical scar tissue and recurrent herniation. Scar tissue is vascularized and will enhance with contrast injection, whilst disc material is avascular and will generally not enhance.[36]

When enhancement occurs in a disc fragment, it will typically be present around the periphery (rim enhancement) and corresponds to diffusion of the contrast medium from the adjacent tissues. The rate of diffusion into a fragment is much slower, allowing for distinction between the scar and fragment. Because of this, it is necessary to perform T1-weighted axial sequence imaging immediately after contrast injection.[30]

In the case of intraspinal tumours, contrast is utilized for the early detection, characterization, localization and extent evaluation of the lesion[10,30]; gadolinium is the modality of choice when investigating primary tumours of the central nervous system.[37–39] When basic MR imaging of an infection is ambiguous, contrast will be used to demonstrate the extent and activity of the lesion and to inform treatment options.[40]

Normal imaging anatomy and common variants

Vertebrae

The vertebral bodies have a high marrow content, which is demonstrated as high signal on T1-weighted images and intermediate to low signal on T2-weighted images. The signal may be slightly non-homogeneous because of the variable amount of fibrous material interlaced within the marrow component. Marrow signal will also vary depending on the age and health status of the patient.[41,42] Before the age of 25, cancellous bone is primarily composed of red marrow; with advancing age, the fatty fraction of marrow will become more important than the red components, leading to an increase in the T1-weighted signal. Any disease leading to an increase in demand of haematopoietic cells (marrow reconversion) will present with signal alterations in the vertebral bodies (increase in T2-weighted signal, decrease in T1-weighted signal).[30] The articular cartilage, cortical bone and endplates are low signal

intensity on both T1-weighted and T2-weighted images. Additional gradient echo sequences will show articular cartilage as intermediate signal intensity, allowing differentiation from the hypointense cortical bone.[43]

Spinal ligaments

Normal ligaments generally appear as low signal intensity structures on all sequences; however, there is one exception of note: the *ligamentum flavum* contains a higher percentage of elastin fibres and will, therefore, appear as an intermediate signal structure on both T1-weighted and T2-weighted sequences.[44]

Spinal canal

The facet joints and capsules, pedicles and discs outline the borders of the spinal canal together with internal ligamentous structures. Hypertrophy of any of these structures can cause impingement on the contents of the canal: the meninges, cerebrospinal fluid, spinal cord, nerve roots, epidural fat and associated vascular network. All of these elements are best visualized on axial, T1-weighted sequences. The cerebrospinal fluid should surround the nerve roots and spinal cord down to the filum terminale. Axial images also allow for evaluation of the shape of the vertebral canal, lateral recess and intervertebral foramina; the normal canal shape is triangular (Figure 4.04).

Intervertebral disc

The intervertebral disc comprises three components: the annulus fibrosus, nucleus pulposus, and cartilaginous vertebral endplate. Under normal circumstances, only the outer third of the annulus fibrosus has a sensory innervation.[45]

The cartilaginous endplate represents the interface between the nucleus, the inner layers of the annulus and the bony vertebral body. Nutrients diffuse from the blood vessels of the vertebral body, through the vertebral endplate, and into the nucleus and inner annulus. This relationship allows for disc nutrition; however, when the endplate becomes compromised, most commonly by injury, a sequence of biochemical events begins that may lead to internal disc disruption, which is considered to be the most common painful disc abnormality.[46,47]

The nucleus pulposus consists of 70%–90% water, while the nuclear tissues consist largely of proteoglycans (65% of dry weight) and type II collagen (15%–20% of dry weight). The remaining tissues are elastic fibres and non-collagenous proteins. The nucleus is normally cohesive and imbibes water due to the negatively charged proteoglycans, which allows it to absorb and disperse compressive loads.[26,45] In the experimental setting, it has been determined that substantial compressive loads do not damage the nucleus; instead, compression may damage the trabecular bone of the adjacent vertebral bodies or the cartilaginous endplates, now recognized as the weak point of the intervertebral disc.[1,27]

The **annular** (or external) component is formed by fibrocartilage and collagen fibres and will therefore display a hypointense signal on most sequences, making it difficult to differentiate from the endplate and articular cartilage. The central **nucleus** is comprised of water and proteinaceous material, which appears as high signal on T2-weighted images. The ideal disc will demonstrate a signal that is isointense to muscle and hypointense to marrow on T1-weighted images. By contrast, the T2-weighted signal should be hyperintense except for the outer annulus. Often, a horizontal band of decreased signal is present on T2-weighted images in the central area of the disc. The aetiology of this phenomenon is unclear; however, it is not considered pathological beyond the age of 40 years.[48]

The ideal disc should also not extend beyond the adjacent vertebral body margins, particularly on the axial planes. There is some 'manoeuvrability' or 'wiggle' room whereby the disc contour on the axial slices can extend slightly beyond the borders of the endplates by up to 2 mm; anything more than this is considered to constitute a disc lesion and, depending on the morphology of the disc in the axial and sagittal plane, particular nomenclature will be applied to indicate the type of disc lesion.[49–51] This is dealt with in more detail later in the chapter.

Spinal cord

The spinal cord and nerve roots will show intermediate T1-weighted and low T2-weighted signal intensity. These structures are best differentiated on T2-weighted sequences, when surrounded by CSF, which will image as hyperintense or bright (Figure 4.08).[30] In the normal adult patient, the spinal cord terminates as the *conus medullaris*, usually situated at the L1–L2 level. This is important to evaluate, as a low-lying cord may be part of a more clinically significant problem such as tethered cord syndrome.

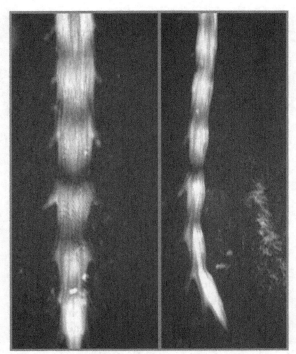

Figure 4.08 • MR imaging of the lumbar spine in the coronal and sagittal planes. A heavily T2-weighted sequence (TR = 3000 / TE = 600) can function as a virtual 'myelogram'; this image is obtained to assess cerebrospinal fluid distribution and to outline the spinal nerves inside the vertebral canal and intervertebral foramen without the need for contrast agents. This can be a useful method for evaluating patients with potential central subarticular or foraminal canal stenosis.

Facet joints

The facet or zygapophyseal joints are formed from the articular processes of two adjacent vertebrae; they are synovial plane joints, complete with a synovial joint capsule and articular cartilage. The facets, along with the laminae, are covered by the ligamentum flavum.[45,52]

Pathological imaging

Disc disease

Endplate damage, due to either macro- or microtrauma, is thought to disrupt the normal homeostasis of the nucleus pulposus. Blood and cellular substances reach the nucleus via the endplate; if this is disrupted, its sets into motion a series of events that leads to the nuclear degradation.[26] Enzymes that degrade the connective tissue, referred to as matrix metalloproteinases (MMPs), are normally present in the healthy nucleus; however, they are dormant. Damage to the endplate leads to the disinhibition of MMPs, which then begin to degrade nuclear proteoglycans and collagen. This degradative process increases the fluidity of the nucleus, reducing its cohesion and ability to resist compression.[53,54] A plain film radiograph may reveal a reduction in disc height and spondylophytes; however, these changes need not be symptomatic.[27,55]

The degenerative process that began in the nucleus may extend into the non-innervated inner layers of the annulus fibrosus. As the MMPs degrade the collagen fibres of the annulus, a radial fissure may begin, which can ultimately extend to the outer annulus. A normal, cohesive nucleus will be unaffected by such a fissure; however, a degraded nucleus can track through radial fissures and delaminated circumferential fibres, which can be visualized on a discogram. Only when the outer annulus becomes sufficiently damaged will the degraded nucleus move into the epidural space. In short, disc lesions occur due to pathological processes beginning with the nucleus and then extending to the periphery of the annulus.[27]

Disc abnormalities have generated controversy amongst radiologists and clinicians for decades. Confusion about the nature of disc pathology was highlighted as early as 1934, when Mixter and Barr published their landmark report of surgery on a 'ruptured' disc,[56] which ushered in the 'dynasty of the disc'.[49,57] At this time, 'herniated' discs were thought to be benign cartilaginous tumours and were called 'chondromas' or 'enchondromas'; since then, defining the nature of disc pathology has been a challenging goal and it was only in 2001 that a consensus paper was finally published.[50,58,59]

It is important to keep in mind that many disc abnormalities are not necessarily associated with pain

generation. In the majority of cases, the disc herniation can be subclassified as either a disc *protrusion* or a disc *extrusion*, the latter being more clinically significant in general, although both are able to contribute to clinical symptomatology, depending on the size of the spinal canal, and their relationship to the nerve roots.[10]

Small tears within the annulus fibrosus can be visualized on T2-weighted sequences as focal hyperintensity areas in the outer annular fibres. For this reason, they are referred to as *high intensity zones* or 'HIZes'. The signal is increased due to the presence of granulation tissue and oedema (Figure 4.09); HIZes are associated with painful annular disruption.[60,61]

Comparison of MR imaging in the supine and upright position shows that the appearance of the HIZ can change; in the standing posture, the HIZ will become more vertically orientated, whereas in the same patient in the supine position, the same HIZ will appear more horizontal. Other interesting observations have been made with the use of upright MR imaging: in the upright position, the central canal size can change, and the surface area of the dural sac has also been seen to alter. Between flexion and extension of the lumbar spine, changes are noted in the contour of the disc, as well as of the contents of the spinal canal and subarticular recess; foramen and extraforaminal region – all of which may play a role in the explanation of the patient's clinical syndrome.[9,62]

Disc bulges are defined as an extension of disc material from the vertebral margin of more than 2 mm; classically, they are circumferential and not commonly associated with pain.[48,58,59]

A general disc bulge may, however, be seen in conjunction with a more focal disc lesion, and the combination may certainly contribute to the patient's clinical syndrome. A common radiological finding is that of degenerative disc disease with a generalized disc bulge causing a reduction in the subarticular foraminal or extraforaminal region in combination with a more focal disc lesion; hypertrophy of the synovial facet joint or ligamentum flavum or even the development

Figure 4.09 • High intensity zone (HIZ) in the outer, posterior annular fibres of L5 seen on T2-weighted MR imaging in the sagittal (**A**) and axial planes (**B**) (arrows). Annular tears are not as easily visible on T1-weighted sequences (**C**) (arrow).

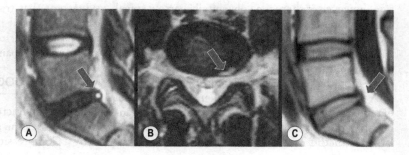

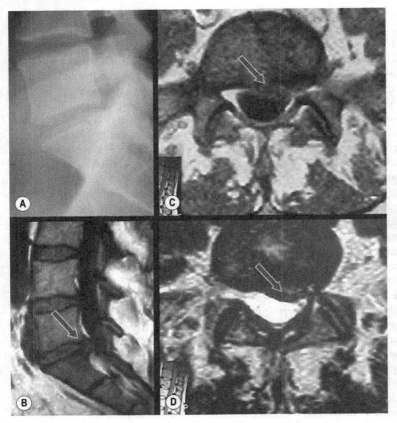

Figure 4.10 • Diagnostic imaging of a patient with low back pain and clinical indications of a left-sided S1 radiculopathy. The plain film radiograph (**A**) shows a mild decrease in the lumbosacral disc space as well as a retrolisthesis at L5. The sagittal T1-weighted MR image of the lumbar spine (**B**) shows a disc extrusion on the left in the central, paracentral, subarticular and foraminal zone at L5–S1 (arrow). The MR image, axial T1-weighted (**C**) and T2-weighted (**D**) sequences demonstrate that the large paracentral, subarticular extrusion is occluding the left lateral recess and compressing the ventral aspect of the thecal sac (arrows).

of a synovial cyst, which then contribute further to impingement of the exiting nerve root or, if extraforaminal, the dorsal root ganglion.[10,30]

Disc protrusions may be broad or focal. A disc protrusion is defined as being present when disc material extends from the vertebral body margin but does not pass the superior or inferior margin of the parent disc and does not extend beneath the posterior longitudinal ligament.[10,11] Functionally, this means that the width of the lesion is larger than the height; this is best assessed on the sagittal slices. Disc protrusions are not commonly directly associated with pain generation; however, if there is a congenitally narrow spinal canal or foramen, or if the patient has compounding factors such as degenerative changes to the joint capsule, then it is possible that a simple disc protrusion may cause an impingement on the traversing or exiting nerve root, thus giving rise to a clinical syndrome.[48,59]

A **disc extrusion** occurs when disc material extends past the margin of the vertebral body, meaning that the anterior-to-posterior diameter will be larger than the medial-to-lateral dimension. There will be continuity in all sections of the disc. Extrusions may extend in any direction but are more commonly seen in the lateral recess in the posterolateral aspect of the spinal canal and are commonly found in symptomatic patients (Figure 4.10).[48,59]

If the herniated disc material lacks continuity or a separate fragment is found, the lesion is defined as a **sequestrated disc** or free fragment. Epidural inflammation often accompanies sequestration and is thought to complicate the epidural mass effect. A posteriorly displaced free fragment is of particular importance, presenting with a bizarre range of clinical symptoms that traditionally has been treated surgically; however, it now appears that spinal manipulation has a better outcome at 1-year follow-up with regard to both pain and functionality.[48,59]

Vertebral body changes

Compression fractures, skeletal tumours and infiltrative processes can all alter the signal of the vertebral body. Compression fractures can present as an altered vertebral body shape and also as decreased T1-weighted and T2-weighted signal intensity adjacent to the area of compression.[10,63] Neoplastic activity typically shows decreased T1-weighted and increased T2-weighted signal, typical of most pathological processes and consistent with marrow replacement by oedema or abnormal cells, or with subchondral marrow changes associated with degenerative disc disease, the so-called *Modic changes* (Figure 4.11). Multiple levels of signal changes raise the suspicion for an infiltrative disease such as osteolytic metastasis or multiple myeloma. Decreased T1-weighted and T2-weighted signal intensity is consistent with sclerotic processes such as osteoblastic metastasis or bone islands.[43,64]

More common causes of altered signal intensity in the vertebral bodies are *haemangiomas* and *fat islands*. Both are well visualized on MR imaging even when radiographs are normal. Haemangiomas will usually be hyperintense on both T1-weighted and T2-weighted images (Figure 4.12). Focal fat islands or deposits in the marrow will display high intensity

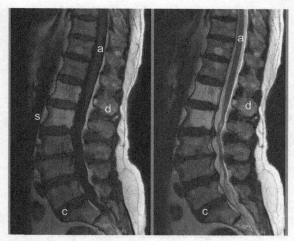

Figure 4.12 • Mid-sagittal T1- and T2-weighted MR images of the lumbar spine in a patient with multiple haemangiomas. Abnormal signal intensity is seen in the vertebral bodies, with increased signal intensity noted on both the T1- and T2-weighted images. The alteration in signal intensity is especially dramatic when compared to the normal bone marrow signal intensity demonstrated in Figure 4.02.

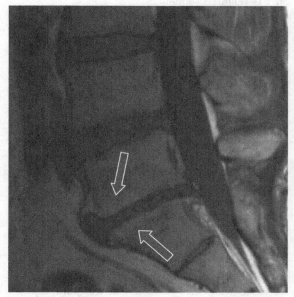

Figure 4.11 • Axial, T1-weighted axial MR imaging of the lumbar spine demonstrating degenerative disc disease at L5–S1. Decreased disc height, anterior and posterior spondylophytes and a posterior degenerative disc lesion are noted. An abnormal area of increased signal is present in the anterior aspect of the adjacent endplates in the subchondral marrow (arrows), findings likely to be Modic type 2 changes, though correlation with the T2-weighted imaging is necessary.

on T1-weighted and virtually disappear on T2-weighted and fat-suppressed techniques.[10,30,65]

Disc disease may affect the vertebral bodies by precipitating the formation of osteophytes; it can also affect the bone marrow. With MR imaging, abnormal signal may be present parallel to the endplates; this can mimic the appearance of infection and can be the cause of unwarranted alarm in the unwary!

Early in the process of these Modic changes, inflammation and granulomatous tissue lead to a decrease in the T1-weighted signal intensity and an increase in the T2 signal intensity; this defines a *Modic type 1* change.[66] Traditionally, this type of change has not been associated with the painful symptoms; however, there now appears to be a closer correlation between pain and this type of Modic change than in the other two types.[67,68]

As the disease progresses, focal fatty marrow conversion may occur and the endplate will demonstrate increased T1-weighted signal intensity; this represents *Modic type 2* change. The T2-weighted signal may stay the same or increase, depending on the degree of change; during the early phase, there is still the remnant of the Modic type 1 change, where a high signal was noted on T2-weighting. As the Modic type 2 changes progress, the signal on T2-weighting will become isointense to the normal endplate signal (Figure 4.11).[66]

Sclerosis parallel to the endplate will be demonstrated by decreased signal intensity on both T1- and T2-weighted sequences and is referred to as *Modic type 3* change.[66] It should be appreciated that Modic changes do not necessarily progress from type 1 to type 3, and may in fact regress with time.

Osteophytes (or spondylophytes) are a very common occurrence and are caused by disc degeneration placing stress on Sharpey's fibres. As they are a continuation of the vertebral body, they will demonstrate signal intensity corresponding to bony marrow and cortical bone, the latter appearing on MR imaging as a low signal on T1- and T2-weighting. There may also be cartilaginous tissue surrounding the osteophyte, which will appear as homogeneous, intermediate signal intensity.[69]

The presence of osteophytes is evidence of degeneration, either of the disc or of the posterior facet joints; however, it is their location – within the central canal, subarticular recess, intervertebral foramen or even in the extraforaminal region – that may be associated with specific clinical syndromes. The advantage of MR imaging over conventional radiographs, which demonstrate the osseous component of osteophytes well, is twofold:

- Osteophytes frequently have a large, radiopaque cartilaginous cap that is often responsible for the actual contact – be it fixed or dynamic – with the adjacent pain-sensitive structures;
- These structures are universally visible with MR imaging; in particular, the relationship between the osteophyte and neural tissue can be assessed.

It is essential for any clinician to assess and correlate these findings with the patient's clinical symptoms in order to best determine their course of management and likely prognosis.

It is also important to consider the relationship not just between osteophyte and soft tissue but also between osteophyte and osteophyte: soft tissue trapped between two opposing impinging structures can prove particularly intractable – this is best assessed on dynamic MR.

Because it is a common condition – and a common cause for MR referral from primary contact practitioners – assessment of lesions within the canal and foramen is something with which even an occasional reader of MR images is likely to rapidly develop familiarity. However, osteophytes extending laterally from the vertebral body may also be associated

with impingement on the dorsal root ganglion (DRG); these are more difficult to detect, possibly because the central and lateral aspects are the ones invariably assessed, particularly on the axial views. It is particularly important not only to 'think outside the box' (or, in this case, the oval) but also to try to always search the sagittal cuts that can occasionally reveal a laterally positioned osteophyte causing damage to the DRG.[70]

Vacuum phenomenon and disc calcification may also appear as a manifestation of disc degeneration. The former, an accumulation of gas within the disc, will be present on MR imaging as a linear zone of low signal intensity on all sequences; however, it is impossible on MR to differentiate gas from other causes of intradiscal low signal on T1- and T2-weighted sequences, including disc calcification. This is one instance where a plain film radiograph may provide better information than MR imaging, and, when clinically indicated, an x-ray may be ordered to differentiate the two conditions. Disc calcification cannot be visualized as well as the vacuum phenomenon and, in the early stages, may present as zone of high intensity on T1-weighted sequences.

Facet arthrosis

Facet (or zygapophyseal) joint arthrosis is usually seen in association with degenerative disc disease.[44] When degeneration occurs, cartilaginous damage, loss of joint space, buckling of the ligamentum flavum, subchondral sclerosis, subchondral cyst formation and osteophyte formation may all be present. Signal intensity changes similar to the one present in the vertebral bodies may be visualized in any of the osseous structures of the posterior elements.[10,66]

If present, subchondral cysts will appear as rounded regions continuous with the articular facets, which display a low signal intensity on T1-weighted sequences and high signal intensity on T2-weighted images; they may also demonstrate peripheral enhancement on contrasted sequences. In addition, increased fluid may be noted in the joint capsule itself. Depending on the amount of facet hypertrophy, the size of the osteophyte and degree of ligamentum flavum buckling, changes in configuration of the spinal canal, lateral recess or foramen may be observed (Figure 4.13).[10,30]

On occasion, particularly on axial supine MR images, collections of high signal on the T2-weighted images will be seen in association with the facet joints

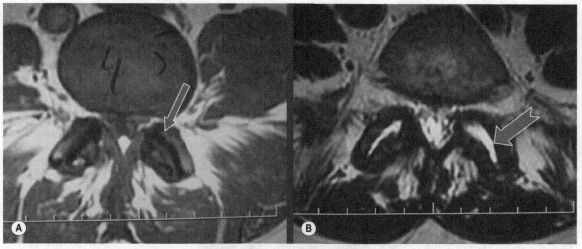

Figure 4.13 • Axial T1-weighted (A) and T2-weighted (B) MR images of the lumbar spine demonstrating signs of degenerative joint disease in the facet joints bilaterally. Irregularities of the joint surfaces and bony proliferation are identified by the arrows; thickening of the ligamentum flavum is also noted. Fluid accumulation inside the articular capsule is indicated by the notched arrow, though it is prudent to confirm a joint effusion with three consecutive axial slices. Of additional interest is the degree of fatty infiltration about the paraspinal musculature bilaterally.

either anteriorly or posteriorly. If these synovial cysts are located anteriorly, they can contribute to the narrowing of the subarticular recess or foramen, contributing to nerve impingement. They are termed *synovial cysts* and are most likely caused by the changes in pressure within the joint, causing a 'herniation' of synovial fluid through a weakened capsule, resulting in the collection of fluid, which may be symptomatic, prompting the need for invasive techniques to remove them.[71,72]

As well as cysts, facet joints may have an increase in the amount of fluid within them: *joint effusion*. This can also result in pain due to the stretching effect on the capsule surrounding the joint. Effusion is best demonstrated on the T2-weighted axial slices, and, although there is no specific measurement to apply to the width of the joint or, indeed, the volume within the joint, joint effusion can be confirmed if there is bright signal coming from the joint on three consecutive slices through the articulation.[30,73]

Spinal stenosis

Degenerative processes such as hypertrophy or osteophyte formation may lead to stenosis and encroachment of the dural sac or neural components; an early sign of this can be effacement of the epidural fat line. In the case of spondylolytic spondylolisthesis, an increase in the anteroposterior dimension is typically visible, decompressing the canal; however, if there is reactive bone formation at the pars interarticularis, this may lead to lateral recess stenosis (Figure 4.14).[10,44,74,75] Perineural (Tarlov) cysts may also widen the canal by constant erosion of bone by the CSF pulse (Figure 4.15).[76]

Whether acquired or congenital, stenosis may involve the spinal canal, the lateral recess or the foramen. Owing to the contrasting effect of CSF, the central canal can be well assessed on T2-weighted images; however, all imaging sequences and planes should be evaluated as nerves may be masked if they take an atypical course or fail to correspond to the angle of the MR imaging plane used. The epidural fat is well visualized on T1-weighted sequences and will facilitate the evaluation of stenosis in the lateral recess or foramen (Figures 4.16, 4.17).

Although various measurements have been published relating to the absolute minimal dimensions of the central canal below which stenosis is guaranteed, an important and yet often-forgotten concept is the fact that what may for one person appear a compromised canal likely to give symptoms, in another will never give rise to problems. This difference can be explained by the relative dimensions of the structures surrounding the central canal, in particular the cord (or conus, depending on the level being considered), the facet capsule and ligamentum flavum. These factors should be taken into account

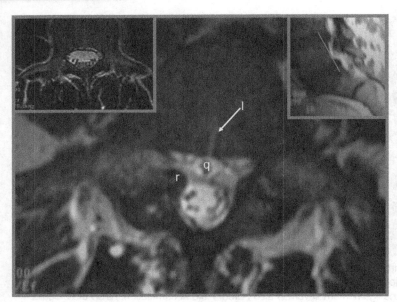

Figure 4.14 • Axial, T2-weighted MR imaging sequence of the lumbar spine demonstrating a spondylolytic spondylolisthesis. The presence of a spondylolytic spondylolisthesis may increase the anterior–posterior diameter of the central canal and usually alters its shape. In the presence of an anterolisthesis, the canal takes on a 'trefoil' appearance. Bony or fibrous proliferation at the pars interarticularis may narrow the central canal size in the transverse plane. A normal axial image is provided for comparison (see left insert). The key to the identification of structures is given in Box 4.01.

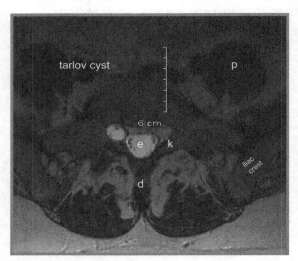

Figure 4.15 • Axial T2-weighted MR imaging of the lumbar spine at the L5–S1 level. A Tarlov (perineural) cyst measuring approximately 1.5 cm and involving the first right sacral nerve root is demonstrated. Note the slight expansion/deformation of the shape of the lateral recess and right foramen. There is mild bony erosion of the posterior vertebral body and pedicle region, likely due to the pressure effect from the cyst.

before referring a patient for surgery and should be correlated with clinical history and examination findings.[77,78]

Treatments for stenosis are variable, with conservative approaches usually being considered first. If these fail to achieve satisfactory improvement, surgical approaches such as laminectomy, discectomy or fasciectomy may be considered (Figures 4.18, 4.19).[79] Fusion, with or without instrumentation, may also be performed concomitantly, depending on the amount of decompression required. This surgical hardware may considerably limit the usefulness of subsequent MR imaging because of the associated artifact; this is example of where CT may be superior to MR imaging in evaluating the outcome of the invention.

The postsurgical spine

Initially on MR imaging, the surgical site will demonstrate an immature scar and haematoma formation. This extradural soft tissue may retain the appearance of the original disc pathology; this finding may be present up to 1 year after the surgical intervention. MR imaging can therefore be ineffective in the evaluation of immediate surgical complications, particularly in the first 4 to 6 weeks and in some instances for up to 6 months, and can be incapable of determining whether persistent potential pain is due to a recurrent disc lesion, to scar tissue or simply to a postoperative soft tissue haematoma.

If a developing infection is suspected, this may warrant MR imaging but with the addition of contrast and perhaps complemented by a CT scan to compensate for the surgical device artifact and also to observe

Figure 4.16 • Sagittal T2-weighted (A) and axial T1-weighted (B) lumbar images of a 25-year-old patient with low back pain and right-sided radiculopathy. A central to right para-central through to extraforaminal disc protrusion is noted, leading to a decrease in the lateral recess and foraminal space on the right compared to that of the left (arrow), which is free and surrounded by fat. The nerve roots are well visualized owing to the contrasting effect of surrounding fat: there is mild displacement of the right nerve root. In (A), the L5 disc demonstrates a hypointense T2-weighted signal consistent with dessication.

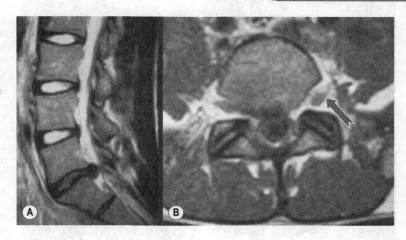

Figure 4.17 • MR imaging of the lumbar spine in a patient with bilateral radiculopathy and leg cramping. A mild disc protrusion and mild degenerative spondylolisthesis associated with facet hypertrophy can be seen on the T2-weighted (A and B are axial, C is a sagittal slice) and T1-weighted sequences (D and E, which are both sagittal slices) (arrow in E). This patient demonstrates central stenosis from the disc protrusion which extends from the posterocentral position to the left extraforaminal zone (notched arrow in A) and lateral recess stenosis from the facet arthrosis bilaterally (arrow in A) and ligamentous hypertrophy also on the right predominantly (striped arrow in B).

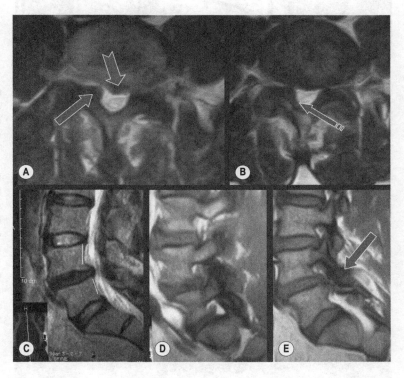

for any subtle bony erosions along the endplate. These should be compared with pre-surgical images; any soft tissue mass will slowly decrease on sequential studies. Over time, scar tissue will also progressively enhance with the addition of contrast; generally, scar tissue enhances earlier on MR imaging and will be hyperintense to adjacent or newly emergent disc material. This determination of whether non-resolving, postsurgical symptoms are arising from a recurrent disc herniation or the development of postoperative scar tissue is important because the management of the patient will differ.[38]

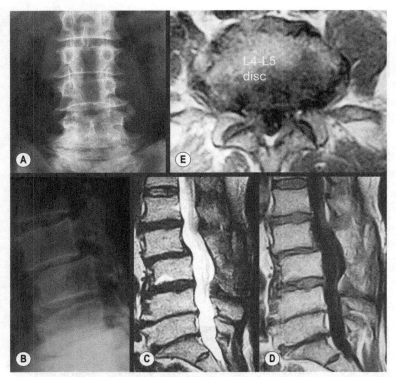

Figure 4.18 • Postsurgical changes associated with laminectomy seen on plain film radiographs, anteroposterior and lateral views (A, B, respectively); sagittal T2-weighted MR imaging (C); and sagittal and axial T1-weighted sequences (D, E). This patient underwent laminectomy at L2–3 and, years later, presented with recurring radiculopathy. Advanced degenerative disc disease can be observed at L4–5 and L5–S1, leading to central, subarticular and foraminal stenosis with an impressive anterolisthesis of L2–3. Modic type 1 endplate changes are present at the anterior aspect of L4 and L5, as well as profuse spondylophyte formation anteriorly and posteriorly at L4 and L5.

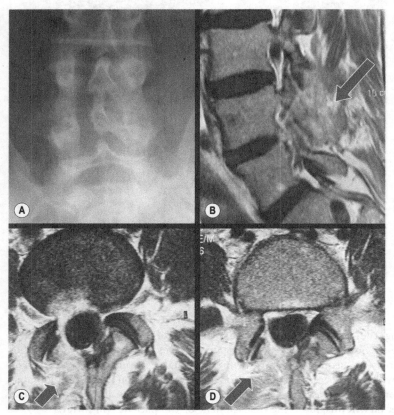

Figure 4.19 • Partial laminectomy defect demonstrated on anteroposterior plain film radiograph of the lumbosacral junction (A), and T1-weighted parasagittal (B) and T1-weighted axial images (C, D). Disorganization and discontinuity of the muscle fibres is indicated by the arrow. The right laminae of L3 and L4 have been removed to allow for canal decompression. There is a mild displacement of the thecal sac to the right into the zone of the defect. Facet arthrosis and ligamentum flavum hypertrophy originally led to the stenosis. Degenerative changes about the left posterior facet are also visible.

Disorganization and lack of continuity of the muscle fibres may be seen in the paraspinal tissues following surgery; this may be due either to lack of use or to denervation. Infection may occur following any surgical intervention. Postoperative discitis will be demonstrated by signal alteration in the vertebral bodies: decreased signal intensity on T1-weighted images, increased signal intensity on T2-weighted images and increased enhancement with contrast. These findings can be similar to normal postoperative changes, making careful correlation with laboratory findings important.[10,51]

And the rest of it . . .

When a clinician requests lumbar MR imaging, their primary concern is to determine the state of the lumbar spine and the surrounding soft tissue and bone structures; however, once the sequences have been obtained, it is important that *all* the information on the images should be fully evaluated, and not just those structures contributing to the immediate differential diagnosis.

This is particularly true of the lower thoracic spine, which is often included in the images, albeit principally on the scout views and sagittal slices. The lower thoracic spine often holds information that may contribute to the clinical picture or reveal changes that warrant further investigation. Often, irregular endplates and altered morphology of the vertebral bodies along with decreased signal in the discs on the T2-weighted images strongly suggests evidence of juvenile discogenic disease, which may be important in the determination of the patient's potential predisposition regarding development of future disc lesions in the lower spine.[80] In other cases, patients may have marrow-based lesions affecting the thoracic spine that may be due to more sinister disorders such as multiple myeloma or metastatic disease.[81] Lower thoracic disc lesions are also readily identifiable on lumbar sagittal slices and, due to the relative dimensions of the spinal cord and conus, a small disc lesion can have a disproportionate impact and cause symptoms that mimic lumbar pathology (see Chapter 3).

Incidental systemic disease can also be identified by the alert radiologist. Kidney lesions are not infrequently present; these may consist of solitary cysts – relatively common in the older patient – or multiple cysts from polycystic kidney disease. The form and size of the kidneys should also be evaluated to determine if there is evidence of any structural abnormality that could lead to functional alterations or the development of significant clinical conditions such as pyelonephrosis. The position and morphology of the uterus is also easily determined and can often result in the detection of leiomyomas that can be subclinical or can often mimic musculoskeletal low back pain.

Clinical pearls

- MR imaging of the lumbar spine in the majority of current cases is performed with the patient supine.
- MR imaging of the lumbar spine is usually performed with continuous slicing from L1 to S1.
- MR imaging of the lumbar spine may be contra-indicated in certain patient populations; for example, those with metallic implants, claustrophobics and, where contrast is to be used, those with sensitivity to contrast agents.
- Pregnancy is a relative contraindication (caution) and should be considered on a case-by-case basis.

References

1. Adams M, Bogduk N, Burton KJ, Dolan P. Epidemiology of low back trouble. In: *The Biomechanics of Back Pain*. 2nd ed. Edinburgh: Churchill Livingstone; 2006:55–72.
2. Bates B, Hoekelman R. Interviewing and the health history. In: Bates B, ed. *A Guide to Physical Examination*. 3rd ed. Philadelphia: JB Lippincott; 1983:1–27.
3. Bates B. The musculoskeletal system. In: Bates B, ed. *A Guide to Physical Examination*. 3rd ed. Philadelphia: JB Lippincott; 1983:324–370.
4. Rowe L, Yochum T. Principles of radiological interpretation. In: Yochum T, Rowe L, eds. *Essentials of Skeletal Radiology*. 2nd ed. Baltimore: Williams and Wilkins; 1996:547–585.
5. Chou R, Fu R, Carrino JA, Deyo RA. Imaging strategies for low-back pain: systematic review and meta-analysis. *Lancet*. 2009;373(9662):463–472.
6. Finch P. Technology insight: imaging of low back pain. *Nat Clin Pract Rheumatol*. 2006;2(10):554–561.
7. Gilbert JW, Wheeler GR, Kreft MP, et al. Repeat upright positional magnetic resonance imaging for diagnosis of disorders underlying chronic noncancer lumbar pain. *J Manipulative Physiol Ther*. 2008;31(8):627–631.

8. Gedroyc WM. Upright positional MRI of the lumbar spine. *Clin Radiol.* 2008;63(9):1049–1050.

9. Alyas F, Connell D, Saifuddin A. Upright positional MRI of the lumbar spine. *Clin Radiol.* 2008;63(9):1035–1048.

10. Stoller D. *Magnetic Resonance Imaging in Orthopaedics and Sports Medicine.* 2nd ed. Philadelphia: Lippincott Williams and Wilkins; 1996.

11. Gundry CR, Fritts HM. Magnetic resonance imaging of the musculoskeletal system. Part 8. The spine, section 2. *Clin Orthop Relat Res.* 1997;(343):260–271.

12. Gundry CR, Fritts HM. Magnetic resonance imaging of the musculoskeletal system. Part 8. The spine, section 1. *Clin Orthop Relat Res.* 1997;(338):275–287.

13. Oostveen JC, van de Laar MA. Magnetic resonance imaging in rheumatic disorders of the spine and sacroiliac joints. *Semin Arthritis Rheum.* 2000;30(1):52–69.

14. Thomas WB. Diskospondylitis and other vertebral infections. *Vet Clin North Am Small Anim Pract.* 2000;30(1):169–182 vii.

15. Chin CT. Spine imaging. *Semin Neurol.* 2002;22(2):205–220.

16. Jinkins JR. Acquired degenerative changes of the intervertebral segments at and suprajacent to the lumbosacral junction. A radioanatomic analysis of the nondiscal structures of the spinal column and perispinal soft tissues. *Eur J Radiol.* 2004;50(2):134–158.

17. Corbett M, Foster N, Ong BN. GP attitudes and self-reported behaviour in primary care consultations for low back pain. *Fam Pract.* 2009;26(5):359–364.

18. Somerville S, Hay E, Lewis M, et al. Content and outcome of usual primary care for back pain: a systematic review. *Br J Gen Pract.* 2008;58(556):790–797, i–vi.

19. Croft PR, Macfarlane GJ, Papageorgiou AC, et al. Outcome of low back pain in general practice: a prospective study. *BMJ.* 1998;316(7141):1356–1359.

20. Savigny P, Watson P, Underwood M. Early management of persistent non-specific low back pain: summary of NICE guidance. *BMJ.* 2009;338:b1805.

21. Kirkaldy-Willis WH. *Managing Low Back Pain.* 4th ed. Edinburgh: Churchill Livingstone; 1999.

22. Eley C. Magnetic resonance imaging for low back injuries: appropriate use in managing workers' compensation claims. *AAOHN J.* 2006;54(10):429–433.

23. Strayer A. Lumbar spine: common pathology and interventions. *J Neurosci Nurs.* 2005;37(4):181–193.

24. Ferri FF. *Ferri's Differential Diagnosis.* Philadelphia: Mosby; 2005.

25. Dudley-Hart F, ed. *French's Index of Differential Diagnosis.* Bristol: Wright; 1985.

26. Bogduk N. *Clinical Anatomy of the Lumbar Spine and Sacrum.* Edinburgh: Churchill Livingstone; 2004.

27. Adams M, Bogduk N, Burton KJ, Dolan P. *The Biomechanics of Back Pain.* Edinburgh: Churchill Livingstone; 2002.

28. Shellock FG, Parker JR, Venetianer C, et al. Safety of gadobenate dimeglumine (MultiHance): summary of findings from clinical studies and postmarketing surveillance. *Invest Radiol.* 2006;41(6):500–509.

29. Li A, Wong CS, Wong MK, et al. Acute adverse reactions to magnetic resonance contrast media – gadolinium chelates. *Br J Radiol.* 2006; 79(941):368–371.

30. Berquist T. *MRI of the Musculoskeletal System.* 4th ed. Philadelphia: Lippincott Williams and Wilkins; 2000.

31. Kanal E, Borgstede JP, Barkovich AJ, et al. American College of Radiology White Paper on MR Safety. *Am J Roentgenol.* 2002;178(6):1335–1347.

32. Kubik-Huch RA, Gottstein-Aalame NM, Frenzel T, et al. Gadopentetate dimeglumine excretion into human breast milk during lactation. *Radiology.* 2000; 216(2):555–558.

33. Beers M, Berkow R. *The Merck Manual.* 17th ed. West Point, PA: Merck & Co; 1999.

34. Kaplan P, Helms C, Dussault R, Anderson M. *Musculoskeletal MRI.* Philadelphia: WB Saunders; 2001.

35. Wigh RE. The thoracolumbar and lumbosacral transitional junctions. *Spine.* 1980;5(3):215–222.

36. Haughton V, Schreibman K, De Smet A. Contrast between scar and recurrent herniated disk on contrast-enhanced MR images. *AJNR Am J Neuroradiol.* 2002; 23(10):1652–1656.

37. Castillo M. Contrast enhancement in primary tumors of the brain and spinal cord. *Neuroimaging Clin N Am.* 1994;4(1):63–80.

38. Bronen RA, Sze G. Magnetic resonance imaging contrast agents: theory and application to the central nervous system. *J Neurosurg.* 1990;73(6):820–839.

39. Dillon WP. Imaging of central nervous system tumors. *Curr Opin Radiol.* 1991;3(1):46–50.

40. Jarvik JG, Bowen B, Ross J. *Practice Guideline for the Performance of Magnetic Resonance Imaging (MRI) of the Adult Spine.* Reston, VA: American College of Radiology; 2006.

41. Vande Berg BC, Lecouvet FE, Galant C, et al. Normal variants of the bone marrow at MR imaging of the spine. *Semin Musculoskelet Radiol.* 2009;13(2):87–96.

42. Hyun SJ, Rhim SC, Kang JK, et al. Combined motor- and somatosensory-evoked potential monitoring for spine and spinal cord surgery: correlation of clinical and neurophysiological data in 85 consecutive procedures. *Spinal Cord.* 2009;47(8):616–622.

43. Helms C, Major N, Anderson MW, et al. Basic principles of musculoskeletal MRI. In: *Musculoskeletal MRI.* 2nd ed. Philadelphia: Elsevier Saunders; 2009:1–19.

44. Grenier N, Kressel HY, Schiebler ML, et al. Normal and degenerative posterior spinal structures: MR imaging. *Radiology.* 1987;165(2):517–525.

45. Standring S, ed. *Gray's Anatomy – The back (Section 45).* Edinburgh: Elsevier; 2009.

46. Muzin S, Isaac Z, Walker 3rd J. The role of intradiscal steroids in the treatment of discogenic low back pain. *Curr Rev Musculoskelet Med.* 2008;1(2):103–107.

47. Sehgal N, Fortin JD. Internal disc disruption and low back pain. *Pain Physician.* 2000;3(2):143–157.

48. Stoller DW, Tirman PF, Bredella MA. *Diagnostic Imaging*

Orthopaedics. Salt Lake City: Amirsys Inc; 2003.

49. Barr JS. Lumbar disk lesions in retrospect and prospect: Joseph S. Barr. Address tape-recorded May 1961. *Clin Orthop Relat Res*. 1977;(129):4–8.

50. Milette PC. The proper terminology for reporting lumbar intervertebral disk disorders. *AJNR Am J Neuroradiol*. 1997;18(10): 1859–1866.

51. Ross JS, Zepp R, Modic MT. The postoperative lumbar spine: enhanced MR evaluation of the intervertebral disk. *AJNR Am J Neuroradiol*. 1996;17(2):323–331.

52. Moore K. The back. In: *Clinically Oriented Anatomy*. 2nd ed. Baltimore: Williams and Wilkins; 1985:565–625.

53. Kokubo Y, Uchida K, Kobayashi S, et al. Herniated and spondylotic intervertebral discs of the human cervical spine: histological and immunohistological findings in 500 en bloc surgical samples. Laboratory investigation. *J Neurosurg Spine*. 2008;9(3):285–295.

54. Bachmeier BE, Nerlich A, Mittermaier N, et al. Matrix metalloproteinase expression levels suggest distinct enzyme roles during lumbar disc herniation and degeneration. *Eur Spine J*. 2009;18(11):1573–1586.

55. Rowe L, Yochum T. Arthritic disorders. In: Yochum T, Rowe L, eds. *Essentials of Skeletal Radiology*. 2nd ed. Baltimore: Williams and Wilkins; 1996:795–974.

56. Mixter WJ, Barr JS. Rupture of the intervertebral disc with involvement of the spinal canal. *N Engl J Med*. 1934;211:210–215.

57. Parisien RC, Ball PA. William Jason Mixter (1880–1958). Ushering in the "dynasty of the disc". *Spine*. 1998;23(21):2363–2366.

58. Milette PC. Reporting lumbar disk abnormalities: at last, consensus!. *AJNR Am J Neuroradiol*. 2001; 22(3):428–429.

59. Fardon DF, Milette PC. Nomenclature and classification of lumbar disc pathology. Recommendations of the Combined Task Forces of the North American Spine Society, American Society of Spine Radiology, and American Society of Neuroradiology. *Spine*. 2001;26(5):E93–E113.

60. Peng B, Hou S, Wu W, et al. The pathogenesis and clinical significance of a high-intensity zone (HIZ) of lumbar intervertebral disc on MR imaging in the patient with discogenic low back pain. *Eur Spine J*. 2006;15(5):583–587.

61. Lim CH, Jee WH, Son BC, et al. Discogenic lumbar pain: association with MR imaging and CT discography. *Eur J Radiol*. 2005; 54(3):431–437.

62. Madsen R, Jensen TS, Pope M, et al. The effect of body position and axial load on spinal canal morphology: an MRI study of central spinal stenosis. *Spine*. 2008; 33(1):61–67.

63. Jung HS, Jee WH, McCauley TR, et al. Discrimination of metastatic from acute osteoporotic compression spinal fractures with MR imaging. *Radiographics*. 2003; 23(1):179–187.

64. Helms C. Trauma. In: *Fundamentals of Skeletal Radiology*. Philadelphia: Elsevier Saunders; 2005:78–112.

65. Ross JS, Masaryk TJ, Modic MT, et al. Vertebral hemangiomas: MR imaging. *Radiology*. 1987;165(1): 165–169.

66. Modic MT, Masaryk TJ, Ross JS, Carter JR. Imaging of degenerative disk disease. *Radiology*. 1988;168(1):177–186.

67. Thompson KJ, Dagher AP, Eckel TS, et al. Modic changes on MR images as studied with provocative diskography: clinical relevance – a retrospective study of 2457 disks. *Radiology*. 2009;250(3): 849–855.

68. Luoma K, Vehmas T, Gronblad M, et al. Relationship of Modic type 1 change with disc degeneration: a prospective MRI study. *Skeletal Radiol*. 2009;38(3): 237–244.

69. Helms C, Major N, Anderson MW, et al. Spine. In: *Musculoskeletal MRI*. 2nd ed. Philadelphia: Elsevier Saunders; 2009:273–323.

70. Grenier JM, Scordilis PJ, Seaman DR, Wessely M. Lumbar MRI. Part 2: Common pathological conditions. *Clinical Chiropractic*. 2006;9(1):39–47.

71. Ayberk G, Ozveren F, Gok B, et al. Lumbar synovial cysts: experience with nine cases. *Neurol Med Chir (Tokyo)*. 2008;48(7):298–303.

72. Kahilogullari G, Tuna H, Attar A. Management of spinal synovial cysts. *Turk Neurosurg*. 2008;18(2): 211–214.

73. Chaput C, Padon D, Rush J, et al. The significance of increased fluid signal on magnetic resonance imaging in lumbar facets in relationship to degenerative spondylolisthesis. *Spine*. 2007;32(17):1883–1887.

74. Grenier N, Kressel HY, Schiebler ML, Grossman RI. Isthmic spondylolysis of the lumbar spine: MR imaging at 1.5 T. *Radiology*. 1989;170(2):489–493.

75. Schiebler ML, Grenier N, Fallon M, et al. Normal and degenerated intervertebral disk: in vivo and in vitro MR imaging with histopathologic correlation. *Am J Roentgenol*. 1991;157(1):93–97.

76. Langdown AJ, Grundy JR, Birch NC. The clinical relevance of Tarlov cysts. *J Spinal Disord Tech*. 2005;18(1): 29–33.

77. Lurie JD, Tosteson AN, Tosteson TD, et al. Reliability of readings of magnetic resonance imaging features of lumbar spinal stenosis. *Spine*. 2008;33(14): 1605–1610.

78. Geisser ME, Haig AJ, Tong HC, et al. Spinal canal size and clinical symptoms among persons diagnosed with lumbar spinal stenosis. *Clin J Pain*. 2007;23(9):780–785.

79. Thalgott JS, Albert TJ, Vaccaro AR, et al. A new classification system for degenerative disc disease of the lumbar spine based on magnetic resonance imaging, provocative discography, plain radiographs and anatomic considerations. *Spine J*. 2004;4(suppl 6):167S–172S.

80. Wood KB, Garvey TA, Gundry C, Heithoff KB. Magnetic resonance imaging of the thoracic spine. Evaluation of asymptomatic individuals. *J Bone Joint Surg Am*. 1995;77(11):1631–1638.

81. Kim HJ, Ryu KN, Choi WS, et al. Spinal involvement of hematopoietic malignancies and metastasis: differentiation using MR imaging. *Clin Imaging*. 1999;23(2): 125–133.

The hip and pelvis

5 (chapter number)

Michelle A. Wessely   Martin Young   Julie-Marthe Grenier

Introduction

Magnetic resonance (MR) imaging of the hip provides a platform to assess the osseous structures and surrounding soft tissues and is thus an invaluable tool in the assessment of both the hip joint and its associated structures. It is therefore important to develop a thorough grounding in the normal anatomical appearance of the pelvis and hip on MR imaging in order to thereafter appreciate the more common disorders that will regularly present in clinical practice.

Because a range of diagnostic modalities is available to the investigating clinician, it is also important that they have an understanding of the applications of each technique and its clinical appropriateness. Often, a patient's principal presenting complaint will be that of low back pain, with associated symptomatology in the hip, groin or thigh.

Depending on the size of the field of view, the hips may be included on MR imaging of the lumbar spine; however, in order to explore the hip's anatomy and pathoanatomy in detail, a focused MR imaging study, initially of both hips followed by a dedicated protocol of the hip in question should be performed, to optimize the detection of any pathology and to help direct the most appropriate clinical management of the patient.

History and examination

As with any patient examination, the eliciting of a detailed and accurate history is paramount and lays the foundation for the performance of an appropriate examination and establishment of a working diagnosis and differential. The most crucial element of the history in this area of the body is the precise localization of the area of pain: many patients who complain of 'hip pain' do not in fact have pain in their hip and, when questioned, will point to their buttock, gluteal fold or iliac crest; similarly, patients who *do* have hip pathology will often complain of symptoms in their groin, or the side or front of their thigh – not infrequently described as 'sciatica'! The use of pain diagrams can help in this regard, but, at the very least, the patient should be asked to point to where they feel pain or discomfort.[1,2]

The nature and precipitation of the pain can also give important clues as to the underlying cause of the patient's complaint. Progressive, insidious pain and stiffness in the groin (often in association with a flexion contracture) and/or the buttock is indicative of arthritis; this will typically be made worse by walking and relieved by sitting. By contrast, a sacroiliac syndrome, which presents with buttock pain that may refer to the groin, will often be acute with an obvious precipitating cause and be relieved by walking and aggravated by sitting.

Sporting injuries often have very localized pain produced by highly specific activities: soccer players may complain of groin pain but only when passing the ball in certain directions; this can help differentiate injury to the adductor longus from rectus femoris or psoas. Increasing pain on repetitive activity is also typical of soft tissue injuries such as bursitis, which commonly affects the greater trochanteric area: often the patient will complain of being unable to sleep on the affected side.

With experience, the clinician will normally be able to recognize the atypical presentation of more

© 2011, Elsevier Ltd.
DOI: 10.1016/B978-0-443-06726-6.00005-6

unusual conditions such as osseous, intrapelvic and spinal lesions. These can, of course, mimic everyday injuries and the clinician should always be alert for an apparently benign condition that fails to respond to normally successful management protocols or is relentlessly progressive. Pain or clicking in the hip of a child is always a cause for concern and usually an indication for diagnostic imaging.[3]

Associated symptoms such as clicking or popping can also be associated with specific conditions[4] and a familial history of pelvic conditions is often very revealing: many conditions such as degenerative coxarthrosis, inflammatory arthropathies, connective tissue disorders and dysplasia have familial tendencies.[5–9]

Examination should commence with observation of the patient both stationary and walking. Obesity (a body mass index greater than 30) is a significant predisposing factor towards coxarthrosis,[10] which will often be accompanied by an obvious flexion contraction causing an inability to stand with a straightened leg on the affected side; other forms of antalgia can also help identify the source of a patient's pain both in posture and gait.

Although there are myriad orthopaedic tests for the hips and sacroiliac joints, few have any proven validity.[11–14] Range of motion, however, often is enough to demonstrate hip pathology, particularly painful reduction of internal rotation. The Patrick/FABER test (external rotation of the hip with the leg in the 'figure-4' position: Flexion, Abduction and External Rotation) has been shown to have good reliability as has digital palpation in the identification of greater trochanteric bursitis – the same is also true of the many myofascial trigger points that frequently coexist with pelvic girdle dysfunction and with the posterior margin of the sacroiliac joint.[12,15,16]

Identification of sacroiliac syndrome is more problematic; however, multiple positive provocation tests have been shown to have a measure of diagnostic reliability; these are detailed in Table 5.01[17–19] along

Table 5.01 Suggested provocation tests for the sacroiliac joint
Provocative tests with evidence of diagnostic reliability

Multiple positives are suggestive of sacroiliac injury; if all tests are negative, injury is diagnostically eliminated	
Gaenslen's test	Sit the patient on the edge of a table, flexing one leg to the chest and dropping the other to the floor
Compression test	The ilium is forced medially against the sacrum; this is usually done with the patient lying on their side (Figure 5.01)
Thigh thrust	The supine patient's hip is flexed to 90° with the knee bent and a posterior shearing force applied to the sacroiliac joint through the femur avoiding hip adduction (Figure 5.02)
Distraction test	With the patient lying supine, the anterior superior iliac spines are pressured from lateral to medial
Sacral thrust	Posterior to anterior pressure is applied to the sacrum immediately adjacent to the sacroiliac joint

Additional sacroiliac joint tests used in combination by the authors with (apparent) success

These tests are not scientifically validated; they do, however, reflect the diagnosis and successful treatment of several thousand sacroiliac joints. The tests have the advantage that they are not all provocative	
Yeoman's test	Forced extension of the sacroiliac joint with the patient lying supine recreating their pain
Leg lift	If the patient is unable to lift both legs together when locked straight, this is indicative of sacroiliac dysfunction
Leg lift with cervical compression	If they are able to perform the above test but find it much more difficult with superior to inferior pressure applied to the top of the head (thus compressing the cervical spine), this is also indicative of sacroiliac dysfunction. Either result is considered as a single positive
Piedallu test	The examiner places their thumbs on the posterior superior iliac spines and watches as the seated patient leans forwards. The failure of the spine to move superiorly in a symmetrical manner indicates sacroiliac dysfunction

Continued

Table 5.01 Suggested provocation tests for the sacroiliac joint—cont'd

Contralateral Kemp's test	Usually Kemp's test (forced lateral flexion with extension) is used as a test for lumbar spine disorder and will produce ipsilateral pain; however, a sacroiliac syndrome will cause *contralateral* pain
Supported Adam's test	Patients with a sacroiliac problem often report pain on slight forward flexion (5°–15°). If the sacrum is braced against the examiner's thigh and the ilia held firmly, the patient can flex with reduced pain and trepidation
Digital palpation	If there is inflammation in the sacroiliac joint, palpation along its easily identified posterior margin will usually be painful

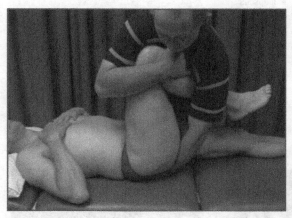

Figure 5.01 • The thigh thrust sacroiliac joint provocation test. (Reproduced from *Manual Therapy*[17] with permission.)

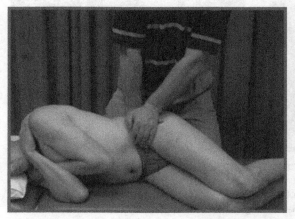

Figure 5.02 • The compression sacroiliac joint provocation test. (Reproduced from *Manual Therapy*[17] with permission.)

with tests that the authors have also found useful when similarly used in combination. It is, however, important not to perform too many tests; if three or four have already proved positive, there is little to be gained from continuing and the patient may well have an adverse reaction – the tests are called provocative for a reason and can eventually aggravate the patient's symptoms. It should also be kept in mind that the pelvis is a closed loop kinematic chain and that comorbidity with lumbosacral facet joint dysfunction is high.[20]

Differential diagnosis

Once the differentiation between intrapelvic conditions, hip pain and sacroiliac syndrome has been made, the diagnosis should be further refined. The main differential with sacroiliac syndrome is with myofascial syndromes in the muscles of the gluteal region and lumbosacral junction and with lumbar spine injury, which can often refer or radiate to the buttock. As these conditions are often comorbid, the clinical challenge is to ascertain the extent of the contribution from each.

When it comes to the hip joint, the main aim of the differential diagnosis is to distinguish between intra-articular pathology, extra-articular pathology, and those conditions that can mimic hip pain. These are summarized in Table 5.02.[3,21,22]

The clinician should also be alert for paediatric cases presenting as knee pain without discernible cause. Two common hip conditions often present in this manner: slipped capital femoral epiphysis and Legg–Calvé–Perthes disease, and both have prognosis directly related to early detection.[23]

Technique and protocols

During any MR imaging evaluation, patient co-operation is critical. For evaluation of the hip, the patient should lie supine with mild internal rotation of the feet. Symmetry of rotation of both feet is important when both joints are examined simultaneously, which they often are to compare the appearance of the trochanters and adjacent muscles.[24–26]

Table 5.02 Causes of pain around the hip joint

Intra-articular	Extra-articular	Mimickers
Avascular necrosis	Adductor strain	Athletic pubalgia
Capsular laxity	Greater trochanteric bursitis	Kidney stones
Chondral damage	Iliopsoas tendinitis	Osteitis pubis
Femoroacetabular impingement syndrome	Iliotibial band	Pubic diastasis
Hip dysplasia	Myofascial syndromes:	Sports hernia
Hydroxyapatite crystal deposition disease (HADD)	• Adductors	
Inflammatory arthropathy	• Glutei	
Labral tears	• Hamstrings	
Legg–Calvé–Perthes disease	• Iliopsoas	
Ligamentum teres injury	• Pelvic floor muscles	
Loose bodies	• Piriformis	
Slipped capital femoral epiphysis	• Quadriceps	
	• Quadratus lumborum	
	• Spinal intrinsics	
	• Tensor fascia lata	
	Piriformis syndrome	
	Sacroiliac joint pathology	
	Stress fracture	

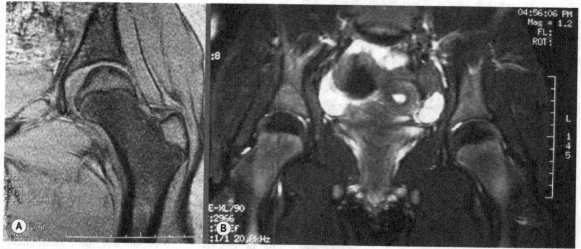

Figure 5.03 • MR imaging of the hip using two different protocols in paediatric patients. In (A), MR imaging of the left hip has been performed using a gradient-weighted sequence in the coronal plane. The specificity of the MR imaging to include just one hip joint allows for the close inspection of this region, particularly with respect to the labrum; however, in (B), an MR image of both hips in the coronal plane using a fluid-sensitive sequence allows for the comparative evaluation of both hips albeit with a reduction in the anatomical detail, but which remains a very useful technique to study the hips. Both techniques have advantages and disadvantages.

Two types of images are available: a screening examination of both hips, or a higher-detail study of a single joint (Figure 5.03).

The study begins with a plan scan (or 'scout' view) through the level of the femoral head and will usually include axial and coronal views (Figure 5.04). T1-weighted and fluid-sensitive images will be obtained in multiple planes. Depending on the pathology suspected, sagittal views may also be acquired (Figure 5.05). Fat-suppression techniques are very

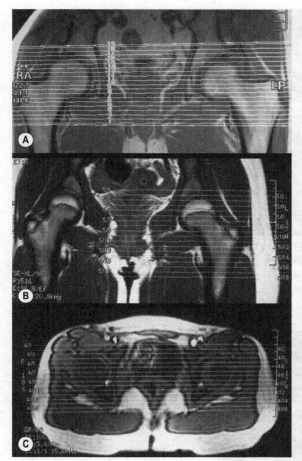

Figure 5.04 • Three MR imaging scout views demonstrating planes of imaging for (A) axial pelvis (T1-weighted), (B) axial hip (T1-weighted in a paediatric patient), and (C) coronal pelvis gradient echo.

commonly used in the hip and pelvis to show early changes in marrow signal.[24,25,27,28]

Intravenous contrast is not routinely utilized but may be helpful to differentiate cystic from solid masses or early ischaemic changes and in the evaluation of labral pathologies that have proven inconclusive on normal MR protocols. In these situations, findings may be accentuated even more if paired with fat-suppression techniques.[25.27,29,30]

Evaluation of the sacrum, sacroiliac joint and superior bony pelvis anatomy requires different positioning for the patient and should be ordered separately. The patient is often asked to lie supine with the knees slightly bent and hip joint mildly flexed; this position precludes good visualization of the iliofemoral joint. The planes of imaging for these areas is also different; in cases where

sacroiliac arthropathy is suspected, images obtained in an oblique coronal plane parallel to the joint may be helpful (Figure 5.06). Intravenous administration of contrast can help identify early sacroiliitis. If pathology is suspected in the posterior soft tissues, imaging in the prone position may be also considered, to limit compression of the soft tissues.[24,25,27,31,32]

Normal anatomy and common variants

MR imaging displays osseous and soft tissue structures with great clarity; the osseous anatomy is best evaluated on the T1-weighted sequences. The acetabular fossa is a deep pocket that covers approximately 40% of the surface of the femoral head. The thick fibrocartilaginous labrum and transverse acetabular ligament completely encircle the acetabulum. Both structures will be demonstrated as low intensity areas on most of the MR sequences.[33]

The femoral head is generally spherical and covered by articular cartilage with the exception of the insertion point of the ligamentum teres: the fovea centralis. Covering the proximal femur is the articular capsule extending from the supra-acetabular region to the femoral neck.[34,35] It is a normal finding to see a small amount of fluid inside the joint space (Figure 5.07). Adjacent to the capsule is one of the largest synovial bursae of the body: the *iliopsoas bursa*. It is seen as a high intensity area on fluid-sensitive images, sandwiched between the muscle and the capsule. In a small percentage of the population, it may even communicate with the joint.[36] MR imaging allows for assessment of the major muscle groups surrounding the hip articulation: the external rotators inserting on the greater trochanter, and iliopsoas attaching to the lesser trochanter and the hip flexors crossing over the large joint (Figures 5.08, 5.09; Box 5.01).[22,33]

In the pelvis and proximal femur, the composition of the bone marrow varies with age, skeletal maturity and health status, and the MR imaging appearance will change accordingly (Figure 5.10). In the adult, bone marrow throughout the pelvis and femoral head will demonstrate intermediate signal intensity, slightly more intense than the muscle, on T1-weighted images; the marrow in adults is generally composed of fatty components. The signal may however be heterogeneous and patchy, interrupted by low signal zones on T1 images, representing residual foci of haematopoietic (red) marrow. These are considered normal findings and are generally bilateral and symmetrical. Abnormality

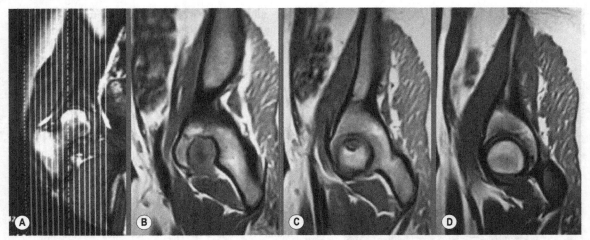

Figure 5.05 • MR imaging using T1-weighted, spin echo images of the hip in the sagittal plane. These sequences are useful in the evaluation of the subchondral bone, in conditions such as avascular necrosis, or in cases of acetabular labral tears. Figure (A) demonstrates the scout view for the resulting sagittal sections (B–D). Note that the anterior aspect of the patient is to the reading left in these figures, which progress from medial to lateral.

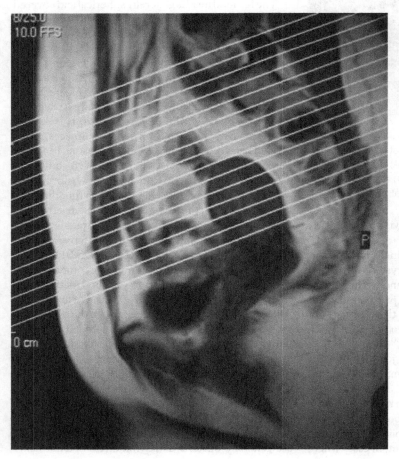

Figure 5.06 • MR imaging depicting scout view of the sacrum. Particularly note the angulation of the plane of imaging which allows this plane to capture not only the sacrum but also a portion of the hip region which may reveal previously occult lesions.

is represented by the persistence of red marrow in the epiphysis and should lead to further investigation. In children, the marrow patterns vary by region. The femoral head and greater trochanter will contain yellow marrow and the intertrochanteric or metaphyseal region will contain haematopoietic marrow (Figure 5.11).[24,28,29,37]

Other causes of marrow signal abnormalities include bone islands. They are easily recognized as decreased signal zones on all sequences and are frequently found in the proximal femur (Figure 5.12).[27,38] Obliquely oriented linear zones of decreased signal intensity in the femoral neck may also be seen and represent the bony weight-bearing trabecular groups. Well-defined areas of abnormal low T1-weighted and high T2-weighted signal intensity may be present in the anterior-lateral portion of the femoral neck. Synovial herniation pit defects are also common in this location and can be recognized by the presence of focal increased signal intensity on T2-weighted images, a sclerotic margin, focal central radiolucency and their characteristic location. Accurate identification is dependent on correlation with other studies such as plain film radiography.[39]

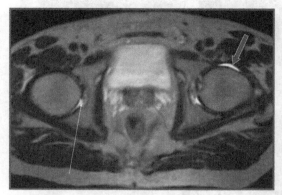

Figure 5.07 • T2/proton-weighted axial MR images of both hips at the level of the femoral head and greater trochanter. Normal synovial fluid is present as a region of increased signal intensity in the right coxofemoral joint space (thin arrow). A mild joint effusion is seen in the left coxofemoral joint space (block arrow). No definitive measurement is accepted to determine the presence of effusion; however, it is generally accepted that only minimal fluid – a barely visible thin film of increased signal – should be seen in the joint space between the femur and acetabulum.

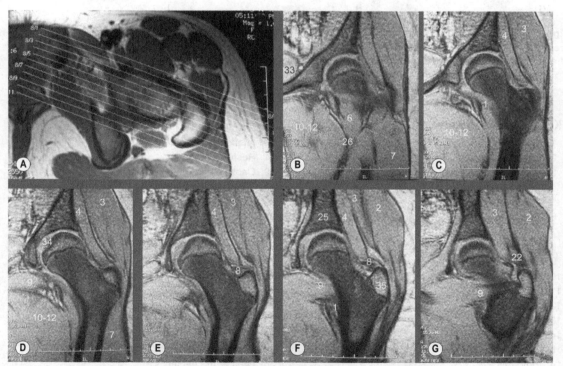

Figure 5.08 • MR imaging demonstrating coronal gradient echo images of the left hip of a 13-year-old girl (A–G). The images are displayed following the scout view (A), from anterior (B) to posterior (G) to depict various normal anatomical structures. Note the degree of detail attained on these images, including the individual muscle groups. The key to the images is detailed in Box 5.01.

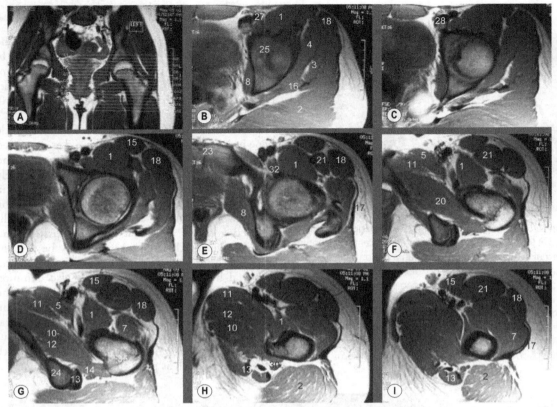

Figure 5.09 • MR imaging demonstrating axial proton density images of the hips of a 13-year-old girl (A–I). The images are displayed from superior (A) to inferior (I) from the supra-acetabular ridge to the diaphysis of the femur. A variety of anatomical structures are depicted on the views. The key to the images is detailed in Box 5.01.

Box 5.01

Key to selected figures

1. Iliopsoas
2. Gluteus maximus
3. Gluteus medius
4. Gluteus minimus
5. Pectineus
6. Vastus intermedialis
7. Vastus lateralis
8. Obturator internus
9. Obturator externus
10. Adductor magnus
11. Adductor longus
12. Adductor brevis
13. Hamstring
14. Quadratus femoris
15. Sartorius
16. Piriformis
17. Iliotibial band
18. Tensor fascia lata
19. Superior gemellus
20. Inferior gemellus
21. Rectus femoris
22. Capsule and transverse ligament
23. Pubic bone
24. Ischium
25. Acetabulum
26. Deep femoral artery
27. Femoral artery
28. Femoral vein
29. Femoral nerve
30. Sciatic nerve
31. Obturator nerve
32. Iliopsoas bursa
33. Bladder
34. Ligamentum teres
35. Greater trochanter
36. Lesser trochanter
37. Greater saphenous vein

Figure 5.10 • MR imaging of the pelvis performed in the coronal plane illustrating the differences in bone marrow patterns between patients of different ages. In (A), T2-weighted imaging with fat suppression of a 56-year-old man demonstrates a predominantly low signal intensity throughout the femoral heads, which is slightly more heterogeneous in the proximal femurs. In (B), T2-weighted imaging with fat suppression in a 13-year-old demonstrates the relatively higher signal intensity throughout the bony pelvis and proximal femoral shafts. In (C), a T1-weighted spin echo image in a 25-year-old woman shows a slightly heterogeneous signal intensity about the proximal femurs. In a younger patient of 13 years old (D), a T1-weighted image demonstrates the overall lower signal intensity seen in the pelvis and proximal femurs except at the level of the epiphyses.

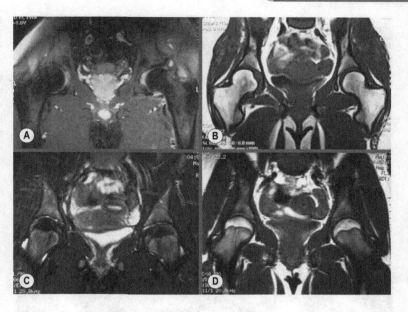

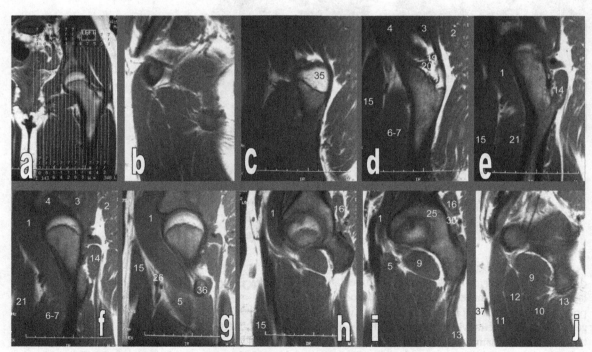

Figure 5.11 • Sagittal, fast spin echo T1-weighted MR images of a 13-year-old girl (A–J). The images are displayed from lateral (A) to medial (J), beginning at the outer aspect of the greater trochanter and continuing medially to the ilium. In this young patient, the femoral head exhibits high signal intensity on the T1-weighted image since it contains yellow marrow and the intertrochanteric or metaphyseal region is of a lower signal intensity since it contains haematopoietic marrow. The key to the images is detailed in Box 5.01.

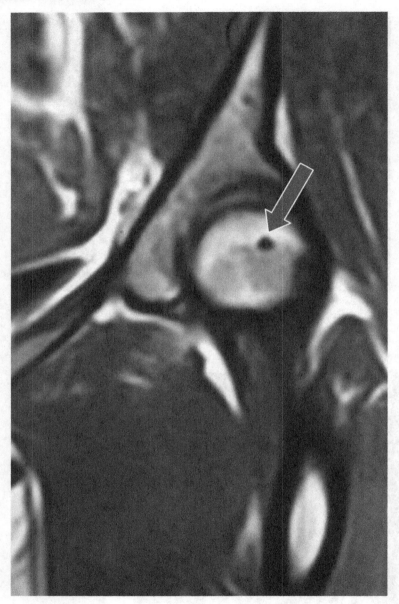

Figure 5.12 • MR imaging: coronal, T1-weighted sequence with a slice taken through the femoral head and acetabulum demonstrating a focal round region of decreased signal intensity at the junction of the femoral head and neck. On T2-weighted imaging this region will normally appear as a region of low signal intensity. This is a small bone island (arrow), a normal variation.

Multiple acetabular labral shapes have been described; however, 66%–80% of normal acetabular labra are triangular other than in the posterosuperior portion, which is typically flat, a finding which is generalized in 9% of individuals. A round labrum appears to be a normal variant and is seen in 11%–13% of individuals, whilst up to 7% have irregular labra. The structure is absent in up to 14% of individuals. No correlation between labral shape and injury or degeneration has been established. The labrum will demonstrate low signal intensity on most MR imaging sequences.[40–43]

Pathological findings

Avascular necrosis

One of the major indications for MR imaging of the pelvis and hip is to investigate the possibility of avascular necrosis (AVN) of the femoral head. MR imaging is very sensitive in the early detection of this condition.[24,25,27]

The risk factors for AVN are multiple and include trauma, corticosteroids (endogenous or exogenous), haemoglobinopathies, alcoholism, pancreatitis, Gaucher's disease, radiation treatment and dysbaric injury. The clinical presentation also varies greatly; however, when suspected, careful examination of *both* hips should be performed since bilateral presentation may be seen in up to 40% of patients (Figure 5.13).[44-46]

Avascular necrosis can be classified using clinical, radiographic or MR criteria (Table 5.03). The changes seen in stage 1, which is almost invariably latent on plain films, represent the hypovascular area surrounding the necrosis. The shape of the femoral head and integrity of the joint space remain intact until stage 3. Although, at this stage, plain films are sufficient to detect AVN,

the degree of bone marrow oedema demonstrated on MR images correlates quite strongly to the levels of reported pain.[47-49] Even though specific measurements are not available, it is important to realize that the normal amount of fluid in the capsule is generally not sufficient to generate signal changes on T2-weighted images, making any high signal intensity area in the joint clinically suspicious.[25,29,50]

Trauma

Dislocations of the hip joint usually only occur following severe trauma and are associated with lesions of the femoral head, labrum and acetabulum. Bone bruises on either the femoral head/neck or acetabulum

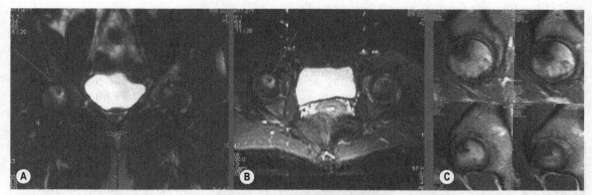

Figure 5.13 • MR imaging of both hips performed in the coronal plane using a short tau inversion recovery (STIR) sequence, demonstrating a focal region of increased signal intensity about the right femoral head, in the subchondral bone, with a central region of decreased signal (arrow (A)). On the axial T2-weighted (B) and sagittal T1-weighted (C) sequences, a focal region of decreased signal intensity is again noted in the centre with associated collapse of the anterior portion of the femoral head, seen particularly well on the sagittal slices (arrow (C)) involving over one-third of the femoral head surface.

Table 5.03 Classification of avascular necrosis

Stage	Clinical features	X-ray features	MR features
0	Often asymptomatic	Absent	Diffuse bone marrow oedema in the femoral neck
1	Mild symptoms	Minimal or absent	Diffuse marrow oedema and concentric lines of low and high T2-weighted signal
2	Pain and stiffness	Mixed osteopenia and sclerosis with cystic changes	Increasing bone marrow oedema with cyst formation
3	Hip stiffness, groin and knee pain	Crescent sign and articular collapse	Crescent sign and articular collapse
4	Hip stiffness, groin and knee pain, antalgic gait	Joint space changes	Joint space changes and effusion

may be visualized as areas of decreased T1-weighted and increased T2-weighted signal zones adjacent to the area of impact (Figures 5.14, 5.15).[24,25,27]

Injuries to the fibrocartilaginous labrum may occur with dislocations or be associated with degenerative processes. They can be difficult to identify on non-contrasted sequences or to differentiate from benign individual variation. Tears may appear as irregularities in the surface as well as focal increases in signal intensities; they may also be associated with cysts. Clicking, snapping, decreased ranges of motion and deep hip pain, aggravated by hip rotation and flexion, are the most common clinical symptoms (Figure 5.16).[51–53]

MR imaging has largely replaced bone scintigraphy as the most effective tool for detecting stress or insufficiency injuries; it can detect changes 24 to 48 hours prior to any other type of imaging modality.[25,54] Insufficiency fractures from biomechanical stresses on weakened bone are common and often radiographically occult. A painful hip in a patient at risk for osteoporosis should always raise clinical suspicion of fracture, even if the patient remains weight-bearing and has no significant history of trauma. In these cases, a limited MR examination may be requested. Coronal and axial T1-weighted and T2-weighted fat-suppressed images of the entire pelvis may show the fracture site as a linear low signal area with surrounding bone marrow oedema. Careful evaluation of the entire pelvis is essential to eliminate concurrent sacral or ischiopubic fractures (Figures 5.17, 5.18).[24,25,27,54–56]

Stress fractures from increased or abnormal stress on normal bone may also be assessed with MR imaging before findings are visible on radiographs. A linear, hypointense zone will be surrounded by a hyperintense bone marrow oedema on T2-weighted images as a response to the stress. Bone marrow oedema and articular irregularities along the pubic symphysis may indicate increased stress in this region; this condition is seen in athletes. It is often referred to as osteitis pubis and will present clinically as groin pain (Figure 5.19).[25,57,58]

Synovial herniation pits

Pit herniation defects (also known as *synovial herniation pits* or *Pitt's pits*) represent a well-rounded abnormality in the cortex of the femoral neck in the upper, outer quadrant and are filled with fibrous and cartilaginous elements. On plain film, their

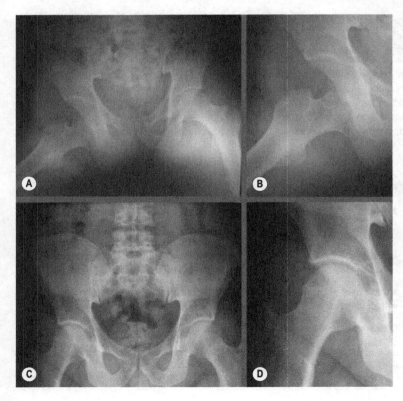

Figure 5.14 • Plain film hip radiographs of a gentleman who sustained a rally car accident involving several rolls of the car. The initial imaging demonstrates dislocation of the right hip (A and B). The patient was recommended to remain immobile for 2 months before resuming normal activities having had the articulation relocated; however, he was still limited by hip pain which was worsening. Follow-up imaging was performed (C and D), which demonstrated an irregularity and deformity about the lateral aspect of the femoral head as well as joint effusion (note the displaced gluteus medius fascial plane). Owing to the previous trauma and the imaging and examination findings, MR imaging was ordered (Figure 5.15). (This case is reproduced courtesy of Vincent Klingelschmitt DC, France.)

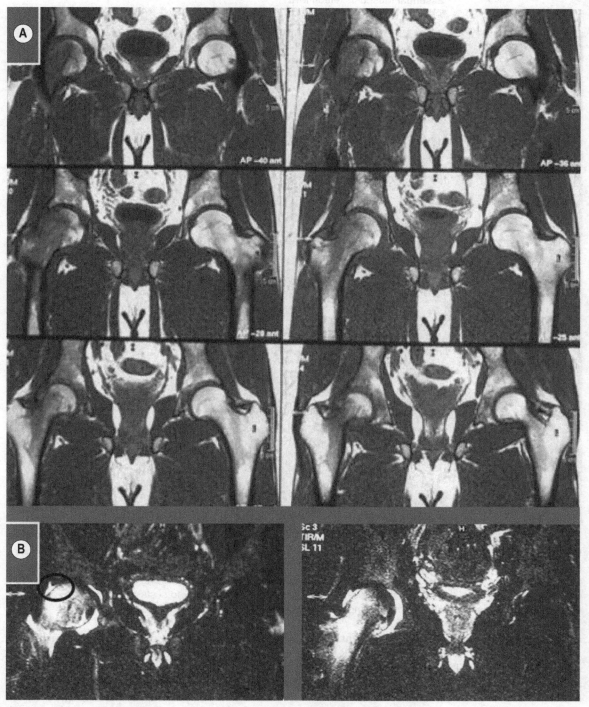

Figure 5.15 • MR imaging of both hips, using coronal T1-weighted (A) and STIR (B) sequences. The T1-weighted sequences demonstrate the large region of decreased signal intensity about the right hip, extending throughout the femoral head to the femoral neck (A). In (B), a large region of increased signal intensity is noted about the right hip extending from the head to the proximal femoral shaft, corresponding to the decreased signal intensity noted on the T1-weighted images and which represents bone marrow oedema which is likely post-traumatic in origin associated with the osteochondral lesion and avascular necrosis of the femoral head. In addition, a large joint effusion is noted about the right hip as well as deformation of the acetabular labrum superolaterally (oval).

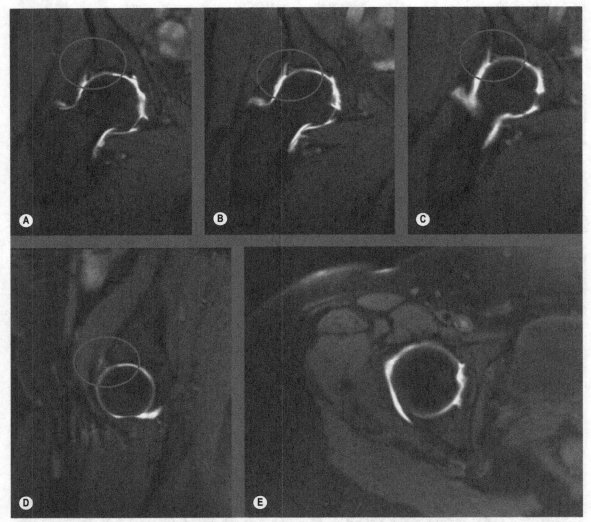

Figure 5.16 • Multiplanar MR imaging of the right hip: a STIR sequence demonstrating the coronal slices (A–C), a sagittal slice (D) and one slice in the axial plane (E). In (A)–(D), the anterosuperolateral labrum, which normally demonstrates a low signal and has a triangular appearance, has a thin high signal intensity line traversing it with a slight deformation of the triangular shape of the labrum; this indicates a small tear, a common injury to sustain during sports activities and which can produce significant clinical symptoms for the patient.

appearance will be of a small, radiolucent lesion with a well-defined sclerotic rim; on MR imaging, a low focus on T1-weighted and high focal signal intensity on T2-weighted images will be seen.[24,25,27,59]

These lesions were thought to be clinically silent and stable; however, there are now multiple reports of expanding, painful lesions and, indeed, synovial herniation pits are now known to be associated with **femoroacetabular impingement syndrome** (Figure 5.20). Clinically, this entity may mimic a labral injury: clicking and pain during normal range of motion, and may predispose to early degenerative changes.[60] Femoroacetabular impingement can be seen in patients with a history of acetabular deformity: developmental dysplasia (Figure 5.21); femoral defects, such as AVN; and slipped capital femoral epiphysis, or in patients with activities involving repetitive hip flexion, rotation and abduction.[61–65] Accessory ossicles such as os acetabulae are also known associated imaging findings (Figure 5.22).[66]

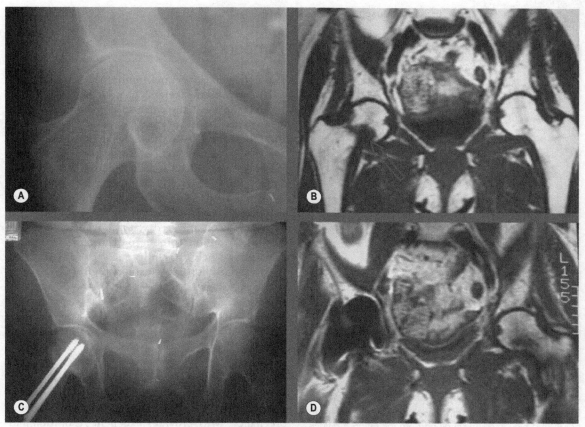

Figure 5.17 • Plain film anteroposterior (AP) spot view of the right hip (**A**) showing an apparent increase in the trabecular pattern in the medial femoral neck and discontinuity of the trabeculae about this region in a patient with general osteopenia, likely due to osteoporosis. On T1-weighted MR imaging, the coronal sequence (**B**) shows a large region of decreased signal intensity in the right femoral neck corresponding to a fracture (arrow). In the follow-up, postsurgical views, the AP radiograph (**C**) demonstrates the presence of two surgical pins fixing the femoral neck fracture. The same MR protocol as previously (**D**) is included to demonstrate that, despite newer surgical materials designed to be compatible with MR units, a large amount of artifact may still be created resulting in a region which is very low signal intensity due to the presence of the surgical pins. This can provide difficulty in the interpretation of such an image, but by manipulating the images, it is possible to evaluate for lesions, such as those affecting the labrum.

Figure 5.18 • MR imaging using a coronal oblique STIR sequence of the sacrum demonstrating the presence of increased signal intensity about the left sacral ala with a region of irregular low signal intensity within (arrow). This represents an insufficiency fracture in a patient with previously diagnosed osteoporosis (detected using DEXA scanning).

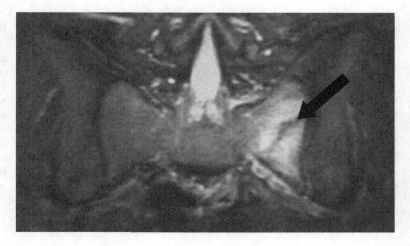

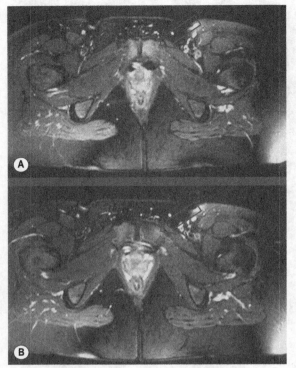

Figure 5.19 • MR imaging, T2-weighted sequences of the pelvis and hips in the axial plane demonstrating a diffuse region of bilaterally increased signal intensity about the pubic symphysis (arrows (A) and (B)). This corresponds to bone marrow oedema in the pubic bone bilaterally due to chronic osteitis, which may be caused by repetitive microtrauma such as sustained in sports injuries, especially in soccer players, or, in rarer cases, local bone infection.

Tumours

The pelvis and proximal femur are common locations for musculoskeletal tumours in patients of any age; these entities can also alter signal patterns. Neoplasms can present as a decreased T1-weighted and increased T2-weighted signal. This represents an inflammatory response but does not differentiate between benign or malignant; primary or secondary. It is generally accepted that the greater value of MR imaging is in the staging of tumours as opposed to their diagnosis, which often can be better accomplished with conventional radiographs. Common tumour or tumour-like conditions in the pelvis include many conditions such as metastatic disease, osteochondroma, fibrous dysplasia, Paget's disease and osteoid osteoma (Figure 5.23).[24,25,27]

Obstetrics

In recent years, applications for obstetrical imaging have been developed. Although ultrasonography remains the imaging modality of choice during pregnancy, MRI provides excellent resolution and tissue contrast for evaluation of both mother and fetus without the use of ionizing radiation (Figure 5.24). The first trimester remains a relative contraindication for MR imaging owing to the lack of information regarding the long-term effects.[67,68]

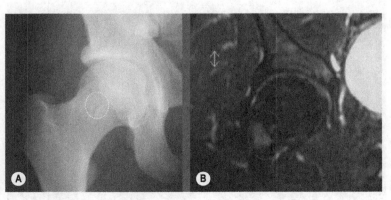

Figure 5.20 • A focal region of decreased density is noted on the anteroposterior (AP) spot radiograph of the right hip (A) corresponding to a synovial herniation pit (Pitt's pit). On the corresponding coronal plane STIR sequence of the right hip (B), a focal region of increased signal intensity is noted; this represents bone marrow oedema in the vicinity of the synovial herniation pit which may be symptomatic.

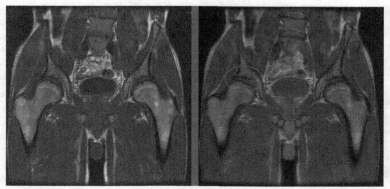

Figure 5.21 • MR imaging of both hips, performed in the coronal plane using T1-weighting. In this patient with bilateral developmental dysplasia of the hips, the sequences were used to study the shape of the hip joint as well as determine associated pathologies such as labral tears, commonly located in the anterosuperior aspect of the labrum. Note the unusual form of the femoral heads bilaterally and the lack of coverage of the femoral heads by the corresponding acetabulum. There is also irregularity noted about the acetabula, particularly on the right (white oval). In addition, there is a list of the lumbar spine to the left, although this may have been due to a positioning error.

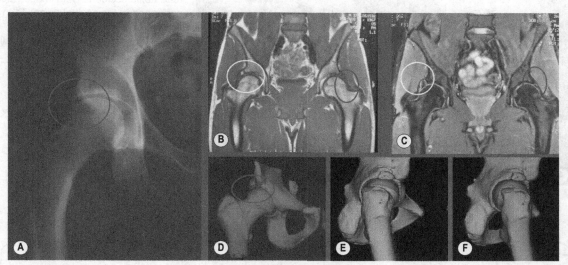

Figure 5.22 • This 37-year-old male presented with a long-standing history of progressive hip pain, worse on the right. On the anteroposterior (AP) radiograph of the right hip (A), an os acetabulum is present with slight remodelling of the lateral femoral neck/head junction (oval), findings associated with femoroacetabular impingement syndrome (FAIS). MR imaging of the hips in FAIS is performed to determine the presence of associated pathologies such as labral tears. Coronal images were performed through both hips, using T1-weighted (B) and T2-weighted (C) sequences. The os acetabulum can be noted in both images (black circles), as well as the alteration in the appearance of the femoral head/neck, noted bilaterally but greater on the right. In addition, an acetabular tear is noted outlined in the white oval on the left side. Three-dimensional CT reconstructions (D–F) were performed to appreciate more fully the change in the junction of the femoral neck and head; this study is normally reserved for those preparing for surgical intervention. The os acetabulum is well defined, as is the unusual shape of the junction (black oval (D)).

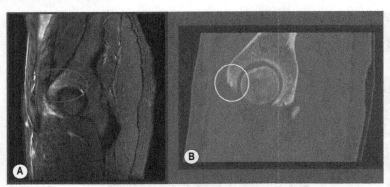

Figure 5.23 • MR imaging, T2-weighted sagittal sequence (A) demonstrating a region of increased signal intensity in the anterior acetabulum, bone marrow oedema (white oval). The corresponding CT sagittal reconstruction image performed, bone window (B), demonstrates a focal region of increased density surrounded by a very small region of radiolucency or nidus (white circle) which is further surrounded by a region of less well defined increase in density that represents reactive sclerosis, the region on the MR image (A) which is affected by the bone marrow oedema.

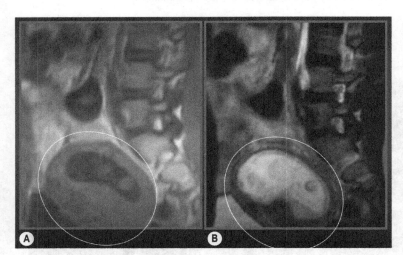

Figure 5.24 • MR imaging of the lumbar spine in a 23-year-old female patient, with low back pain following a road traffic accident. Both images are performed in the sagittal plane, T1 in figure A and T2 in figure B. In both images, it is noted that the uterus (oval) is enlarged and that there is a small focus of altered signal, in figure A intermediate and in B decreased signal intensity. This represents a foetus in a patient who did not know that they were pregnant at the time of the imaging study.

Clinical pearls

- Avascular necrosis of the hip is a relatively common disease process with multiple associated risk factors. It may present as deep joint pain or even pain referred to the knee.
- Avascular necrosis is bilateral in approximately 40% of cases.

- Acute onset of hip pain in a patient at risk for osteoporosis should prompt rapid and thorough evaluation to exclude femoral neck fractures.
- Groin pain is one of the most difficult presentations to evaluate and treat. In athletes, osteitis pubis or other stress reactions should be considered as a possible diagnosis.

References

1. Bates B. The musculoskeletal system. In: Bates B, ed. *A Guide to Physical Examination*. 3rd ed. Philadelphia: JB Lippincott; 1983: 324–370.

2. Bates B, Hoekelman R. Interviewing and the health history. In: Bates B, ed. *A Guide to Physical Examination*. 3rd ed. Philadelphia: JB Lippincott; 1983:1–27.

3. Tibor LM, Sekiya JK. Differential diagnosis of pain around the hip joint. *Arthroscopy*. 2008;24(12): 1407–1421.

4. Blankenbaker DG, Tuite MJ. Iliopsoas musculotendinous unit. *Semin Musculoskelet Radiol*. 2008;12(1):13–27.

5. Beers M, Berkow R. Temporomandibular disorders. In: *The Merck Manual*. 17th ed. West Point, PA: Merck & Co; 1999: 772–776.

6. Valdes AM, Spector TD. The contribution of genes to osteoarthritis. *Med Clin North Am*. 2009;93(1):45–66, x.

7. Malagon V. Development of hip dysplasia in hereditary multiple exostosis. *J Pediatr Orthop*. 2001;21(2):205–211.

8. Pailthorpe CA, Benson MK. Hip dysplasia in hereditary motor and sensory neuropathies. *J Bone Joint Surg Br*. 1992;74(4):538–540.

9. Mau H. Familial hip dysplasia with short acetabular roofs. *Z Orthop Ihre Grenzgeb*. 1988;126(2):156–160.

10. Andersen RE, Crespo CJ, Bartlett SJ, et al. Relationship between body weight gain and significant knee, hip, and back pain in older Americans. *Obes Res*. 2003;11(10):1159–1162.

11. Martin RL, Irrgang JJ, Sekiya JK. The diagnostic accuracy of a clinical examination in determining intra-articular hip pain for potential hip arthroscopy candidates. *Arthroscopy*. 2008;24(9):1013–1018.

12. Martin RL, Sekiya JK. The interrater reliability of 4 clinical tests used to assess individuals with musculoskeletal hip pain. *J Orthop Sports Phys Ther*. 2008;38(2):71–77.

13. Dreyfuss P, Dreyer SJ, Cole A, Mayo K. Sacroiliac joint pain. *J Am Acad Orthop Surg*. 2004;12(4): 255–265.

14. Weksler N, Velan GJ, Semionov M, et al. The role of sacroiliac joint dysfunction in the genesis of low back pain: the obvious is not always right. *Arch Orthop Trauma Surg*. 2007;127(10):885–888.

15. Travell J, Simons D. *Myofascial Pain and Dysfunction*. Baltimore: Williams and Wilkins; 1992.

16. Paydar D, Thiel H, Gemmell H. Intra and interexaminer reliability of certain palpatory procedures and the sitting flexion test for sacroiliac joint mobility and dysfunction. *J Neuromusc Sys*. 1994; 2(2):65–69.

17. Laslett M, Aprill CN, McDonald B, Young SB. Diagnosis of sacroiliac joint pain: validity of individual provocation tests and composites of tests. *Man Ther*. 2005;10(3): 207–218.

18. Laslett M, Williams M. The reliability of selected pain provocation tests for sacroiliac joint pathology. *Spine*. 1994;19(11): 1243–1249.

19. Kokmeyer DJ, Van der Wurff P, Aufdemkampe G, Fickenscher TC. The reliability of multitest regimens with sacroiliac pain provocation tests. *J Manipulative Physiol Ther*. 2002;25(1):42–48.

20. Young MF. The physics of anatomy. In: *Essential Physics for Musculoskeletal Medicine*. Edinburgh: Elsevier; 2009.

21. Ferri FF. *Ferri's Differential Diagnosis*. Philadelphia: Mosby; 2005.

22. Eustace S, Johnston C, O'Neill P, O'Byrne J. *Sports Injuries: Examination, Imaging and Management*. Edinburgh: Churchill Livingstone; 2007.

23. Beers M, Berkow R. *The Merck Manual*. 17th ed. West Point, PA: Merck & Co; 1999.

24. Stoller D. *Magnetic Resonance Imaging in Orthopaedics and Sports Medicine*. 2nd ed. Philadelphia: Lippincott Williams and Wilkins; 1996.

25. Berquist T. *MRI of the Musculoskeletal System*. 4th ed. Philadelphia: Lippincott Williams and Wilkins; 2000.

26. Mirowitz S. *Pitfalls, Variants And Artifacts in Body MR Imaging*. St Louis: Mosby; 1996.

27. Kaplan P, Helms C, Dussault R, Anderson M. *Musculoskeletal MRI*. Philadelphia: WB Saunders; 2001.

28. Dawson KL, Moore SG, Rowland JM. Age-related marrow changes in the pelvis: MR and anatomic findings. *Radiology*. 1992;183(1):47–51.

29. Stoller DW, Tirman PF, Bredella MA. *Diagnostic Imaging Orthopaedics*. Salt Lake City: Amirsys Inc; 2003.

30. Docherty P, Mitchell MJ, MacMillan L, et al. Magnetic resonance imaging in the detection of sacroiliitis. *J Rheumatol*. 1992; 19(3):393–401.

31. Hodler J, Yu JS, Goodwin D, et al. MR arthrography of the hip: improved imaging of the acetabular labrum with histologic correlation in cadavers. *Am J Roentgenol*. 1995; 165(4):887–891.

32. Braun J, Golder W, Bollow M, et al. Imaging and scoring in ankylosing spondylitis. *Clin Exp Rheumatol*. 2002;20 (6 suppl 28):S178–S184.

33. Standring S, ed. *Gray's Anatomy – Pelvic girdle and lower limb – pelvic girdle, gluteal region and hip joint* (Section 111). Edinburgh: Elsevier; 2009.

34. Moore K. The perineum and pelvis. In: *Clinically Oriented Anatomy*. 2nd ed. Baltimore: Williams and Wilkins; 1985:298–395.

35. Green J, Silver P. The pelvis. In: *An Introduction to Human Anatomy*. Oxford: Oxford University Press; 1981:224–253.

36. Wunderbaldinger P, Bremer C, Schellenberger E, et al. Imaging features of iliopsoas bursitis. *Eur Radiol*. 2002;12(2):409–415.

37. Levine CD, Schweitzer ME, Ehrlich SM. Pelvic marrow in adults. *Skeletal Radiol*. 1994;23(5): 343–347.

38. Greenspan A. Bone island (enostosis): current concept – a review. *Skeletal Radiol*. 1995;24(2):111–115.

39. Nokes SR, Vogler JB, Spritzer CE, et al. Herniation pits of the femoral neck: appearance at MR imaging. *Radiology*. 1989; 172(1):231–234.

40. Lecouvet FE, Vande Berg BC, Malghem J, et al. MR imaging of the acetabular labrum: variations in 200 asymptomatic hips. *Am J Roentgenol.* 1996;167(4):1025–1028.

41. Hachiya Y, Kubo T, Horii M, et al. Characteristic features of the acetabular labrum in healthy children. *J Pediatr Orthop B.* 2001; 10(3):169–172.

42. Aydingoz U, Ozturk MH. MR imaging of the acetabular labrum: a comparative study of both hips in 180 asymptomatic volunteers. *Eur Radiol.* 2001;11(4):567–574.

43. Abe I, Harada Y, Oinuma K, et al. Acetabular labrum: abnormal findings at MR imaging in asymptomatic hips. *Radiology.* 2000;216(2):576–581.

44. Watson RM, Roach NA, Dalinka MK. Avascular necrosis and bone marrow edema syndrome. *Radiol Clin North Am.* 2004;42(1):207–219.

45. Bachiller FG, Caballer AP, Portal LF. Avascular necrosis of the femoral head after femoral neck fracture. *Clin Orthop Relat Res.* 2002; (399):87–109.

46. Mirzai R, Chang C, Greenspan A, Gershwin ME. The pathogenesis of osteonecrosis and the relationships to corticosteroids. *J Asthma.* 1999;36(1):77–95.

47. Ito H, Matsuno T, Minami A. Relationship between bone marrow edema and development of symptoms in patients with osteonecrosis of the femoral head. *Am J Roentgenol.* 2006;186(6):1761–1770.

48. Mitchell DG, Rao VM, Dalinka M, et al. Hematopoietic and fatty bone marrow distribution in the normal and ischemic hip: new observations with 1.5-T MR imaging. *Radiology.* 1986;161(1):199–202.

49. Huang GS, Chan WP, Chang YC, et al. MR imaging of bone marrow edema and joint effusion in patients with osteonecrosis of the femoral head: relationship to pain. *Am J Roentgenol.* 2003;181(2):545–549.

50. Mitchell DG, Rao V, Dalinka M, et al. MRI of joint fluid in the normal and ischemic hip. *Am J Roentgenol.* 1986;146(6): 1215–1218.

51. Blankenbaker DG, Tuite MJ. The painful hip: new concepts. *Skeletal Radiol.* 2006;35(6):352–370.

52. Toomayan GA, Holman WR, Major NM, et al. Sensitivity of MR arthrography in the evaluation of acetabular labral tears. *Am J Roentgenol.* 2006; 186(2):449–453.

53. Schmid MR, Notzli HP, Zanetti M, et al. Cartilage lesions in the hip: diagnostic effectiveness of MR arthrography. *Radiology.* 2003; 226(2):382–386.

54. Lubovsky O, Liebergall M, Mattan Y, et al. Early diagnosis of occult hip fractures MRI versus CT scan. *Injury.* 2005;36(6): 788–792.

55. Verbeeten KM, Hermann KL, Hasselqvist M, et al. The advantages of MRI in the detection of occult hip fractures. *Eur Radiol.* 2005;15(1): 165–169.

56. Frihagen F, Nordsletten L, Tariq R, Madsen JE. MRI diagnosis of occult hip fractures. *Acta Orthop.* 2005; 76(4):524–530.

57. Rodriguez C, Miguel A, Lima H, Heinrichs K. Osteitis pubis syndrome in the professional soccer athlete: a case report. *J Athl Train.* 2001;36(4):437–440.

58. Brennan D, O'Connell MJ, Ryan M, et al. Secondary cleft sign as a marker of injury in athletes with groin pain: MR image appearance and interpretation. *Radiology.* 2005; 235(1):162–167.

59. Rowe L, Yochum T, eds. *Essentials of Skeletal Radiology.* 2nd ed. Baltimore: Williams and Wilkins; 2004.

60. Kassarjian A, Belzile E. Femoroacetabular impingement: presentation, diagnosis, and management. *Semin Musculoskelet Radiol.* 2008;12(2):136–145.

61. Kassarjian A, Brisson M, Palmer WE. Femoroacetabular impingement. *Eur J Radiol.* 2007;63(1):29–35.

62. Murphy S, Tannast M, Kim YJ, et al. Debridement of the adult hip for femoroacetabular impingement: indications and preliminary clinical results. *Clin Orthop Relat Res.* 2004;(429): 178–181.

63. Beall DP, Sweet CF, Martin HD, et al. Imaging findings of femoroacetabular impingement syndrome. *Skeletal Radiol.* 2005; 34(11):691–701.

64. Hart ES, Metkar US, Rebello GN, Grottkau BE. Femoroacetabular impingement in adolescents and young adults. *Orthop Nurs.* 2009; 28(3):117–124; quiz 25–26.

65. Allen D, Beaule PE, Ramadan O, Doucette S. Prevalence of associated deformities and hip pain in patients with cam-type femoroacetabular impingement. *J Bone Joint Surg Br.* 2009;91(5):589–594.

66. Hergan K, Oser W, Moriggl B. Acetabular ossicles: normal variant or disease entity? *Eur Radiol.* 2000; 10(4):624–628.

67. Brown MA, Birchard KR, Semelka RC. Magnetic resonance evaluation of pregnant patients with acute abdominal pain. *Semin Ultrasound CT MR.* 2005; 26(4):206–211.

68. Thompson SK, Goldman SM, Shah KB, et al. Acute non-traumatic maternal illnesses in pregnancy: imaging approaches. *Emerg Radiol.* 2005;11(4):199–212.

6

The knee

Martin Young Michelle A. Wessely Julie-Marthe Grenier
Nicholas Green

Introduction

Before magnetic resonance (MR) imaging became readily available in the 1990s, comprehensive imaging of the frequently injured internal structures of the knee joint was primarily accomplished with arthroscopy. In comparison to MR imaging, this procedure is both invasive and expensive and, in modern clinical practice, arthroscopies are no longer routinely performed; they do, however, still have a role in clarifying inconclusive findings and, of course, for therapeutic benefits. Magnetic resonance is now considered the gold standard for intra-articular imaging of the knee[1,2]; indeed, the knee is the joint most commonly imaged using this modality, partly because the joint is particularly vulnerable to both acute and chronic injury and partly because of the accuracy and detail afforded to both the surgeon and the physician.[3,4]

Since the first successful nuclear resonance experiment on biological tissue in 1946,[5] there have been tremendous improvements in equipment, computer software, protocols and clinical interpretation. These advances have helped to improve image quality and diagnostic accuracy (including the appearance of normal variants) and reduce the effects of imaging artifacts.

History and examination

Perhaps more than any other joint, the knee has an embarrassment of recognized orthopaedic tests, usually eponymous and often of unproven sensitivity and reliability[6,7]; however, a standard examination routine need contain no more than a handful of such tests if the history and examination are properly structured.

As with any conscious and articulate patient, obtaining a full and competent history should form the backbone of the clinician's diagnostic work-up. There are several factors that are of particular importance in the knee; these are detailed in Box 6.01 and should be capable of guiding the physician to the most likely involved structures, informing their differential diagnosis and guiding their physical examination.[8,9]

This should commence not with the knee itself but with general observation of the patient and their height, weight and somatotype, with calculation of the body mass index (BMI) if necessary; more than in any other joint, the incidence of degenerative change in the knee is linked to obesity.[10–14] Evaluation of gait can give a good indication of the severity of the injury and the degree of disability, and assessment of stance can direct the clinician to asymmetries of alignment; genu varum or genu valgum; and tibial torsion.[9] Pes planus, which can significantly increase valgus knee stress, can also be readily identified at this stage. This observation can be extended to the local area about the knee, wherein any discoloration, swelling, atrophy or displacement should be noted and investigated further.[15]

This should be augmented by palpation, which should assess any areas of abnormal temperature and the quality of any swelling as well as attempting to elicit specific site tenderness and identify trigger points; in particular, the hypertonic popliteus muscle is a commonly overlooked cause of pain and perpetuation of knee pathomechanics.[16] The femoral, popliteal and dorsalis pedis pulses should all be checked and compared. Many conditions, such as vascular disease, bursitis, tendonitis, ligamentous sprain, patellar

DOI: 10.1016/B978-0-443-06726-6.00006-8

Important historical considerations in the knee

The injury

- Precise mechanism of injury
- Onset and progression of symptoms
- Location and type of pain
- Aggravating and relieving factors

Background

- Previous injuries to the lower extremity, pelvis and low back
- Surgical history
- Sporting activities
- Employment history
- History of obesity
- Familial history

subluxation, Baker's cyst, neuroma and some osteo-chondral defects, can be identified, if not positively confirmed, by history, observation and expert palpation, and local joint line tenderness has been shown to be a sensitive and reliable test for determining a meniscal lesion.[17]

In the younger patient, where symptoms allow, there is a range of functional tests that can be performed; these are particularly useful in assessment of the high-performance athlete with persistent yet subtle lesions and of knee laxity or instability[9] and are detailed in Table 6.01. In the less able patient, active and passive ranges of motion will suffice: flexion, extension plus valgus and varus stress, which can best assess collateral ligament injury; these should be compared to the unaffected side. Movement of the knee may also elicit clicking, popping

Table 6.01 Functional knee tests

Test	Ask the patient to...
Stationary jog	Jog gently on the spot
Fast jog	Increase the tempo and increase their knee lift
'Housemaid's knee'	Kneel upright
'Parson's knee'	Kneel whilst leaning backwards
'Duck waddle'	'Walk' whilst fully squatting
Hopping	Hop on the affected limb with the toe pointing inwards and then outwards

or grating, suggestive of a foreign body or meniscal tear; this can be further assessed using McMurray's test, which consists of flexing and extending the knee in neutral, then with internal and external tibial rotation whilst the thumb and fingers are placed over the joint line.

Special tests are also needed to assess the cruciate ligaments. The more commonly injured anterior cruciate ligament is evaluated using the modified Lachman's test whereby the supine patient lies with their hip and knee flexed to approximately 20° and the examiner, thumbs on the proximal tibia, draws the distal extremity anteriorly; instability is noted if the excursion is greater than on the unaffected side. The posterior drawer test is used to assess the posterior cruciate ligament and involves the same position for both patient and examiner but this time the tibia is drawn posteriorly.[9]

Although there is a plethora of special tests and measurements for assessment of the patella in the patient with patellofemoral pain syndrome, many of these are of dubious or, at best, unproven value.[18] A competent assessment of the patella consists mainly of observation of the structure both statically and dynamically. Conditions involving frank abnormalities of the patella such as luxation, patella alta, patella baja or agenesis are usually immediately obvious[19]; palpation can also readily determine bipartite patellae, the absence of pain or previous trauma will usually be sufficient to differentiate this from fracture or non-union.

Although radiographs may be required to precisely determine the *quadriceps angle* or *Q-angle* (Figure 6.01), the experienced practitioner should be able to determine when this falls outside the normal range of 10–15° for men and 15–23° for women[9,20,21]; an increased Q-angle is strongly linked to patellofemoral pain.[20]

Assessment of muscle bulk can also be a key indicator of patellar tracking syndrome. Unless bilateral MR images have been acquired, this assessment will not generally be aided by specialist imaging. Although protocols have been developed for kinematic MR imaging, enabling the patella motion to be captured during early flexion, the expense involved coupled with technical difficulties in reliably acquiring the sequences have severely restricted the application of MR imaging to patellar tracking assessment.[18,22]

The diagnosis can best be checked by the squat test; in healthy subjects the patella will rotate medially at 90° of knee flexion, whilst in patient with abnormal patellar function the rotation will be lateral.[23] During

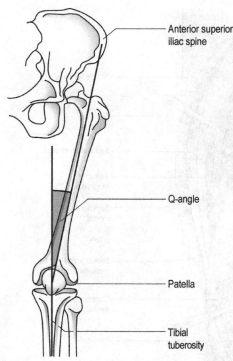

Anterior superior
iliac spine

Q-angle

Patella

Tibial
tuberosity

Figure 6.01 • The Q-angle lies between an imaginary line drawn from the anterior superior iliac spine (ASIS) through the centre of the patella and a line from the centre of the patella to the centre of the tibial tuberosity.

the squat, it is also possible to ascertain and, with practice, source any crepitus or clunking which may be associated with patellar subluxation or degeneration or with intra-articular pathology.[9,15]

Finally, any assessment of the knee articulation should include a thorough neurological assessment[24]; not only can lumbar radiculitis refer pain to the knee, it can also disrupt the functionality of the major muscle groups attaching about the joint. Local nerve damage also needs to be eliminated; the peroneal nerve is vulnerable as it passes superficially over the head of the fibula and the popliteal fossa houses the tibial, common peroneal, sural and posterior femoral cutaneous nerves as well as an articular branch from the obturator nerve (Figure 6.02).[25–27]

Differential diagnosis

Several challenges face the clinician seeking to establish and refine a differential diagnosis for the patient with knee pain. Although the history can give strong

clues from the mechanism of injury, the onset of pain can often be insidious or inconclusive: the symptoms can often be due to dysfunction elsewhere in the kinematic chain either from biomechanical consequence or by referred pain. This latter is particularly crucial when considering paediatric cases; both slipped capital femoral epiphysis and Legg–Calvé–Perthes disease can present as knee pain with no hip symptoms – and the cost of a missed diagnosis can be serious for the patient. The age of the patient should help to direct the clinical thinking.[28–30]

Knee pain can also be a symptom of systemic disease: crystal disease, or inflammatory or septic arthropathy. A list of common conditions causing knee pain is given in Table 6.02.[28,31] As well as the history, the location of the knee pain should also help to guide and clarify the clinician's thinking; a list of conditions that can be suggested by location alone is given in Box 6.02.[28]

Protocols

The biggest advantage of MR imaging is its ability to obtain high soft tissue contrast without use of ionizing radiation. Depending on the sequences used, and on the field of view, exquisite detail of the knee's articular cartilage and ligamentous structures can be obtained.

In order to requisition an MRI examination, a clinician must have a good understanding of the presenting symptoms and diagnostic differential so that the examination protocol can be tailored to the anatomy or pathology in question. For example, suspicion of meniscal pathology may require different slices and sequences compared to a suspected injury to the lateral collateral ligament. A good working diagnosis can also save imaging time by reducing the number of sequences necessary, which helps to reduce the time required to acquire the images. The relatively slow image acquisition time is one of the main disadvantages of the MRI technique, with a non-contrast knee evaluation taking up to 45 minutes.

Most imaging centres have pre-established protocols for evaluation of the knee, making the referrals easier for the clinician. When protocols are determined, factors such as magnet strength need to be considered. High-field magnets (generally more than 1.0 Tesla [T]) may perform better than intermediate- or low-field magnets (less than 0.7 T) for some sequences, especially in the case of fat

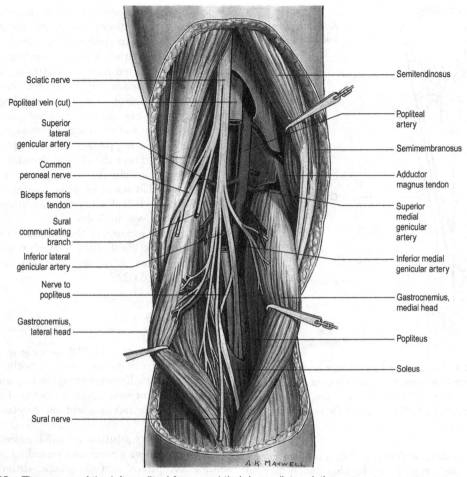

Sciatic nerve

Popliteal vein (cut)

Superior lateral genicular artery

Common peroneal nerve

Biceps femoris tendon

Sural communicating branch

Inferior lateral genicular artery

Nerve to popliteus

Gastrocnemius, lateral head

Sural nerve

Semitendinosus

Popliteal artery

Semimembranosus

Adductor magnus tendon

Superior medial genicular artery

Inferior medial genicular artery

Gastrocnemius, medial head

Popliteus

Soleus

A.K. MAXWELL

Figure 6.02 • The nerves of the left popliteal fossa and their immediate relations. Reproduced, with permission, from Gray's Anatomy for Students, Drake R, Vogl W and Mitchell A, eds (Elsevier, 2009)

suppression. Sequence names vary greatly according to the manufacturer and software type and can be confusing for the clinician. For example, a General Electric (GE) scanner will use different terminology than a Siemens or Philips model. Patient and scan information is also displayed differently on the printed images, depending on the software used.

Most imaging protocols for the knee include sagittal, axial and coronal images with the field of view ranging from 14 cm to 16 cm, depending on patient size. The slice thickness usually varies from 3 mm to 5 mm with an interstitial gap of about 0.5 mm. Gaps, or areas of non-imaged anatomy in between the slices, are used to decrease 'cross-talk' in two-dimensional imaging acquisition;[32–35] cross-

talk is the presence of unwanted signals coming from adjacent anatomy.

Normal anatomy and common variants

Numerous false positive findings have explanations in variants of anatomy or technical artifacts; a thorough understanding of normal anatomy and its appearance on MR imaging is therefore essential in order to accurately identify the abnormal.

The knee is often described as a synovial hinge joint;[27,36,37] however, this is a gross simplification from both an anatomical and biomechanical

Table 6.02 Differential diagnosis of knee pain by age

Children and adolescents	Adults	Older adults
Patellofemoral pain syndrome	Patellofemoral pain syndrome	Osteoarthritis
Osgood–Schlatter disease	Medial plica syndrome	Crystal-induced inflammatory arthropathy: gout, calcium pyrophosphate crystal deposition disease (pseudogout)
Jumper's knee (patellar tendonitis)	Pes anserine bursitis	Popliteal cyst (Baker's cyst)
Referred pain: slipped capital femoral epiphysis, Legg–Calvé–Perthes disease	Trauma	Neoplasm: metastatic cancer
Osteochondral defect	Inflammatory arthropathy: rheumatoid arthritis, Reiter's syndrome (reactive arthritis), pigmented villonodular synovitis	Trauma
Juvenile rheumatoid arthritis (Still's disease)	Tendonitis/bursitis	Synoviochondrometaplasia
Trauma	Septic arthritis	
Neoplasm: Ewing's sarcoma, osteosarcoma	Stress fracture/Stress reaction	
	Referred pain: neurogenic, hip and leg pathology	
	Neoplasm: osteochondroma, aneurysmal bone cyst	

Box 6.02

Differential diagnosis of knee pain by location
Anterior knee pain

Patellar subluxation or dislocation
Osgood–Schlatter lesion
Jumper's knee (patellar tendonitis)
Patellofemoral pain syndrome (chondromalacia patellae)

Medial knee pain

Medial collateral ligament sprain
Medial meniscal tear
Pes anserine bursitis
Medial plica syndrome

Lateral knee pain

Lateral collateral ligament sprain
Lateral meniscal tear
Iliotibial band tendonitis

Posterior knee pain

Popliteal cyst (Baker's cyst)
Posterior cruciate ligament injury

perspective; the femorotibial joint is the largest in the body and also one of the most complicated (Figure 6.03). The presence of the menisci make the joint complex and, of course, the knee consists of more than just this single joint; the proximal tibiofibular joint, a synovial plane joint, and the patellofemoral articulation make the knee, functionally, a compound joint, most correctly defined as a *bicondylar joint*.[25,38,39] Unlike a true hinge joint, the knee demonstrates limited rotation about two other orthogonal axes, it can increase its valgus and varus angles passively and is reliant on femoral rotation to obtain its highly stable close packed position.[38,39]

In general, the menisci can be evaluated using single echo proton density images. Spin echo T1-weighted images and gradient echo techniques can also be very useful. When assessing ligaments, tendons or other soft tissues, the preferred techniques will be fluid-sensitive, or T2-weighted, sequences. Hyaline cartilage and loose bodies can be best evaluated using gradient echo techniques, with or without fat suppression, and fat-suppressed spin echo sequences.[32–34]

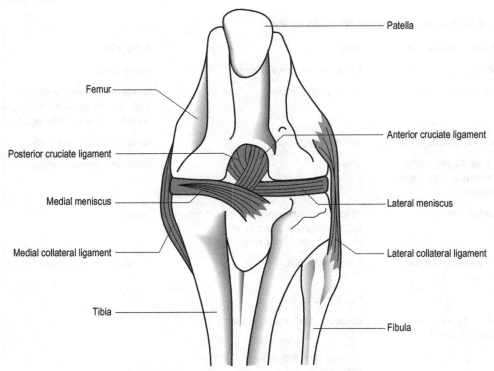

Figure 6.03 • Principal components of the left knee.

Menisci

The menisci of the knee are well visualized and commonly evaluated with MR imaging. The normal meniscus is a semicircle of cartilage and collagen fibres, thicker peripherally and thinner centrally; they display low signal intensity on all sequences (Figure 6.04).

The medial meniscus is slightly bigger and has a larger radius than its lateral counterpart. The 'horns' of the latter are usually of equal size; in the medial meniscus, the anterior horn is larger than the posterior.[3,25,27]

On the sagittal slices, each meniscus has a 'bow-tie' appearance (Figures 6.05, 6.06). Towards the midline, the menisci have the appearance of two triangles.[32–34,40] In some individuals, the morphology of the meniscus is more representative of a disc. 'Discoid' menisci are variable in appearance; many are not true discs but merely have wider-than-normal bodies.[41,42] The incidence of discoid meniscus is estimated at being between 3% and 4.5%; they are nearly always found in the lateral meniscus.[43–45] On the sagittal views, the meniscus will not demonstrate the typical 'bow-tie' appearance; the pathological

implication of this morphological variant will be discussed later in the chapter.

Intrasubstance signal may be present on the peripheral edge, representing vascularity; this finding is more prominent in younger patients and may be mistaken for a tear. The popliteus tendon adjacent to the lateral meniscus and the normal attachments of the meniscofemoral ligaments on both the medial and lateral side are other structures occasionally mimicking tears.[32–35]

A common normal variant that can mimic pathology is a 'speckled' anterior horn lateral meniscus. Present in as many as 60% of normal patients, this appearance is due to fibres of the anterior cruciate ligament inserting into the meniscus; it can present an appearance similar to that of a macerated anterior horn.[46]

Ligaments

Cruciate ligaments

The anterior and posterior cruciate ligaments are two other structures very commonly evaluated with MR imaging. Both ligaments are intra-articular but extrasynovial structures linking the femur and tibia (Figure 6.07).[25,36]

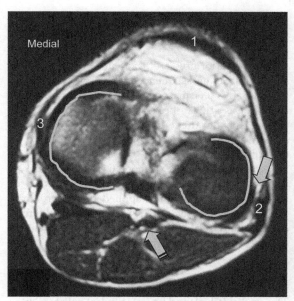

Figure 6.04 • Axial T2-weighted MR image of the right knee of a 27-year-old. The different morphology of the two menisci can be well visualized. The relationship between the menisci and the capsule/collateral ligaments is also demonstrated. The lateral meniscus is not attached to the capsule or lateral collateral ligament (LCL), as demonstrated by the area of high signal between the two structures (arrow). Other areas of interest are the quadriceps tendon (1), the LCL (2) and the medial collateral ligament (MCL) (3) and the neurovascular bundle (striped arrow).

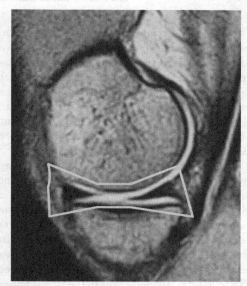

Figure 6.06 • Sagittal T1-weighted MR image of the right knee of a 27-year-old male at the level of the medial compartment demonstrates the 'bow-tie' appearance of the medial meniscus. Notice the wider configuration of the medial meniscus compared with that of the lateral meniscus noted in Figure 6.05.

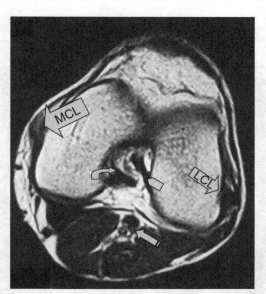

Figure 6.07 • Axial T2-weighted MR image of the right knee of a 27-year-old male. The proximal attachment of the anterior cruciate ligament (arrow head) and posterior cruciate ligament (curved arrow) are demonstrated in the intercondylar groove. The lateral collateral ligament and medial collateral ligament cannot be well visualized in this plane. Indirect evaluation is possible by the lack of adjacent effusion. The neurovascular bundle comprising the popliteal artery, vein and tibial nerve can be seen surrounded by the gastrocnemius muscle (striped arrow).

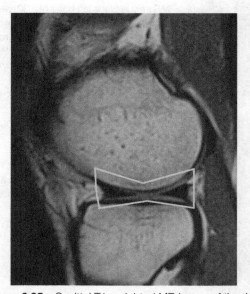

Figure 6.05 • Sagittal T1-weighted MR image of the right knee of a 27-year-old male demonstrating the normal 'bow-tie' appearance of the lateral meniscus (outlined to illustrate the two components, the anterior and posterior horns).

The anterior cruciate ligament (ACL), which is frequently injured during athletic activities, is a very important structure providing stability to the knee and preventing anterior translation of the tibia. It also prevents excessive internal rotation and hyperextension. The ACL attaches at the posterior aspect of the lateral femoral condyles and on the medial anterior aspect of the tibial plateau. It does not, contrary to popular belief, insert on the tibial spines.[25,27] The ACL is best visualized on sagittal images (Figures 6.08, 6.09). On some scans, the small anteromedial and larger posterolateral fibre bundles can be differentiated, especially if the patient's lower extremity is placed with approximately 5° of external rotation in order to align the fibres with the plane of the scan; this can give the structure a striated appearance.[3] On the coronal slices, the ACL appears as a flattened structure adjacent to the lateral femoral condyles. There can often be some high signal within the ligament, most particularly near its insertion on the tibia.[2]

In approximately 1% of cases, the ligament can contain a cyst; whilst normally clinically insignificant – if sufficiently large, it can occasionally cause a feeling of stiffness – this can mimic the appearance of a tumour.[47–49]

The posterior cruciate ligament (PCL) is seen in all MRI planes and sequences as a band of low signal intensity. It is seen in its entirety on the sagittal slices, appearing as a thick fibrous band originating from the medial aspect of the femoral condyle. From the condyle, it extends inferiorly to the posterior aspect of the tibial plateau, taking the appearance of an 'inverted hockey stick' (Figure 6.10A).[50] Injury to the PCL, which classically occurs as a result of an anterior-to-posterior force applied to the proximal tibia, such as may occur with contact of the femur against the dashboard in an automobile accident, is relatively rare in comparison to ACL injuries.[32–34]

Collateral ligaments

The medial (tibial) and lateral (fibular) collateral ligaments are slightly more difficult to evaluate than the cruciate ligaments. The medial collateral ligament (MCL) is a flat band running from the epicondyles of the femur and attaching into the medial tibia. The MCL fibres are continuous with the joint capsule

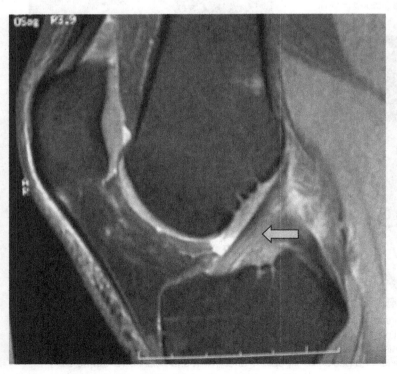

Figure 6.08 • Sagittal T2-weighted MR image of the left knee of a 30-year-old male. The course of the anterior cruciate ligament can be traced from the tibial to femoral surfaces; the fibre bundles can be appreciated (arrow). This ligament consists of multiple collagen fascicles, with two prominent bundles, posterolateral and anteromedial. Specific MR imaging protocols can be performed to visualize the anterior cruciate ligament, which can at times be difficult to image due to its oblique course related to the position of the patient's knee.

Figure 6.09 • Sagittal T1-weighted MR image of the right knee demonstrating the anterior cruciate ligament (arrow head) and distal portion of the posterior cruciate ligament (curved arrow). The fibre bundles of the anterior cruciate ligament are not easily distinguishable in this patient. Other structures of interest are the quadriceps tendon (1a), infrapatellar tendon (ligament) (1b), and the posterior femorotibial articular capsule (2).

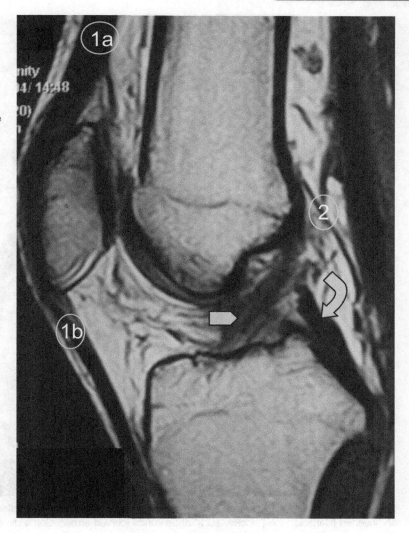

in its entirety; they also insert into the medial meniscus.[25,51] The MCL is, however, extrasynovial; it prevents valgus angulation.[9,27] Isolated injuries to this ligament are rare because of the close contact with the other medial structures.[25,32–35] This ligament is best visualized on coronal slices, appearing as an area of dark signal typical of most ligaments and tendons.

The lateral or fibular collateral ligament (LCL) is a round, cord-like structure joining the distal femur to the fibular head conjointly with the biceps femoris; it is also intimately related to the iliotibial band. Unlike the medial ligament, the LCL is not in contact with the meniscal surface; these structures are separated by the popliteus tendon. The LCL is only continuous with the articular capsule along the femur.[25,51] The

LCL resists varus angulation and some internal rotation.[9,25] Injuries to the LCL are associated with trauma to other posterolateral structures such as the capsule and cruciate ligaments.[32–34]

Other ligaments

One of the commonest normal variants of the knee is the presence of a **transverse (geniculate) ligament**, which runs between the anterior horns of medial and lateral menisci, within **Hoffa's fat pad** (Figure 6.10C,D). Its purpose remains unknown; however, it is present in 58% of knees and, importantly, can frequently mimic a tear at the point of its insertion on the anterior horn of the lateral meniscus.[52–54]

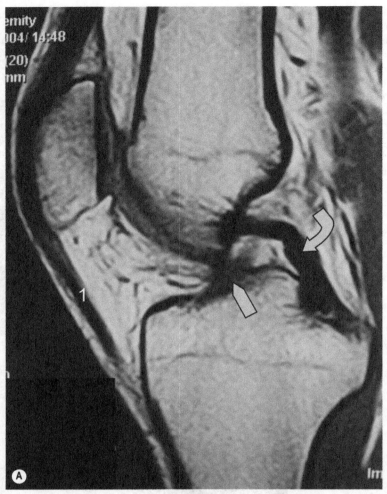

Figure 6.10 • (A) Sagittal T1-weighted MR image of the right knee. The posterior cruciate ligament demonstrates an 'inverted (Canadian ice-) hockey stick' appearance (curved arrow). Some distal fibres of the anterior cruciate ligament can also be seen near the tibial attachment (arrow head). The normal appearance of the infrapatellar tendon/ligament (1) is well visualized in the proximal portion.

Continued

There are two other common meniscal ligamentous variants that can mimic tears: the **ligament of Humphrey**, the anterior branch of the meniscofemoral ligament, is present in 37% of patients; the posterior **meniscofemoral ligament** (the ligament of Wrisberg) in 84%.[55,56] The meniscofemoral ligament runs from the medial femoral condyle via the intracondylar notch to the posterior horn of the lateral meniscus, where is can give rise to the appearance of a (pseudo)tear. The ligament of Humphrey passes anteriorly to the posterior cruciate ligament; the ligament of Wrisberg, posteriorly.[3,25]

Bursae

Other important soft tissue structures identified on MR imaging are bursae, of which there is a wealth about the knee. These are detailed in Table 6.03;[32–34] inflammation of these structures (bursitis) can mimic other intra-articular pathologies. Clinical data as well as a good knowledge of the location and morphology of the bursae are again very useful in establishing an accurate diagnosis and evaluating comorbidities. The **popliteal bursa**, located between the medial head of the gastrocnemius and the

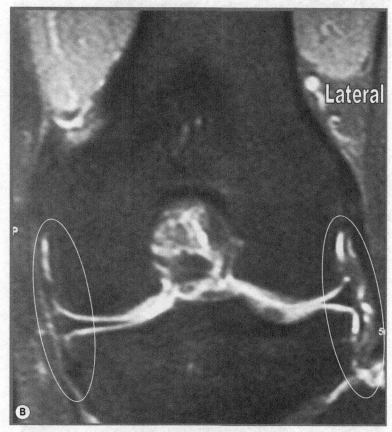

Figure. 6-10—cont'd • (B) MR imaging of the right knee, coronal T2-weighted fat-saturated image, where the medial and lateral collateral ligaments are visible, the fibres of which extend proximally and distally from the respective menisci (ovals).

Continued

semimembranosus muscle, is usually the most vulnerable to injury and may be seen even when asymptomatic as an area of increased T2-weighted signal in the posterior aspect of the knee.[3,25] As fluid accumulation increases, secondary problems such as compartment syndromes may arise. The other bursae are not easily visualized unless inflammation is present, when they become prominent on the fluid-sensitive sequences.

Synovial plicae

Another frequently seen variant is the presence of a thin, fibrous band running between the facet of the patella and medial joint capsule. Most easily noted on the axial sequences, this represents an embryological remnant, the **medial patella plica**. Although superior and inferior plicae can also be found, it is the medial plica, an inward fold of the synovial lining, that is most commonly noted; one or more plicae can be found in over half of all knees.[57,58]

The plicae are only clinically significant if they become thickened or stiffen; in *medial patella plica syndrome*, the structure can become entrapped between the femur and patella, causing pain, clicking and locking. There is no definitive measurement for a thickened plica; the diagnosis is a matter of correlation with clinical presentation and radiological judgment.[3,57]

Pathology

Internal derangements of the knee are common in a wide group of the population. Injuries range from those related to sports activities to consequences of degeneration. In addition to providing superb soft tissue detail, MR is also a useful tool for gathering

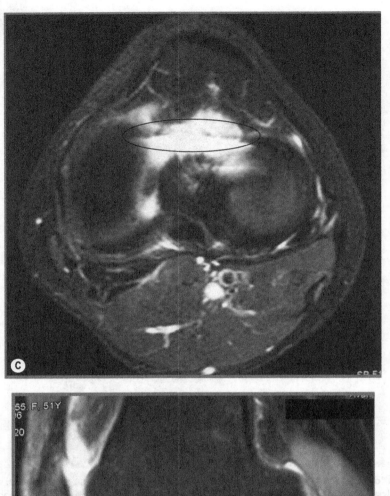

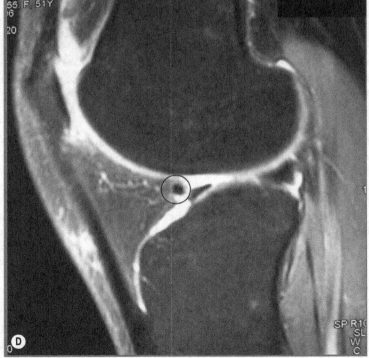

Figure. 6-10—cont'd • (C) MR imaging of the right knee, axial plane, using T2-weighted fat-saturated imaging, where, between the two anterior cornu of the menisci, a vague horizontal low signal region is noted, representing the transverse ligament, which in this patient is complete (oval). (D) MR imaging of the right knee in the sagittal plane, T2-weighted fat-saturated image, demonstrating the low-signal round focus seen just anterior to the medial anterior horn of the meniscus which represents a well-developed transverse ligament (circle).

Table 6.03 The bursae of the knee

Location between …	Comment
Anterior	The anterior bursae are the most clinically important
Lower patella and skin	Prepatellar bursa. Inflammation causes 'housemaid's knee'
Tibia and infrapatellar tendon	Deep infrapatellar bursa
Distal tibial tuberosity and skin	Superficial infrapatellar bursa. Inflammation causes 'parson's knee'
Superior extension of synovium	Suprapatellar bursa
Posterior	Most posterior bursae are variable
Medial tendon of gastrocnemius and semimembranosus	Popliteal bursa
Lateral	
Joint capsule and lateral head of the gastrocnemius muscle	This bursa can be continuous with the joint cavity and thus contain synovial fluid
The tendon of biceps femoris and the lateral collateral ligament	
The tendon of popliteus and the lateral collateral ligament The tendon of popliteus and the lateral femoral condyle	These bursae often communicate
Medial	There may be variable bursae lying deep to the medial collateral ligament
The medial head of gastrocnemius and the tendon of semimembranosus	Semimembranosus bursa (This bursa also connects with the fibrous capsule and usually communicates with the joint)
The tendon of semimembranosus, the medial tibial condyle and the medial head of gastrocnemius	This bursa may communicate with the semimembranosus bursa
The medial collateral ligament and the tendons of sartorius, gracilis and semitendinosus	Pes anserine bursa
The tendons of semimembranosus and semitendinosus	This variable bursa is frequently absent

information about the subchondral and marrow components of bone.

Bone marrow patterns vary with age. In children of 12 years and under, most of the marrow space is usually filled with haematopoietic cells or red marrow, typically of intermediate signal intensity on both T1- and T2-weighted images. In adults, the bone marrow signal is usually high on T1-weighted images and intermediate on T2-weighted images, consistent with yellow or fatty marrow.[32–35]

Marrow signal changes, or reconversion, can be indicative of systemic diseases and may be found as an incidental finding in the work-up of an orthopaedic condition (Figure 6.11).[59,60] Injuries to bone, such as contusions or stress fractures, are easily detected with MRI as a change in bone marrow signal (Figure 6.11B). When the signal from the marrow is eliminated by fat suppression, bone marrow oedema becomes more evident. It can be demonstrated on fluid-sensitive and fat-suppressed images by focal areas of increased signal.[32–34]

Osseous structures

Bone contusions

Many injuries to the soft tissue structures of the knee are associated with osseous damage. Blunt fractures are usually well visualized on conventional radiography; however, bone bruising requires MR imaging to

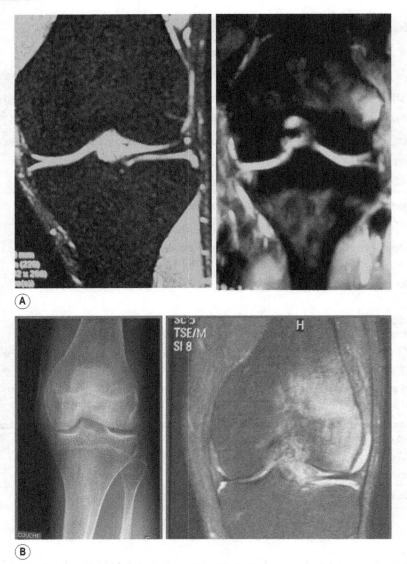

Figure 6.11 • (A) MR imaging, coronal slice of the left knee representing the normal marrow pattern found in a 27-year-old male (left image). This is an example of a fat-suppressed technique called short tau inversion recovery (STIR). This technique is useful in the detection of marrow reconversion, demonstrated by inhomogeneous signal intensity of the bone marrow in the distal femur and proximal tibia in the image on the right. This image was acquired from a 50-year-old obese female who was also a heavy smoker. (B) Imaging of a 24-year-old male patient with a previous history of spontaneous fractures, of various bones, due to osteogenesis imperfecta. Due to a recent history of a fall, the patient had imaging performed, initially digital imaging, of which the anteroposterior view is provided (left) where the reduced density of bone can be appreciated. However, it is only on the coronal T2 fat-saturated MR image (right), performed within a week of the radiograph, that the large region of increased signal intensity (bone marrow oedema) involving the distal lateral femoral condyle and the supracondylar region is noted, likely due to a partial, lateral patella subluxation, not reported clinically by the patient.

be identified. Bone bruises, microfractures or trabecular injuries are characterized principally by bone marrow oedema and will present as decreased signal areas on T1-weighted images and increased signal areas on T2-weighted and on fat-suppressed images (Figure 6.12).[32-34]

The identification of bone bruises can help in predicting the presence of concurrent soft tissue injuries. For example, acute tears of the ACL are often associated with bone bruises at the lateral femoral condyles and the posterolateral aspect of the tibial plateau. Examples of bone bruising can be seen in the images associated with ligamentous tears below.

Chondromalacia patellae

Softening of the articular cartilage of the deep surface of the patella can lead to crepitus, foreign body sensation and retropatellar pain, typically aggravated during flexion. A typical complaint will be of pain when descending stairs or walking downhill.[30,61]

Chondromalacia patellae is common and affects almost every age group but with a variety of aetiologies. Idiopathic chondromalacia patellae is seen in growing children and teenagers; degenerative chondromalacia patellae is more likely to be seen in a middle to older age population.[62] For both groups, imaging features will be similar (Figure 6.13A,B). In the beginning stages of the disease, areas of high signal will be present on fluid-sensitive sequences. This finding may be associated with an increase in overall cartilage thickness and represents oedema.[61] As the disorder progresses, the articular surface will appear more irregular with focal thinning that can expand to and expose the subchondral bone.

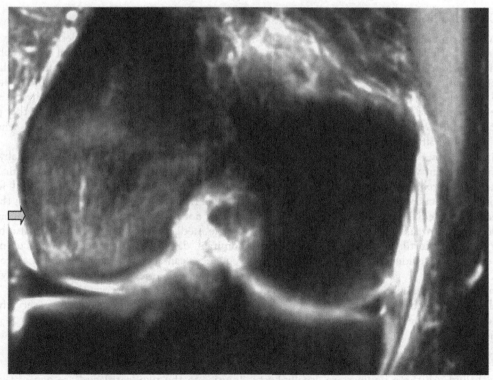

Figure 6.12 • MR imaging, sagittal STIR sequence demonstrating a large region of heterogeneous increased signal intensity located in the distal lateral femur due to a sizeable bone contusion involving the femoral condyle (straight arrow). The patient also suffered from a torn anterior cruciate ligament, medial collateral ligament sprain and a moderate joint effusion.

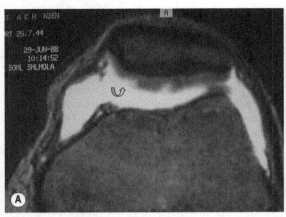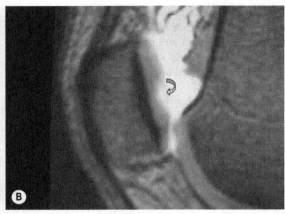

Figure 6.13 • MR imaging of the knee. (A) Axial T1-weighted image of the patellofemoral articulation with the addition of intra-articular contrast, demonstrating chondromalacia patella. Focal irregularity and frank loss of the articular cartilage surface is illustrated by the curved arrow. (B) Sagittal T1-weighted image with the addition of contrast, demonstrating chondral fissuring and erosion (curved arrow) along the articular cartilage of the patella due to chondromalacia patella.

Osteochondral injuries

Osteochondral injuries (osteochondritis dissecans) predominantly affect younger individuals. These injuries are considered the result of an accumulation of microtraumatic events at the level of the osteochondral region leading to a series of avascular events. They are characterized by bone necrosis, subsequent re-ossification and healing.[63–65] A history of trauma is found in about half of those patients affected.[3,61] Depending on the extent of the involvement, patients may present with deep joint pain and locking, clicking or a catching sensation.[30,33] In the knee, osteochondral defects are most common at the lateral aspect of the medial femoral condyle at the most convex area of the articular surface (Figure 6.14).[61] If the injury is purely cartilaginous, plain films will be normal except for evidence of mild soft tissue swelling.

MR imaging is very sensitive in the early stages of the development of an osteochondral injury; depending on the severity of the disease, the imaging presentation can range from a focal thin rim of abnormal signal intensity in the cartilage (on the fluid-sensitive images) to a well-visualized fragment surrounded by synovial fluid. All these findings are usually best visualized on T2-weighted or fat-suppressed images. Changes can be bilateral in approximately 25% of patients. The treatment options range from conservative pain management to debridement and grafting.[30,33,61]

Patella

Although roughening of the underside of the patella can be evaluated using conventional radiography, MR imaging comes into its own in assessing patella dislocation. This diagnosis can be impossible to arrive at clinically in the 50% of cases where the patella has instantly and spontaneously reduced; the patient themselves is usually unaware as to what has happened.

The diagnosis with MR images is usually quite straightforward: there will be a characteristic contusion on the anterior aspect of the lateral femoral condyle from the impaction of the patella; this may or may not be accompanied by a 'kissing' contusion on the medial patella itself. There will also be concomitant damage to the medial retinaculum. The sequences can also be used to establish a prognosis: the presence of a piece of loose cartilage usually necessitates arthroscopic intervention; an intact patella cartilage can normally be managed conservatively.[66]

Meniscal injuries

Injuries to the two 'cartilages' are one of the most common causes of knee pain and disability and are well visualized on MR images. Presumably in response to mechanical stress or degeneration, the chemical composition of the meniscus changes, resulting in intrasubstance signal alterations, referred

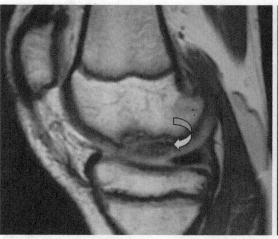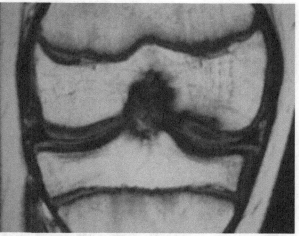

Figure 6.14 • MR imaging of the knee, sagittal (left) and coronal (right) T1-weighted images in a 15-year-old patient with knee pain. Gross irregularity about the lateral surface of the medial femoral condyle surface is well illustrated. A large fragment is noted adjacent to the irregular surface, the osteochondral fragment (curved arrow), which in this patient has not displaced further than 2 mm away from the donor site on the distal femur.

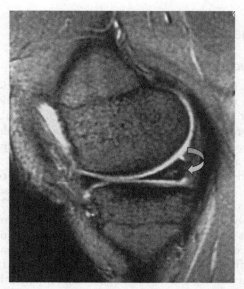

Figure 6.15 • Sagittal T2-weighted MR image of the knee demonstrating intrameniscal substance high signal intensity (curved arrow) which does not extend to the articular surface and is not associated with deformation of shape of the meniscus. This is an example of myxoid degeneration, although it would be necessary to review all planes available to confirm that there is no articular surface contact.

to as *myxoid degeneration* (Figure 6.15).[67] This change is generally asymptomatic and is not linked to a higher incidence of meniscal tearing[61]; it can, however, be mistaken for a tear.[3]

In the acute patient, the mechanism of injury usually involves rotation combined with a varus or valgus stress. This mechanism is also likely to compromise collateral and cruciate ligaments, explaining in part the common association and comorbidity between these structures.[9] Degenerative changes are usually as the result of repetitive microtrama and are also commonly associated with dysfunction elsewhere in the lower kinematic chain and with obesity.

Patients with meniscal damage usually present with pain, a sensation of their knee 'giving way', swelling and locking. The swelling may be sporadic, influenced by the activity level.[30,33,61]

Meniscal tears have multiple imaging presentations and grading systems related to the imaging features.[30,33,61] The definition of a true meniscal tear is an area of increased signal intensity in the meniscus extending to one or more articular surfaces; therefore, high signal regions that do not extend to the articular surface or communicate with the joint should not generally be considered as true tears.[68–70]

Tears of the menisci are described with reference to their orientation, length, location and presence of any free fragment.[71,72] The most common location for an isolated meniscal tear is the posterior horn of the medial meniscus (Figure 6.16); the most common types of tear are oblique (or horizontal), radial (free edge or 'parrot-beak') and 'bucket-handle'.[3]

Tears are also often seen as an element in more complex knee injuries involving capsular or ligamentous disruption.[30,33,61] When associated with

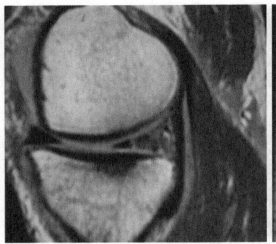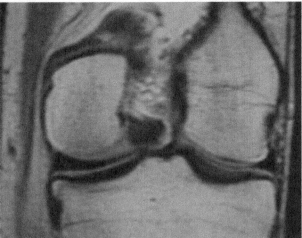

Figure 6.16 • MR imaging of the knee, sagittal (left) and coronal (right) T1-weighted images demonstrating abnormal signal intensity in the posterior horn of the medial meniscus with deformation of the contours of the meniscus, with altered signal intensity reaching the articular surface and blunting of the anterior surface, due to a tear of the posterior horn of the medial meniscus.

injuries to structures such as the anterior cruciate ligament, meniscal tears may often be overlooked because they tend to be located in atypical areas such as the posterior horn of the lateral meniscus or in the periphery of the medial meniscus.[61] It is also worth recalling the normal variants discussed above that may simulate the presence of a meniscal injury.[43–45]

Depending on the type of tear, the location of the defect and the condition of the patient, various treatment options are available. Comprehensive rehabilitation programmes, suturing and meniscectomy (partial or total) are the most common treatment options.[30] When evaluating images of a postoperative patient, correlation with preoperative films is usually essential as the signal intensity of the repaired area can remain high for years after.[33,61] MR arthrography may be helpful in postoperative knees to differentiate scar tissue from a re-tear of the meniscus.[73]

Discoid menisci are often enlarged and can therefore be symptomatic; they are also more prone to tears, degeneration and cyst formation. Meniscal cysts develop from accumulation of fluid in an existing tear. On examination, a palpable, painful mass may be found, especially if the cyst is very large. The mucinous and proteinaceous mass may fluctuate in size according to the degree of knee flexion.[30,61] On MR images, the cyst appears as high signal intensity on fluid-sensitive sequences and is situated adjacent to the articular space (Figures 6.17, 6.18).[74]

Ligamentous injuries

Cruciate ligaments

Cruciate ligament tears are also common, particularly those to the anterior ligament, which are typically caused by anterior translation of the tibia, external rotation of the femur on the tibia with valgus stress on a weight-bearing leg. It is a common injury for athletes practising sports involving constant acceleration and deceleration whilst changing direction, such as football (in all of its forms and variations), basketball, downhill skiing and tennis.[61,75–82]

Owing to the mechanism of injury, mid-substance tears are by far the most common type of injury. Discontinuity and an alteration of the orientation of the fibres are two direct signs of a tear (Figure 6.19). Joint effusion and haemarthrosis are non-specific but useful indicators of joint pathology; however, these findings can obscure the ligament fibres, so other indirect signs may be needed to confirm the diagnosis. These include anterior tibial subluxation (the *floppy sign*), deepening of the lateral femoral condylar notch (to more than the normal limit of 2 mm) and specific patterns of bone bruises (Figure 6.20).[3,61]

Partial tears of the ACL can be seen as intrasubstance high signal zones. They can be post-traumatic or chronic in nature. Secondary signs such as bone bruises, prominent joint effusion or the presence of associated meniscal injuries can be once again

Figure 6.17 • Coronal, T2-weighted MR image of the knee demonstrating a large multi-loculated meniscal cyst (arrow). Note the abnormal signal involving the adjacent meniscus extending to the lateral articular surface denoting a partial tear (arrow head) of the posterior horn.

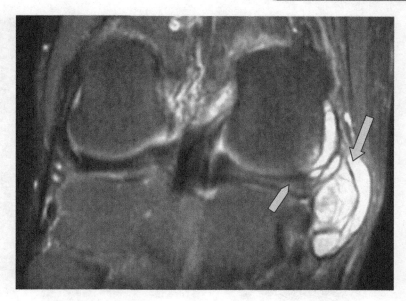

Figure 6.18 • Axial T2-weighted MR image of the knee demonstrating a large multi-loculated meniscal cyst (arrow). Note the abnormal signal involving the adjacent meniscus extending to the lateral articular surface denoting a partial tear (arrow head).

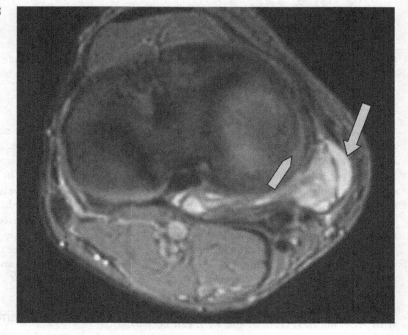

helpful to establish a diagnosis. Chronic tears may be associated with mild effusion but the main differential feature is the prominent fibrosis and associated scar tissue formation.[61]

Different treatment options for ACL injuries result in different postoperative imaging presentations. Again, observation of the preoperative images is very helpful. Reconstructed ligaments, especially when using autografts, have a tendency to remain avascular (low signal intensity) for years after implantation. The fibrous appearance will not be maintained postoperatively but rather there will be an irregular appearance.[61]

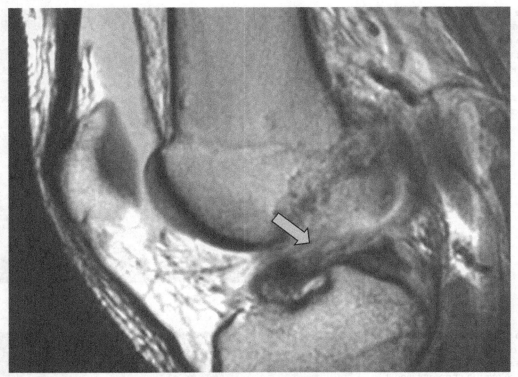

Figure 6.19 • Sagittal T1-weighted MR image of the knee demonstrating an acute high-grade tear affecting the anterior cruciate ligament. There is discontinuity of the ligament fibres (arrow). Effusion and haemarthrosis are also present which can exaggerate the grade of anterior cruciate ligament tear.

A common cause of postsurgical pain following ACL reconstruction is the development of scar tissue in Hoffa's fat pad. Although this can present in different ways, depending on its precise location, it most commonly affects knee extension and/or patellar motion. The MR appearance can also vary; however, the classic presentation is that of a *Cyclops' lesion* (Figure 6.21).[83,84]

Injuries to the posterior cruciate ligament are very rarely seen as isolated incidents. The most common mechanism of injury is by direct blunt force to the anterior knee as in a severe motor vehicle accident where the flexed knee hits the dashboard.[9,61] As with ACL injuries, tears of the PCL can be partial or complete. Partial tears can present as focal zones of increased signal intensity and disruption of the normal 'inverted hockey stick' appearance of the PCL (Figure 6.22)[50]; however, the PCL is unusual in that damage to it often involves stretching without overt disruption of its fibres and the fluid-sensitive sequences are therefore normal although the T1-weighted and proton density images will have a subtly increased signal. The width of the ligament will also increase; greater than 7 mm is regarded as being clinically significant.[3]

Management of isolated PCL injuries commonly includes conservative measures. Aggressive rehabilitation plans including strengthening of the hamstring are preferred since increased tone in the large muscle group in the posterior thigh can act as a substitute for the injured ligament by providing pull on the tibia and removing stress from the compromised PCL.[33]

Collateral ligament injuries

Excessive valgus and varus stress are the main causes of injury to the medial and lateral collateral ligaments, respectively. Damage to the medial and lateral collateral ligaments can be grouped according to the severity of the sprain.[30,33]

Low-grade injuries (grade 1) present as oedematous areas of increased T2-weighted signal and haemorrhagic changes (mixed signal) extending

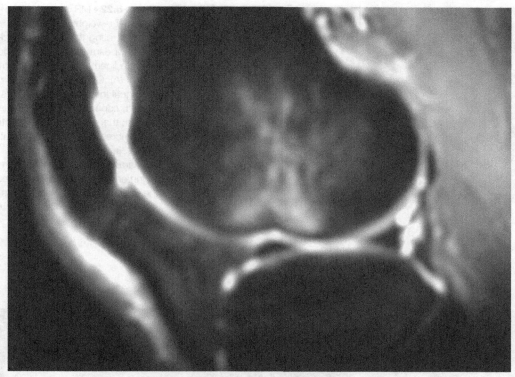

Figure 6.20 • MR imaging of the knee, sagittal STIR (short tau inversion recovery) image in a patient with an acute anterior cruciate ligament tear. This image demonstrates the deep lateral femoral notch, joint effusion and a large bone bruise extending to the supracondylar region of the distal femur and is the same patient as seen in Figure 6.18.

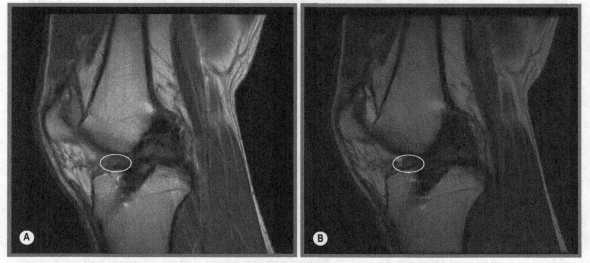

Figure 6.21 • MR imaging of the knee, post ACL reconstructive surgery, demonstrating (A) a T1 weighted sagittal MR of the knee with a region of oval intermediate signal located just anterior to the ACL graft (oval). (B) Again a region of oval abnormal signal is identified, this time of lower signal (see oval). This lesion seen in both figures is a cyclops lesion.

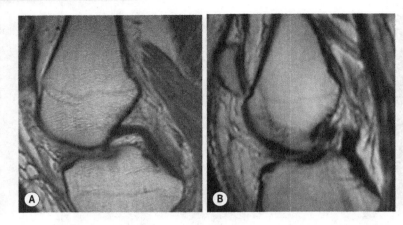

Figure 6.22 • MR imaging of the knee, sagittal T1-weighted images demonstrating the 'inverted hockey stick' appearance of the posterior cruciate ligament (PCL) in a normal patient (A). Compare this to (B), where the signal intensity of the PCL is altered, especially in the proximal portion; there is also lack of continuity of the fibres. The PCL has lost its typical 'inverted hockey stick' appearance. Note also the altered alignment of the tibia with respect to the distal femur. This represents a chronic tear of the PCL, which was confirmed by arthroscopy.

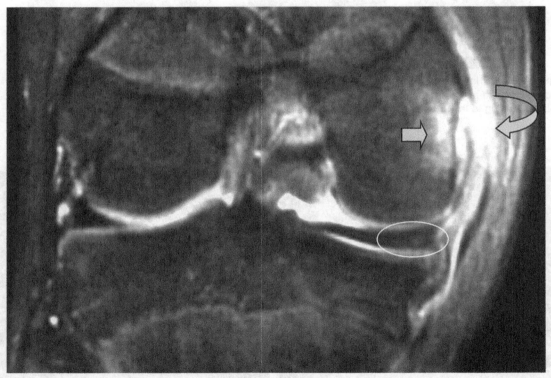

Figure 6.23 • MR imaging of the knee, coronal STIR (short tau inversion recovery) image demonstrating extensive increased signal intensity in the soft tissues about the medial collateral ligament (curved arrow) with discontinuity of the fibres. In addition, high signal intensity is also noted about the medial femoral condyle suggesting a bone contusion (straight arrow) and horizontal high signal intensity in the medial meniscus (oval). The appearance of high signal intensity at the level of the growth plates in the distal femur and proximal tibia is normal in this young patient.

into the subcutaneous tissues. Haemarthrosis and joint effusion are not as common in LCL sprains because of the extracapsular location of the structure.[32-34]

High-grade injuries are associated with discontinuity of the fibres and loss of the normal contours of the ligament (grade 2) or complete disruption of the fibres (grade 3). These are demonstrated in Figure 6.23. Once again, isolated collateral injury is a rare phenomenon and, if found, close attention should be paid to the adjacent bone marrow signal and status of the capsulomeniscal complex, especially about the medial compartment, owing to the high risk of collateral damage in these areas.[32-34]

Damage to the LCL and, indeed, the lateral meniscus, can be difficult to differentiate clinically from *iliotibial band syndrome*; the only clue may be weakness of the tensor fascia lata muscle.

However, with MR imaging, the diagnosis is relatively straightforward: if there is fluid on both sides of the iliotibial band on the T2-weighted images, the diagnosis is confirmed.[85,86]

Clinical pearls

- Always try to view the T2 or STIR sequences first, to locate where the lesion is, and then use the T1-weighted sequence to determine the precise anatomy involved in the process.
- Verify the presence of any lesion using a minimum of two (or preferably three) planes.
- Always correlate the clinical history and examination with the imaging findings to determine appropriate clinical management of the patient.

References

1. Galea A, Giuffre B, Dimmick S, et al. The accuracy of magnetic resonance imaging scanning and its influence on management decisions in knee surgery. *Arthroscopy*. 2009;25(5):473–480.

2. Crawford R, Walley G, Bridgman S, Maffulli N. Magnetic resonance imaging versus arthroscopy in the diagnosis of knee pathology, concentrating on meniscal lesions and ACL tears: a systematic review. *Br Med Bull*. 2007;84: 5–23.

3. Helms C, Major N, Anderson MW, et al. The knee. In: *Musculoskeletal MRI*. 2nd ed. Philadelphia: Elsevier Saunders; 2009:353–383.

4. Rowe L, Yochum T. Principles of radiological interpretation. In: Yochum T, Rowe L, eds. *Essentials of Skeletal Radiology*. 2nd ed. Baltimore: Williams and Wilkins; 1996:547–585.

5. Bloch F, Hansen W, Packard M. Nuclear induction. *Phys Rev*. 1946;69:127.

6. Smith TO, Davies L, Donell ST. The reliability and validity of assessing medio-lateral patellar position: a systematic review. *Man Ther*. 2009;14(4):355–362.

7. Smith TO, Davies L, O'Driscoll ML, Donell ST. An evaluation of the clinical tests and outcome measures used to assess patellar instability. *Knee*. 2008;15(4):255–262.

8. Bates B, Hoekelman R. Interviewing and the health history. In: Bates B, ed. *A Guide to Physical Examination*. 3rd ed. Philadelphia: JB Lippincott; 1983:1–27.

9. Eustace S, Johnston C, O'Neill P, O'Byrne J. The knee and calf. In: *Sports Injuries: Examination, Imaging and Management*. Edinburgh: Elsevier Churchill Livingstone; 2007:135–218.

10. Grotle M, Hagen KB, Natvig B, et al. Obesity and osteoarthritis in knee, hip and/or hand: an epidemiological study in the general population with 10 years follow-up. *BMC Musculoskelet Disord*. 2008;9:132.

11. Lohmander LS, Gerhardsson de Verdier M, Rollof J, et al. Incidence of severe knee and hip osteoarthritis in relation to different measures of body mass: a population-based prospective cohort study. *Ann Rheum Dis*. 2009;68(4):490–496.

12. Zeng QY, Zang CH, Li XF, et al. Associated risk factors of knee osteoarthritis: a population survey in Taiyuan, China. *Chin Med J (Engl)*. 2006;119(18):1522–1527.

13. Holmberg S, Thelin A, Thelin N. Knee osteoarthritis and body mass index: a population-based case-control study. *Scand J Rheumatol*. 2005;34(1):59–64.

14. Andersen RE, Crespo CJ, Bartlett SJ, et al. Relationship between body weight gain and significant knee, hip, and back pain in older Americans. *Obes Res*. 2003;11(10):1159–1162.

15. Bates B. The musculoskeletal system. In: Bates B, ed. *A Guide to Physical Examination*. 3rd ed. Philadelphia: JB Lippincott; 1983:324–370.

16. Travell J, Simons D. *Myofascial Pain and Dysfunction*. Baltimore: Williams and Wilkins; 1992.

17. Meserve BB, Cleland JA, Boucher TR. A meta-analysis examining clinical test utilities for assessing meniscal injury. *Clin Rehabil*. 2008;22(2): 143–161.

18. Wilson T. The measurement of patellar alignment in patellofemoral pain syndrome: are we confusing assumptions with evidence? *J Orthop Sports Phys Ther*. 2007;37(6):330–341.

19. Seron M, Yochum T, Barry M, Rowe L. Skeletal dysplasias. In: Yochum T, Rowe L, eds. *Essentials of Skeletal Radiology*. 2nd ed. Baltimore: Williams and Wilkins; 1996:858–1652.

20. Emami MJ, Ghahramani MH, Abdinejad F, Namazi H. Q-angle: an invaluable parameter for evaluation of anterior knee pain. *Arch Iran Med.* 2007;10(1):24–26.

21. Omololu BB, Ogunlade OS, Gopaldasani VK. Normal Q-angle in an adult Nigerian population. *Clin Orthop Relat Res.* 2009;467(8):2073–2076.

22. Shellock FG, Stone KR, Crues JV. Development and clinical application of kinematic MRI of the patellofemoral joint using an extremity MR system. *Med Sci Sports Exerc.* 1999;31(6): 788–791.

23. Wilson NA, Press JM, Koh JL, et al. In vivo noninvasive evaluation of abnormal patellar tracking during squatting in patients with patellofemoral pain. *J Bone Joint Surg Am.* 2009;91(3):558–566.

24. Bannister R. Disorders of the nerve roots and peripheral nerves. In: *Brain and Bannister's Clinical Neurology.* 7th ed. Oxford: Oxford University Press; 1992:420–458.

25. Standring S, ed. *Gray's Anatomy - Pelvic girdle and lower limb – knee (Section 113).* Edinburgh: Elsevier; 2009.

26. Standring S, ed. *Gray's Anatomy - Pelvic girdle and lower limb – thigh (Section 112).* Edinburgh: Elsevier; 2009.

27. Moore K. The lower limb. In: *Clinically Oriented Anatomy.* 2nd ed. Baltimore: Williams and Wilkins; 1985:396–564.

28. Calmbach WL, Hutchens M. Evaluation of patients presenting with knee pain: Part II. Differential diagnosis. *Am Fam Physician.* 2003;68(5):917–922.

29. Calmbach WL, Hutchens M. Evaluation of patients presenting with knee pain: Part I. History, physical examination, radiographs, and laboratory tests. *Am Fam Physician.* 2003;68(5):907–912.

30. Hammer WI. *Functional Soft Tissue Examination and Treatment by Manual Methods.* Riverwoods, IL: Aspen; 1999.

31. Rowe L, Yochum T. Arthritic disorders. In: Yochum T, Rowe L, eds. *Essentials of Skeletal Radiology.* 2nd ed. Baltimore: Williams and Wilkins; 1996:795–974.

32. Kaplan P, Helms C, Dussault R, Anderson M. *Musculoskeletal MRI.* Philadelphia: WB Saunders; 2001.

33. Stoller D. *Magnetic Resonance Imaging in Orthopaedics and Sports Medicine.* 2nd ed. Philadelphia: Lippincott Williams and Wilkins; 1996.

34. Berquist T. *MRI of the Musculoskeletal System 4th ed.* Philadelphia: Lippincott Williams and Wilkins; 2000.

35. Mirowitz S. *Pitfalls, Variants And Artifacts in Body MR Imaging.* St Louis: Mosby; 1996.

36. Green J, Silver P. The muscles and joints of the lower limb. In: *An Introduction to Human Anatomy.* Oxford: Oxford University Press; 1981:128–146.

37. Joseph J. Bones of the leg and knee joint. In: Hamilton W, ed. *Textbook of Human Anatomy.* 2nd ed. London: MacMillan; 1976:123–129.

38. Palastanga N, Field D, Soames R. The lower limb. In: *Anatomy and Human Movement: Structure and Function.* 5th ed. Edinburgh: Elsevier Butterworth Heinmann; 2006:235–470.

39. Young MF. The physics of anatomy. In: *Essential Physics for Musculoskeletal Medicine.* Edinburgh: Elsevier; 2009.

40. Grenier J-M, Green N, Wessely M. Knee MRI part 1: basic overview. *Clinical Chiropractic.* 2004;7(3): 147–150.

41. Youm T, Chen AL. Discoid lateral meniscus: evaluation and treatment. *Am J Orthop.* 2004; 33(5):234–238.

42. Klingele KE, Kocher MS, Hresko MT, et al. Discoid lateral meniscus: prevalence of peripheral rim instability. *J Pediatr Orthop.* 2004;24(1):79–82.

43. Kocher MS, Klingele K, Rassman SO. Meniscal disorders: normal, discoid, and cysts. *Orthop Clin North Am.* 2003;34(3): 329–340.

44. Tachibana Y, Yamazaki Y, Ninomiya S. Discoid medial meniscus. *Arthroscopy.* 2003;19(7): E12–E18.

45. Rohren EM, Kosarek FJ, Helms CA. Discoid lateral meniscus and the frequency of meniscal tears. *Skeletal Radiol.* 2001;30(6):316–320.

46. Shankman S, Beltran J, Melamed E, Rosenberg ZS. Anterior horn of the lateral meniscus: another potential pitfall in MR imaging of the knee. *Radiology.* 1997;204(1):181–184.

47. Fernandes JL, Viana SL, Mendonca JL, et al. Mucoid degeneration of the anterior cruciate ligament: magnetic resonance imaging findings of an underdiagnosed entity. *Acta Radiol.* 2008;49(1):75–79.

48. Drosos GI, Pozo JL. Large extrasynovial intracapsular ganglia of the knee: a report of 3 cases. *Arthroscopy.* 2005;21(11): 1362–1365.

49. Dinakar B, Khan T, Kumar AC, Kumar A. Ganglion cyst of the anterior cruciate ligament: a case report. *J Orthop Surg (Hong Kong).* 2005;13(2):181–185.

50. Regatte RR, Akella SV, Borthakur A, et al. In vivo proton MR three-dimensional T1rho mapping of human articular cartilage: initial experience. *Radiology.* 2003;229(1):269–274.

51. Joseph J. Muscles and fascia of the lower limb. In: Hamilton W, ed. *Textbook of Human Anatomy.* 2nd ed. London: MacMillan; 1976:179–195.

52. Sintzoff Jr SA, Stallenberg B, Gillard I, et al. Transverse geniculate ligament of the knee: appearance and frequency on plain radiographs. *Br J Radiol.* 1992;65(777):766–768.

53. Watanabe AT, Carter BC, Teitelbaum GP, et al. Normal variations in MR imaging of the knee: appearance and frequency. *Am J Roentgenol.* 1989;153(2): 341–344.

54. Watanabe AT, Carter BC, Teitelbaum GP, Bradley Jr WG. Common pitfalls in magnetic resonance imaging of the knee. *J Bone Joint Surg Am.* 1989;71(6): 857–862.

55. Ranalletta M, Rossi W, Paterno M, et al. Incidence of the anterior meniscofemoral ligament: an arthroscopic study in anterior cruciate ligament-deficient knees. *Arthroscopy.* 2007;23(3):275–277.

56. Nagasaki S, Ohkoshi Y, Yamamoto K, et al. The incidence and cross-sectional area of the

meniscofemoral ligament. *Am J Sports Med*. 2006;34(8):1345–1350.

57. Sznajderman T, Smorgick Y, Lindner D, et al. Medial plica syndrome. *Isr Med Assoc J*. 2009;11(1):54–57.

58. Griffith CJ, Laprade RF. Medial plica irritation: diagnosis and treatment. *Curr Rev Musculoskelet Med*. 2008;1(1):53–60.

59. Hartman RP, Sundaram M, Okuno SH, Sim FH. Effect of granulocyte-stimulating factors on marrow of adult patients with musculoskeletal malignancies: incidence and MRI findings. *Am J Roentgenol*. 2004;183(3):645–653.

60. Ollivier L, Gerber S, Vanel D, et al. Improving the interpretation of bone marrow imaging in cancer patients. *Cancer Imaging*. 2006;6:194–198.

61. Stoller DW, Tirman PF, Bredella MA. *Diagnostic Imaging Orthopaedics*. Salt Lake City: Amirsys Inc; 2003.

62. Zhang H, Kong XQ, Cheng C, Liang MH. A correlative study between prevalence of chondromalacia patellae and sports injury in 4068 students. *Chin J Traumatol*. 2003;6(6):370–374.

63. De Smet AA, Fisher DR, Graf BK, Lange RH. Osteochondritis dissecans of the knee: value of MR imaging in determining lesion stability and the presence of articular cartilage defects. *Am J Roentgenol*. 1990;155(3):549–553.

64. Fritz RC. MR imaging of osteochondral and articular lesions. *Magn Reson Imaging Clin N Am*. 1997;5(3):579–602.

65. Bhosale AM, Richardson JB. Articular cartilage: structure, injuries and review of management. *Br Med Bull*. 2008;87:77–95.

66. White BJ, Sherman OH. Patellofemoral instability. *Bull NYU Hosp Jt Dis*. 2009;67(1):22–29.

67. Ferrer-Roca O, Vilalta C. Lesions of the meniscus. Part I: Macroscopic and histologic findings. *Clin Orthop Relat Res*. 1980;(146):289–300.

68. Kaplan PA, Nelson NL, Garvin KL, Brown DE. MR of the knee: the significance of high signal in the meniscus that does not clearly extend to the surface. *Am J Roentgenol*. 1991;156(2):333–336.

69. De Smet AA, Tuite MJ. Use of the "two-slice-touch" rule for the MRI diagnosis of meniscal tears. *Am J Roentgenol*. 2006;187(4):911–914.

70. De Smet AA, Norris MA, Yandow DR, et al. MR diagnosis of meniscal tears of the knee: importance of high signal in the meniscus that extends to the surface. *Am J Roentgenol*. 1993;161(1):101–107.

71. Widuchowski W, Widuchowski J, Trzaska T. Articular cartilage defects: study of 25, 124 knee arthroscopies. *Knee*. 2007;14(3):177–182.

72. Christoforakis J, Pradhan R, Sanchez-Ballester J, et al. Is there an association between articular cartilage changes and degenerative meniscus tears? *Arthroscopy*. 2005;21(11):1366–1369.

73. Ciliz D, Ciliz A, Elverici E, et al. Evaluation of postoperative menisci with MR arthrography and routine conventional MRI. *Clin Imaging*. 2008;32(3):212–219.

74. Tyson LL, Daughters Jr TC, Ryu RK, Crues 3rd JV. MRI appearance of meniscal cysts. *Skeletal Radiol*. 1995;24(6):421–424.

75. Alentorn-Geli E, Myer GD, Silvers HJ, et al. Prevention of non-contact anterior cruciate ligament injuries in soccer players. Part 1: Mechanisms of injury and underlying risk factors. *Knee Surg Sports Traumatol Arthrosc*. 2009;17(8):859–879.

76. Meyer EG, Haut RC. Anterior cruciate ligament injury induced by internal tibial torsion or tibiofemoral compression. *J Biomech*. 2008;41(16):3377–3383.

77. Davies H, Tietjens B, Van Sterkenburg M, Mehgan A. Anterior cruciate ligament injuries in snowboarders: a quadriceps-induced injury. *Knee Surg Sports Traumatol Arthrosc*. 2009;17(9):1048–1051.

78. Krosshaug T, Nakamae A, Boden BP, et al. Mechanisms of anterior cruciate ligament injury in basketball: video analysis of 39 cases. *Am J Sports Med*. 2007;35(3):359–367.

79. Hewett TE, Myer GD, Ford KR. Anterior cruciate ligament injuries in female athletes: Part 1, mechanisms and risk factors. *Am J Sports Med*. 2006;34(2):299–311.

80. Brooks JH, Fuller CW, Kemp SP, Reddin DB. Epidemiology of injuries in English professional rugby union: part 2 training injuries. *Br J Sports Med*. 2005;39(10):767–775.

81. Brooks JH, Fuller CW, Kemp SP, Reddin DB. Epidemiology of injuries in English professional rugby union: part 1 match injuries. *Br J Sports Med*. 2005;39(10):757–766.

82. Brown JR, Trojian TH. Anterior and posterior cruciate ligament injuries. *Prim Care*. 2004;31(4):925–956.

83. Papakonstantinou O, Chung CB, Chanchairujira K, Resnick DL. Complications of anterior cruciate ligament reconstruction: MR imaging. *Eur Radiol*. 2003;13(5):1106–1117.

84. Wang J, Ao Y. Analysis of different kinds of cyclops lesions with or without extension loss. *Arthroscopy*. 2009;25(6):626–631.

85. Stabler A, Glaser C, Reiser M. Musculoskeletal MR: knee. *Eur Radiol*. 2000;10(2):230–241.

86. Vasilevska V, Szeimies U, Stabler A. Magnetic resonance imaging signs of iliotibial band friction in patients with isolated medial compartment osteoarthritis of the knee. *Skeletal Radiol*. 2009;38(9):871–875.

The ankle and foot

Michelle A. Wessely   Martin Young

Introduction

Non-invasive imaging of the ankle and foot can comprise a variety of approaches including plain film radiography, ultrasound, computed tomography (CT) and magnetic resonance (MR) imaging, depending on the clinician's suspicions and the available resources. Whilst the basic imaging techniques may be useful in many circumstances, an increasing number of patients undergo MR imaging owing to the unsurpassed detail that it provides, particularly of the ligamentous complexes around the ankle.

In cases of ankle trauma, MR imaging also gives useful information regarding the bone marrow and allows assessment of the effect of the injury on joint biomechanics – altered weight-bearing can result in areas of bone marrow oedema in other areas of the mid- and forefoot that may contribute to the patient's clinical syndrome.

For most primary contact healthcare providers, it would be a rare month that did not see at least a couple of patients attend having 'turned' their ankle; it is therefore important to have a good knowledge of the basic anatomical appearance of the ankle and foot on MR images and to be aware of the arrangement of the ligamentous complexes about the ankle, the intricate path of muscle tendons through the ankle and foot, and the normal and pathological appearance of the tibiofibular syndesmosis, which can help considerably with the classification of an ankle injury and its resulting prognosis and management.

It is also necessary to appreciate the importance of accurate diagnosis and prompt treatment of conditions in this area; disorders affecting this region, such as Morton's neuroma or intermetatarsal bursitis, can have a far-reaching effect on the patient due to the disruption of lower kinematic chain mechanics.[1,2] Although orthopaedic testing can provide some information as to the range of diagnostic possibilities, further imaging, particularly MR imaging, can often prove key in identifying the pain-producing structure. Although ultrasonography is being increasingly utilized, this modality can be very operator-dependent, which makes it less reliable and prone to producing false negative results.[3,4]

History and examination

Much of what holds true for the knee also applies to the ankle and foot; this should not be surprising as they are directly connected elements in what, in standing posture, is a closed-loop kinematic chain.[2] Because of this, the knee, ankle and foot often need to be assessed as a unit and the reader should direct themselves to Chapter 6 in order to review this material.

Obviously, the orthopaedic tests specific to the knee are not appropriate for those of the ankle and foot; however, apart from range of motion and digital palpatory pressure, there are far fewer such tests for this region. Those that there are will be dealt with on a condition-by-condition basis later in the chapter.

Differential diagnosis

The foot is susceptible to many conditions; these can mimic each other and exist as comorbidities. Although a thorough history will help to direct the

© 2011, Elsevier Ltd.
DOI: 10.1016/B978-0-443-06726-6.00007-X

Table 7.01 Differential diagnostic considerations for the foot and ankle

Vascular	Diabetes mellitus, thrombophlebitis, Raynaud's syndrome
Infection/ Inflammation	Osteomyeltis/gout, Reiter's syndrome/ plantar fasciitis, bursitis, tendinitis, cellulitis
Neoplasm	Primary or secondary cancers
Dermatological	Complex regional pain syndrome (Sudek's atrophy)
Iatrogenic	Drug interactions, postsurgical syndromes
Congenital	Morton's toe, talipes
Anatomical	Accessory muscles, Morton's neuroma, calcaneal spur
Trauma	Acute or chronic
Endocrine/ Environmental	Syndromes related to footwear

clinician's thinking, more than any other joint, the 'V-I-N-D-I-C-A-T-E' mnemonic will help to avoid the missed diagnosis (Table 7.01).

Clinical indications for imaging

The clinical indications for MR imaging of the ankle and foot are varied and may also depend on the clinical protocols established by the imaging centre and the availability of resources. Based on current evidence, MR imaging of the ankle and foot is considered the imaging modality of choice for conditions such as internal derangements (for example, impingement syndromes or tarsal tunnel syndrome) that commonly affect the distal lower extremity or for postoperative evaluation.[5–7] MR imaging gives the anatomical detail needed to identify both the pathology and the effect on the surrounding structures; this is important to evaluate since it will affect both the clinical management of the patient and their prognosis.

Although more basic imaging studies can imply a disorder and, indeed, demonstrate the dynamic effects of the condition, it is the soft tissue detail that MR imaging affords that sets it apart. Not only is it possible to have 3-mm slices in the sagittal, axial and coronal planes but also it is relatively simple to angle these planes obliquely in order to analyse the course of tendons or to position the foot with different angulations to optimize the visualization of specific structures; this ability gives MR imaging unsurpassed flexibility. As with other areas of the body, the correlation of the clinical presentation and examination findings to the MR images is the skill that leads to effective diagnosis and management. Proper evaluation of the imaging sequences can also identify other areas of clinical interest: contributory causative factors, secondary pathologies or incidental findings, all of which enhance the clinician's understanding of their patient.

An example of the benefits offered by MR imaging can be easily seen if you consider a common clinical entity such as **os trigonum syndrome** in which the flexor hallucis longus tendon may be compromised by the aberrant ossicle, leading to a posterior impingement syndrome. Although the os trigonum itself is demonstrated well on plain film images, the tendinous involvement can only be inferred from the partial or complete obliteration of *Kager's fat pad*, a triangular region of decreased density noted posterior to the tibia and fibula and superior to the calcaneus on the lateral view in most well-exposed digital radiographic images. Just anterior to this fat pad lie various structures, which, if irritated (as is the case in os trigonum syndrome), can cause partial or complete obliteration of the anterior margin of Kager's fat pad. This, however, is an inference; by comparison, MR images will show clearly the precise location and severity of the soft tissue involvement.

Likewise, in cases of trauma, bony and associated soft tissue lesions can be easily identified, and monitored throughout the patient's clinical management. This is particularly so when surgery is needed, when MR imaging can be used to determine the postsurgical response and evaluate intermediate- to long-term complications, including avascular necrosis and osteochondral injuries, which may remain undetected with other imaging modalities.

Procedure and sequences

MR imaging of the ankle requires that the patient lies supine with the ankle perpendicular to the lower leg; however, if the course of a particular tendon requires analysis, the position of the ankle may need to be modified in order to avoid technical artifacts such as the *magic angle effect* (explained in detail in Chapter 8). A support may be used to immobilize the patient and maintain the position during the imaging study.

A surface coil is usually used to increase the signal capture; a skin marker may be added to signal to the person reading the image the region of clinical interest (Figure 7.01). The sequences usually consist of all three planes: sagittal (Figures 7.02–7.04), axial (Figures 7.05–7.07) and coronal (Figures 7.08–7.10), using a combination of T1- and T2-weighted (or STIR) sequences, depending on the clinical scenario.

Contrast is used where a mass or infection is suspected, in order to determine the character and behaviour of the lesion and therefore aid the diagnosis; if this is the case, a T1-weighted, fat-suppressed image is used with the addition of gadolinium. Contrast can be given to the patient either via intravenous injection or directly into the articulation. Intra-articular injection is used to better visualize the state of the articular surface of the tibiotalar joint and to determine more completely the presence of any intra-articular body, which may be difficult to confirm on regular MR studies. Each contrasted slice is 4 mm in thickness, usually with an overlap of 0.5 mm.

MR imaging of the foot is ordinarily performed with the patient in the prone position. Although this position may be difficult for some patients, it allows for the toes to be maintained in the anatomically neutral position, and for the patient to be as immobile as possible during the imaging study, therefore limiting motion artifact, which can degrade the final

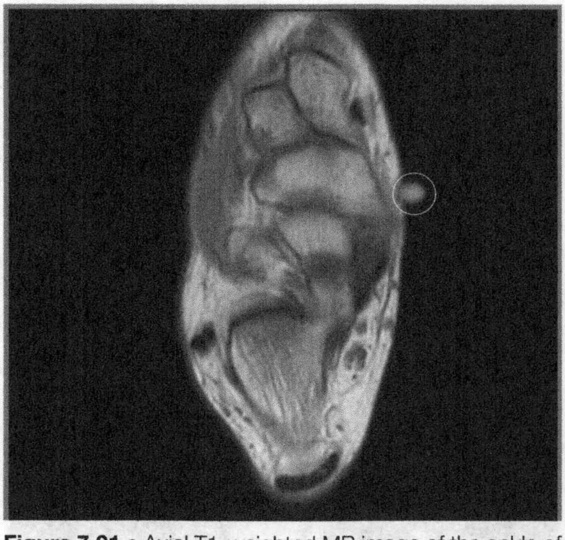

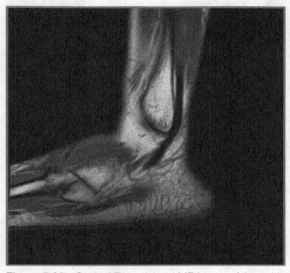

Figure 7.02 • Sagittal T1-weighted MR image of the ankle of a 33-year-old female with hind- and midfoot pain demonstrating the fibula with the tendons of the peronei wrapping around the distal aspect. When interpreting the sagittal plane, by identifying the fibula, the laterality of the slice is more easily determined.

Figure 7.01 • Axial T1-weighted MR image of the ankle of a 33-year-old female with pain on the medial aspect of the midfoot. A region of high signal intensity is noted on the medial aspect of the skin, just medial to the navicular. This is a skin marker to indicate the epicentre of pain or swelling noted by the patient and is useful to note when interpreting the final image.

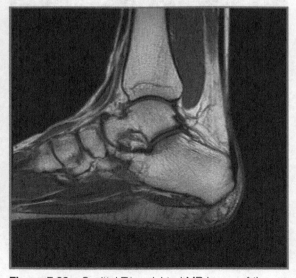

Figure 7.03 • Sagittal T1-weighted MR image of the ankle of a 33-year-old female with hind- and midfoot pain. This image is in the midsagittal plane and demonstrates well the bone and soft tissue detail.

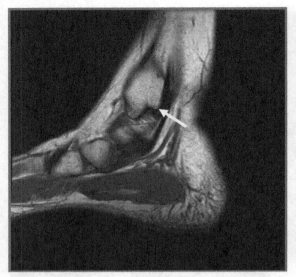

Figure 7.04 • This sagittal T1-weighted MR image of the ankle of a 33-year-old female with hind- and midfoot pain is one of the most medial slices that was captured during this study; notice the position of the medial malleolus (arrow).

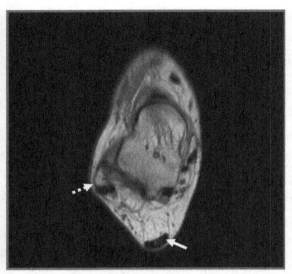

Figure 7.06 • MR imaging of the ankle of a 33-year-old female with hind- and midfoot pain. This axial T1-weighted image is slightly more inferior than in the previous figure. It is useful to start from superior and to work inferiorly to retain an orientation to the image. Note the most distal tip of the lateral malleolus (dashed arrow) and the sickle-shaped Achilles tendon (arrow).

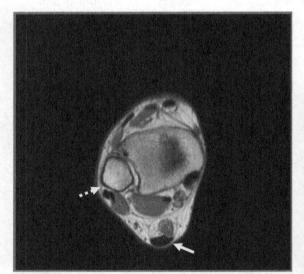

Figure 7.05 • Axial T1-weighted MR image of the left ankle of a 33-year-old female with hind- and midfoot pain. This slice is taken in the region of the distal tibia and fibula. Orientation to this image can be made by using the Achilles tendon (arrow) to determine the posterior, and then, opposing this, the anterior aspects. The fibula, with the peronei tendons wrapping around it (dashed arrow), help determine the lateral aspect of the ankle and, therefore, by elimination, the medial aspect.

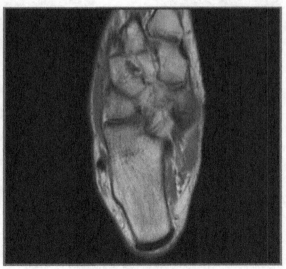

Figure 7.07 • Axial T1-weighted MR image of the ankle of a 33-year-old female with hind- and midfoot pain. This is one of the more distal slices; note the insertion of the Achilles tendon on the calcaneus.

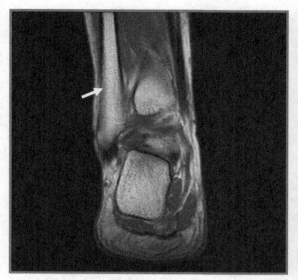

Figure 7.08 • MR imaging of the ankle of a 33-year-old female with hind- and midfoot pain. This is one of the most posterior slices in the coronal plane. On this T1-weighted image, one's orientation is based around the fibula, a lateral structure (arrow); once found, the remaining structures are more easily identified.

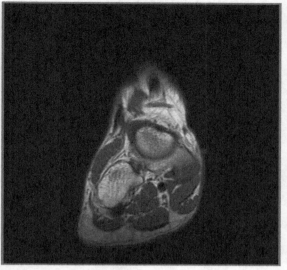

Figure 7.10 • MR imaging of the ankle of a 33-year-old female with hind- and midfoot pain. This is the most anterior slice of a coronal T1-weighted series. It is useful to start with the most posterior slice and then work forward to remain orientated to the image. This slice is performed in the posterior aspect of the midfoot.

image quality and therefore reduce the diagnostic quality. The sequences are the same as in the ankle; however, the sagittal image is performed along the long axis of the metatarsals, and may be referred to as the long axis; the axial slice perpendicular to the second or third metatarsal long axis and which may be referred to as the short axis; and the coronal image in a plane connecting the second and fifth metatarsals. These slight variations are useful to know in order to better orientate the anatomical structures when interpreting the final MR image.

Normal imaging appearance

Although there are a variety of methods to evaluate imaging of the ankle and foot, it is useful to approach the interpretation by identifying individual anatomic structures; from the first, it is important to be aware that there can be a wide variation in appearances, further complicated by the number of potential anomalies. These can be divided into those comprising the soft tissues, including tendons, ligaments and synovial capsules, and fascia; neural; and osseous structures. Our emphasis will be placed primarily on those structures that are commonly implicated in the development of clinical syndromes.

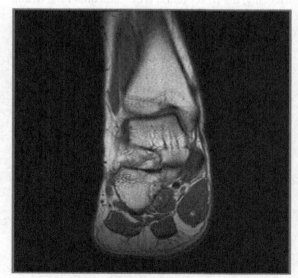

Figure 7.09 • MR imaging of the ankle of a 33-year-old female with hind- and midfoot pain. This image is also in the coronal plane, slightly more anterior than the previous slice. Note the changing form of the bony structures, and the appearance of the sustentaculum tali.

In order to help identify the different structures, the ankle and foot may be divided anatomically into four sections – anterior, posterior, medial and lateral; this helps with both orientation and systematic evaluation.

Tendons

Posterior

The posterior tendons include the Achilles (calcaneal) and plantaris, both of which have associated bursae (Figure 7.11). The **Achilles tendon** has a broad insertion along the posterior aspect of the calcaneus, which is often irregular in this region due to the development of degenerative changes associated with soliciting the tendon during the activities of daily living. The tendon is best seen on the sagittal and axial cuts. Normally, on the

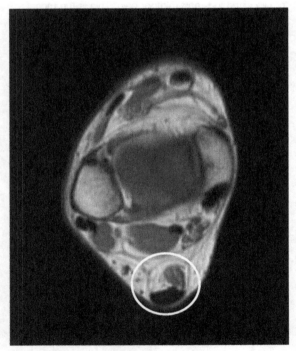

Figure 7.11 • Axial T1-weighted MR image of a patient with ankle discomfort. The posterior tendon structures can be identified (circle) with the most posterior structure representing the Achilles tendon with its low signal intensity. The tendon may demonstrate a small focus of increased signal in its centre, though this is not visible in this patient. Just medial to the Achilles tendon, located anteriorly, is a region of grey, intermediate signal; this represents the soleus muscle.

sagittal imaging, it is noted as a long, relatively thick, low signal intensity structure that courses from the intermediate signal of the gastrocnemius muscle to its insertion on the calcaneus. It thickens somewhat just above this insertion; this should not be interpreted as a focal tendinosis. The tendon should be evaluated on both the T1- and T2-weighted images; on both sequences, it should be seen as a low signal intensity structure.

On axial images, the normal Achilles tendon may contain small regions of slightly brighter signal within it. These are seen on both the T1- and T2-weighted sequences and are due to the internal architecture of the tendons, representing areas where the fibres are gathered together in small pockets. This appearance is normal and should not be confused with the small foci of high signal arising from small micro-tears in the tendon representing degenerative changes or overuse. These are only seen on the T2-weighted images, will be visible on all planes, and suggest a diagnosis of tendinosis. This makes it important to verify the tendon in at least two planes in order to differentiate the normal appearance of the tendon from pathology; correlation with clinical presentation can also help the clinician considerably in this aspect.

Medial

Medially, the flexor tendons descend under the flexor retinaculum; these comprise the tibialis posterior, flexor digitorum longus and flexor hallucis longus (mnemonically referred to as 'Tom, Dick and Harry'). The **tibialis posterior tendon** is prone to rupture, though not as frequently as that of the Achilles tendon.[8]

As the tendon descends to its insertion on the navicular and metatarsals, the shape of the tendon changes on the axial slices from an oval structure to a flatter configuration as it courses past the medial aspect of the talus. As the tendon continues to descend, it divides into smaller bundles as it approaches the navicular and metatarsals.[9] The appearance of this normal fibrous division may be confused with a distal tear; however, tears in the insertions of the tendon are rare and the normal appearance can be confirmed by the lack of high-signal oedema on the fluid-sensitive sequences (Figure 7.12).

The **flexor digitorum longus tendon** runs alongside and superficial to that of the tibialis posterior. It is rarely injured in isolation and is more commonly associated with a generalized regional tendinopathy. The **flexor hallucis longus tendon** has a rather unusual course that can render it susceptible to

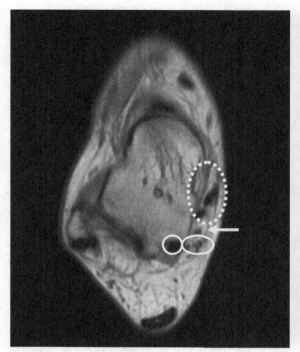

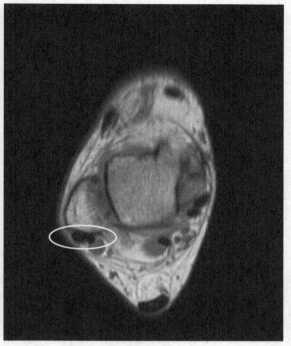

Figure 7.12 • Axial T1-weighted MR image demonstrating the medial soft tissue structures. The hatched oval represents the tibialis posterior tendon located anteriorly, with the flexor digitorum longus tendon lying more posteriorly (hint – use the Achilles tendon to orientate to the image). The arrow points to a small, intermediate signal intensity structure, which represents the posterior tibial vein. Directly posterior to this is an oval within which are located two small round structures, the most medial of these is the posterior tibial artery; the tibial nerve lies laterally. The small circle surrounding the low signal intensity structure represents the flexor hallucis longus.

Figure 7.13 • Axial T1-weighted MR sequence of the ankle demonstrating two small low signal intensity structures enclosed within a white oval. These structures represent the peronei tendons. The most lateral structure (hint – note the lateral malleolus) represents the peroneus longus tendon and the more medial structure, the peroneus brevis tendon. Note their intimate association with the posterior aspect of the lateral malleolus.

Lateral

The **peroneus longus** and brevis tendons are located laterally (Figure 7.13). Both these muscles share the action of eversion and dorsiflexion of the foot.[11] As both tendons descend, they are located posterolaterally to the lateral malleolus. As the tendons pass this region, they are stabilized in part by the superior peroneal retinaculum, which, depending on the imaging quality, can be identified. At this level, the tendon of the peroneus longus is seen as a rounded structure in the axial plane; this helps distinguish it from the flatter appearance of the **peroneus brevis** tendon. As it passes further distally, the peroneus brevis is located anterior to the peroneal tubercle of the calcaneus. Both tendons may be surrounded by a thin layer of fluid on the fluid-sensitive sequences, which is normal. Although there is no formal measurement for the quantification of fluid, more than just a thin layer may be considered as tenosynovitis.

injury. As it passes behind the talus, in those patients who have an os trigonum, friction may be created between the tendon and the accessory ossicle; this can lead to symptoms of posterior impingement, including discomfort and pain on plantar flexion and perhaps focal swelling palpable behind the ankle joint. In the same region, the tendon changes its course from being a predominantly vertical to a more horizontal orientation; during this transition, it can be more prone to injury. The tendon of the flexor hallucis longus is well depicted in its proximal course in both the sagittal and axial planes; as it turns to become more horizontal, it is initially well visualized on the axial and then the sagittal/long axis images as it approaches its insertion.[10]

Anterior

The tendons in this region comprise the tibialis anterior, which lies most medially, then the extensor hallucis longus, extensor digitorum longus and peroneus tertius (Figure 7.14).[12] The tendons pass inferiorly to the superior and inferior divisions of the extensor retinaculum, which may be identifiable on MR imaging. These structures are only occasionally affected by pathology; of the anterior tendons, the **tibialis anterior** tendon is most frequently involved. In particular, the tibialis anterior tendon course is straight with limited opportunity to be impinged by surrounding structures, unlike the posterior compartment structures. The appearance of the tendon on axial slices is that of a round or oval structure, which, as it approaches the insertion points on the first metatarsal and medial cuneiform, becomes flatter. The normal thickness of the tendon within 3 cm of these insertion points is that of no more than 5 mm.[13] Injuries are usually either of a direct nature, which may occur at any age and which may be associated with fractures of soft tissue lesions, or as a result of degenerative processes, in which case the patient is often 60 to 70 years old with chronic symptoms.[14]

Ligaments

The ankle and foot ligaments may also be well visualized using MR imaging; this modality is particularly useful in evaluation of complex or refractory ankle sprains or in those patients who solicit their ankles regularly.[15] However, for routine ankle sprains, clinical examination alone, augmented if necessary by diagnostic ultrasound, is usually sufficient. The ligaments most frequently involved in clinical syndromes are the medial ligament complex (deltoid ligament) and lateral ligament complex. These ligaments are best evaluated using axial MR images, although the sagittal and coronal planes complement these sequences. Generally, ligaments are thin, low signal intensity structures; their identification is relatively straightforward if their anatomical relations are familiar to the examiner.

The ankle ligaments can be divided in to three regions: the lateral ligamentous complex, which is the most prone to injury; the medial group, consisting of the deltoid complex; and the central syndesmosis, or tibiofibular complex, which is important for retaining the stability of the ankle and which may be injured in high-grade ankle traumas,

resulting in instability of the ankle.[16] Often, there is a predominant group of ligaments involved with a secondary or tertiary group affected by means of the 'contre coup' mechanism, so, as the patient rolls over the ankle into inversion, often, a rapid eversion will occur following this, thereby resulting in lateral and medial involvement. The physical examination and diagnostic imaging should take this into consideration.

Lateral

The lateral ligamentous complex comprises the anterior talofibular (ATAF), calcaneofibular and posterior talofibular (PTAF) ligaments. The ATAF is the most commonly injured ankle ligament and is commonly the victim of the typical ankle sprain, whereby the patient has 'turned over' on their ankle.

These ligaments are best seen on the axial projection, where they appear as a low signal intensity linear structure forming the anatomical boundary of the ankle joint capsule. Normally, they appear as a regular structure, posterior to which synovial fluid is contained; this is well depicted on the T2-weighted or STIR images.

The calcaneofibular ligament can be evaluated on the axial slice but, in the opinion of the authors, the coronal oblique fluid-sensitive sequences work best for depicting this ligament, normally seen as a small, thin low signal band extending from the calcaneus to the medial inferior aspect of the lateral malleolus.

The PTAF ligament is a sturdy structure which is rarely damaged, and, when affected, tends to be part of a significant ankle injury. It is well depicted on the axial slices where it is seen as a thick, irregular band of low signal intensity.

Medial

The medial complex of ligaments is composed predominantly of the deltoid ligament, which, from the standpoint of anatomy and imaging, can be subdivided (from anterior to posterior) into tibionavicular, tibiocalaneal and tibiotalar ligaments. The posterior aspect of the tibiotalar ligament is the thickest and is in proximity to the descending tibialis posterior tendon.

The deltoid ligament may be injured as an isolated phenomenon but, more commonly, it occurs in conjunction with a lateral ankle sprain, most probably due to the transfer of forces from one side of the joint to the other – this is why it is always important to test all ligament groups in a patient with an ankle sprain.

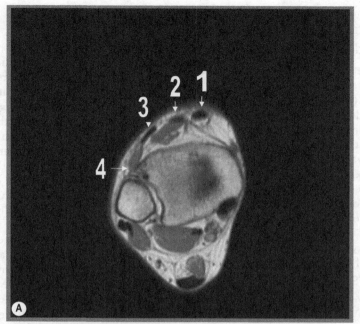

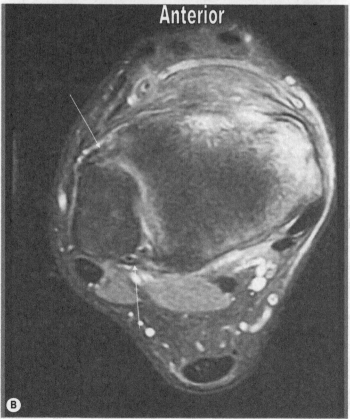

Figure 7.14 • (A) Axial T1-weighted MR image demonstrating the anterior tendon structures. Using the lateral malleolus and Achilles tendon to orientate to the ankle, note that there are a number of low signal intensity structures lying anterior to the tibia and fibula. From medial to lateral, these represent the tibialis posterior (1), the extensor hallucis longus (2), the extensor digitorum longus (3) and the position of the peroneus tertius (4). (B) Axial T2-weighted sequence demonstrating laterally the anterior and posterior tibiofibular ligaments (white arrows). Notice the bright signal in the anteromedial aspect of the distal tibia due to recent trauma, sustained during a rugby match.

Tibiofibular syndesmosis

The syndesmosis between the tibia and fibula is a combination of three anatomical structures: the anterior tibiofibular (ATIF) ligament, behind which the tibiofibular syndesmosis proper is noted as the lower limit of the interosseous membrane; behind this, the posterior tibiofibular (PTIF) ligament is located. The best way to evaluate this region is to work from the most cephalad slice on the axial sequence, where the lower end of the interosseous membrane can be located as a region of relatively thick but regular low signal intensity connecting the tibia and fibula. The ATIF ligament is also well seen on the axial slices as a thin, low signal intensity structure; because of its oblique path, it is necessary to follow it on consecutive slices to be certain that it is fully intact. The PTIF ligament is also nicely demonstrated on the axial slice.

Foot

As with the ankle, ligaments abound in the foot; of particular clinical relevance are the *Lisfranc* and *Chopart* ligaments. The Lisfranc ligament is seen as a band of low signal intensity, connecting the medial cuneiform to the base of the second metatarsal; it confers stability to the midfoot. The Chopart ligament, which also helps stabilize the midfoot, is also known as the *bifurcate ligament*, and is composed of the lateral calcaneonavicular and medial calcaneocuboid ligaments.

Normal variants and developmental anomalies

Osseous variants and paediatric considerations

A number of common variations in the osseous and soft tissue structures may be encountered about the foot and ankle. It is important for the clinician to be familiar with these and their clinical significance.

A frequent cause of foot and ankle pain is the development of accessory ossicles. In the ankle, the two most common accessory ossicles are the *os trigonum* and the *accessory navicular* (or *os tibiale externum*) *bone* (Figure 7.15). An **os trigonum** will be found immediately posterior to the talus and is not usually palpable; therefore, its existence can only be determined by diagnostic imaging. It arises from the failure to fuse of an accessory ossification centre located just posterior to the lateral talar tubercle ossification centre. Normally, this will occur at around 13 years of age; however, in about 10% of the population it remains separated and forms a separate bone (Figure 7.15). In some patients, a pseudoarticulation with the talus may occur.

Although many patients with an os trigonum will be asymptomatic, some will complain of pain in the posterior aspect of the ankle that is worsened by plantar flexion, thus those who dance, run downhill or play football are particularly affected, although even activities of general daily living may be enough to provoke the development of pain. Pain may develop with onset of the condition or remain dormant until later life when altered regional biomechanics create stress between the bony structure and the surrounding soft tissues, most significantly the adjacent tendon of the flexor hallucis longus muscle; this is termed *os trigonum syndrome* or *posterior impingement syndrome*.[17,18]

Posterior impingement syndrome may also develop as a result of a large *talar process* (also known as the *Stieda process*), located on the posterolateral surface of the talus. Both an os trigonum and a long talar process may be detected on routine radiography, particularly on the lateral view. The inflammatory process itself may also be suggested by the obliteration of the posterior margin of Kager's fat pad; however, MR imaging is easily superior in the depiction of the precise location of the bony structure and its effect on the surrounding structures. This allows for the specific grading of any lesion located in the flexor hallucis longus and, with this, the prognosis of the patient. Although MR imaging in any of the three main planes will assist in the precise anatomic location of the bony structure, the sagittal sequence is particularly helpful as it allows for determination of the relative positions of both the osseous structures and the flexor hallucis longus tendon.

In the case of an **accessory navicular**, the patient may complain of discomfort and pain on the medial side of the midfoot and exhibit swelling in the region. With larger accessory navicular bones, the patient may even remark on the presence of a hard mass on the inside of the midfoot, which may cause pressure on the inside of their shoes. On radiographs, a prominent or accessory navicular may be demonstrated just medial to the parent navicular bone. Although an accessory navicular is considered by some to be a post-traumatic lesion – an avulsive fracture of the cartilaginous growth plate – the fact that it is so frequently found bilaterally suggests otherwise.[19]

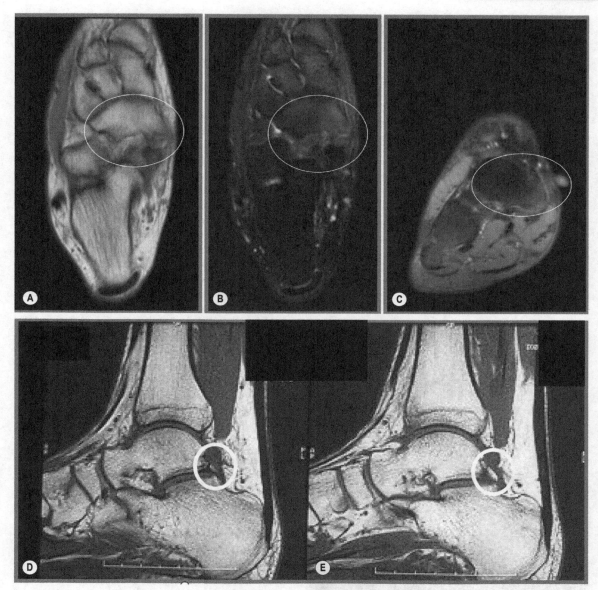

Figure 7.15 • MR imaging of the ankle in the axial plane in T1-weighted (A) and STIR (B) sequences, and in the coronal plane in STIR (C), in a 33-year-old female with pain along the medial aspect of her midfoot, which had begun after wearing new shoes. The ovals enclose the region of abnormality, demonstrating a large navicular with an accessory navicular just medial and posterior to the navicular bone. In (B), a homogeneous region of increased signal is noted in the navicular and accessory navicular, which is also seen in (C). This is due to oedema created by the altered mechanics in this region, and the irritation created by the presence of the accessory navicular bone. By comparison, (D) and (E) represent sagittal slices using T1-weighted sequences and show a separate, marrow-filled structure posterior to the talus, which represents an os trigonum (white circle).

With MR imaging, the relationship of the accessory bone with the surrounding soft tissue structures can again be appreciated to a fuller extent; in particular, the posterior tibialis tendon is particularly vulnerable to tears in the presence of an accessory navicular. Other pathologies that may arise include the development of a painful bursa, or the development of bone marrow oedema in either the accessory navicular or parent navicular bone.[20]

Although diagnostic ultrasound can also be used to detect the dynamic relationship of the soft tissue structures, the detail that is achieved with MR imaging provides a higher degree of accuracy and a better overview of the region in question; musculoskeletal ultrasound is limited in the depth to which it can penetrate and cannot readily demonstrate conditions such as bone marrow oedema that can add considerably to the clinician's clinical thinking.

Muscular variations

The most common and clinically significant muscular variant is the presence of a fourth peroneus muscle, peroneus quartus. Although small, this supplementary muscle can have clinical consequences (Figure 7.16).

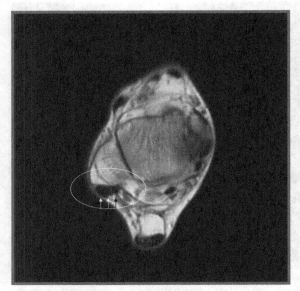

Figure 7.16 • Axial T1-weighted MR sequence of a 57-year-old male who complained of discomfort in the posterior aspect of his ankle; the region outlined by the white oval contains three low signal intensity structures. The lateral two, indicated by the white arrows, represent the tendons of peroneus longus (left arrow) and brevis; however, there is a third region of low signal intensity noted, marked by a black arrow. This represents the peroneus quartus, which may on occasion be associated with peroneus brevis tears, owing to the increased pressure on the peroneal retinaculum, which is stretched around the tendons.

Pathological conditions

Osseous conditions

Trauma

Trauma to the ankle and foot constitutes a major proportion of injuries to the musculoskeletal system as a whole; which of us has not, at some time, turned our ankle or stubbed our toe, even if the consequences are usually no more than a few days' discomfort? Although radiography is useful in identifying the basic injury in many cases, further imaging may be necessary if symptoms persist or complications develop or, in the case of an athlete, to determine exactly the degree of injury sustained.[14] MR imaging is ideal to assess such injuries, being able to determine the osseous and soft tissue relationships, aiding in the development of clinical management strategies and in establishing the patient's prognosis.

Although a slightly simplistic approach, it is helpful to divide foot and ankle trauma into acute and chronic presentations (some patients will of course present with an acute clinical syndrome following recent trauma on top of a pre-existing chronic injury, as in the case of a new ankle sprain in a patient who has had a previous clinical history of multiple sprains).

Acute trauma

Acute trauma represents a common presenting complaint, such as that relating to a sporting activity whereby an acute twisting injury results in impaction between the osseous structures (particularly of the ankle) and tears of the soft tissue structures surrounding the region. In such cases, regions of high signal intensity within the osseous structures may be detected soon after the injury; this represents bone marrow oedema. The pattern of this oedema may assist in determining the direction of injury and therefore help to identify the associated soft tissue structures that may be implicated.[14]

A common complication of such an injury is fragmentation of a piece of articular cartilage, which may be attached to the underlying bone, forming a *chondral* or *osteochondral defect* respectively. The talar dome is a particularly common site for such injuries to occur. In addition to a history of recent ankle trauma, the patient may also report a sensation of the articulation being 'blocked' during normal activity or, at times, sudden immobility or 'locking' following simple movement. The patient may also notice that the joint becomes intermittently swollen; the physical examination will often confirm this through visual observation or a related reduction in the joint's range of motion.[21,22]

Whilst routine radiography is often used in the first instance to assess the osseous and articular aspects of the ankle, avascular necrosis in its early stages is usually negative on these studies. MR imaging allows identification of such injuries at a much earlier stage and can give much more detail regarding the level of the articular cartilage damage, the extent of displacement of the fragment and the viability of the donor site. Osteochondral defects are particularly well demonstrated using MR imaging and intra-articular contrast is not normally required (Figure 7.17).[15]

This makes the acquisition of images non-invasive, as compared with computed tomography (CT), wherein iodinated contrast is normally necessary to evaluate the articular cartilage, carrying a risk of complications and potential discomfort for a patient who is already in pain. MR imaging is also superior in providing an overall view of the articulation, identifying other factors that may affect the clinical management of the patient, such as bone marrow oedema or injury to surrounding soft tissue structures.[23]

If there is less than 10 mm of fragment displacement and no rotation of the fragment with respect to the donor site, treatment may simply involve partial or complete immobilization; however, surgery may be required to return the fragment to the donor site if there is significant displacement or an awkward positioning of the fragment. If there is an associated chondral injury (for example fibrillation), grafting, autologous or otherwise, may be considered.[24,25]

On MR imaging, the view that is particularly useful in determining the presence of an intra-articular fragment and assessing cartilage damage is the STIR or T2-weighted coronal images; the sagittal and axial images will provide the dimensions of the donor site and, therefore, the extent of the lesion. MR imaging can also provide further information regarding associated injuries. These lesions are often associated with ankle sprains; consequently, a careful evaluation of the ligaments about the ankle is an important part of the evaluation routine.[17,26]

Chronic trauma

Chronic trauma may also be well visualized on MR imaging and may result from repeated injuries such as those sustained in consecutive ankle sprains, or be related to abnormal biomechanics. This may be intrinsic (congenital, developmental or acquired) or extrinsic, for example from ill-fitting footwear (Figure 7.18).

An example of a clinical syndrome related to inappropriate shoes is *Haglund's syndrome* (or deformity), whereby wearing high heels or poorly fitting 'basketball shoes' causes chronic irritation to the posterior aspect of the ankle. The patient, often a woman, will complain of pain and swelling around the posterosuperior aspect of the calcaneus and demonstrate a noticeable lump in the same region. The condition is often complicated by retrocalcaneal bursitis, retro-Achilles bursitis and thickening of the distal Achilles tendon (Figure 7.19).[27,28]

Although a number of treatment options are available, first and foremost to correct the precipitating cause, surgery is often required to modify the surrounding bony structures and to reduce the thickening of the tendon. Similar effects may occur in the other bones of the ankle and of the foot, either due to poor-fitting footwear or in those who place a high demand on their feet, such as long-distance runners.[29,30]

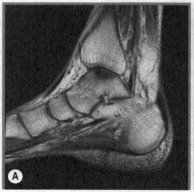
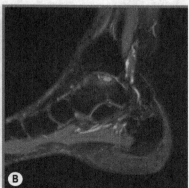

Figure 7.17 • MR images of a 57-year-old male suffering with ankle pain and a sensation of the joint catching on occasion. T1-weighted (A) and STIR (B) sequences in the sagittal plane demonstrate an abnormality of the dome of the talus. In (A), a region of low signal is noted involving the majority of the articular surface of the talus. This is well visualized as a region of high signal intensity on the STIR sequence, where, in addition, irregularity of the articular surface of the talus is noted.

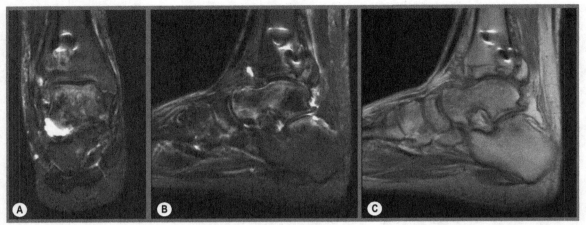

Figure 7.18 • A 33-year-old female presenting with pain in the ankle and foot following surgery for ligamentous tears about the ankle (the low signal intensity regions in the distal tibia are bony screws). MR imaging of the ankle and midfoot was performed in the coronal plane (**A**) and sagittal plane (**B, C**); these demonstrate that, on the T2-weighted images of (**A**) and (**B**), regions of diffuse heterogeneous increased signal intensity are noted in the talus, navicular and cuneiformis. This represents bone marrow oedema, which, on a T1-weighted image (**C**), is visible as a heterogeneous decrease in signal intensity. The patient is thought to have developed the regions of bone marrow oedema secondary to the altered mechanical stress placed on the ankle and foot following surgery. No associated soft tissue swelling was noted.

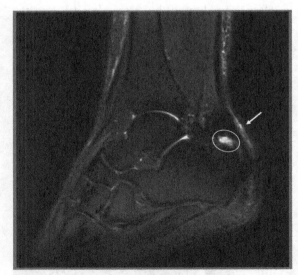

Figure 7.19 • A 40-year-old female presented with discomfort about the posterior aspect of her ankle, which was worsened when using high heels. Sagittal STIR imaging of the ankle demonstrates a retrocalcaneal (oval) and retro-Achilles (arrow) bursitis. The Achilles tendon is thickened at its most distal aspect due to chronic irritation. This imaging triad of bursitis in the retrocalcaneal and retro-Achilles bursa and thickening of the Achilles tendon has been referred to as Haglund's deformity.

Such patients are also at risk of developing stress fractures, which usually present with diffuse pain that is difficult to localize. Eventually, particularly if the precipitating activity is not curtailed, the pain will focus over the affected region, most commonly the diaphysis of the second or third metatarsal. Although routine radiography may demonstrate a local periosteal response and a bone scan may demonstrate focal increased uptake corresponding to a local increase in bone metabolic activity, the MR images will be able to grade the stress fracture from a simple local periostitis to a complete, though often radiographically subtle, fracture.[3]

The T2-weighted images will demonstrate oedema in the periosteum, perhaps in the medullary cavity and in the surrounding periosteal tissues, whilst the T1-weighted sequences can be used to determine the degree of cortical thickening due to the periostitis and the actual fracture line. Clinical management includes reducing or eliminating the causative activity, modifying footwear and, if necessary, the use of an air cast. Further evaluation of underlying bone density issues is important to eliminate osteopenia, which can cause an insufficiency fracture.

Avascular necrosis

Both the foot and ankle can be affected by avascular necrosis, although the condition has a predilection for the head of the second or third metatarsal and for the talus. In the foot, the major predisposing factor appears to be increased biomechanical stress, often associated with footwear; in particular, high heels. By contrast, the condition when seen in the ankle, usually follows specific, identifiable trauma.[31]

Routine radiography can demonstrate the classic changes of avascular necrosis: increased density in the subarticular region, subchondral fracture and, eventually, articular surface collapse; however, MR imaging will show these findings at a significantly earlier stage. It can also be used to detect any associated bone marrow oedema, which may perpetuate the patient's symptoms, and evaluate the local structures for any associated injury. MR imaging will normally demonstrate avascular necrosis of the heads of the metatarsals as a high signal on the fluid-sensitive sequences in all planes, with focal low signal intensity just under the head of the metatarsal involved.[32,33]

Ligaments

The most commonly injured ligaments in the region are the lateral ligaments of the ankle; often, the patient will have a history of repetitively turning over on their ankle with the development of pain, swelling and perhaps discoloration about the anterolateral aspect of the ankle. Although ankle sprains may be the result of the application of altered stress to the ankle, conditions such as tarsal coalition may predispose the patient to repetitive sprains. Coalition should be evaluated during the clinical examination, where a stiff midfoot will be detected, perhaps associated with a pes planus deformity.

Radiographs are useful in identifying coalition, which tends to occur between the calcaneus and navicular or calcaneus and talus. Although MR imaging is not necessarily systematically used in those patients with coalition, if the patient has a clinical history of repeated ankle sprains and pain or limitation of activity, MR imaging can be useful to determine the presence of a fibrous synchondrosis, and associated bone marrow oedema that may accompany this, as well as for the evaluation of the effects of the coalition, in determining the most appropriate management of the patient.[34,35]

In cases of a partial or complete rupture, this ligament is most easily assessed using the axial images. By placing the patient's foot in slight dorsiflexion, the whole ligament will be included in a single slice, making the interpretation easier. If this is not possible, it is important to trace the ligament in its entirety as it courses obliquely from its origin on the medial aspect of the lateral malleolus to its insertion on the lateral aspect of the talus. If this ligament is torn, either partial or complete disruption of the fibres will be noted on MR images; in addition, on the fluid-sensitive sequences, the high-signal synovial fluid will be seen tracking out anterior to the normal position of the ligament, indicating that the synovial capsule has been broached.[34,35]

In patients with a history of repeated sprains, the ligament may appear irregular and thickened with small foci of increased signal within it on the fluid-sensitive sequences; this is due to chronic inflammatory changes. The ATAF ligament may be injured as an isolated phenomenon, or be a component of more complex sprains. Depending on anatomical factors and the position of the ankle during the injury event, the calcaneofibular and, to a lesser extent, the PTAF may also be involved.

The calcaneofibular ligament is also often involved clinically; again, fluid may be noted surrounding the ligament in cases of partial or complete rupture, which helps to confirm the presence and severity of injury.

When injured, the posterior tibiotalar ligament may be associated with a small amount of fluid, which extends to surround the descending tibialis posterior fibres, suggesting a tendinopathy of this tendon, when in fact it is just the result of the inflammation associated with the damaged tibiotalar ligament.

Although the PTIF ligament is rarely injured in isolation, when damaged, as may be the case following a severe trauma to the ankle, which may be accompanied by fractures affecting the ankle complex, loss of the normally well-defined low signal intensity linear ligament as well as noting surrounding high signal owing to the leakage of the synovial fluid is useful to determine injury.[10,36]

Both the Lisfranc and Chopart ligaments may be involved in disruption following a direct or indirect trauma and may be associated with fracture/dislocations of the articulations contributing to the region in question. This is the case particularly with patients affected by diabetes where the Lisfranc fracture/dislocation injury may occur, causing either an adduction or abduction injury as well as dorsal subluxation of the base of the second metatarsal.[37,38]

Tendons

Tears of the tendons about the ankle and foot may also be evaluated well with MR imaging, especially when associated bony injuries and additional soft tissue structures need to be evaluated. If small foci of high signal are noted within tendons on T2-weighted images, a diagnosis of tendinosis should be considered. This appearance is caused by small micro-tears in the tendon, arising from degenerative changes or overuse. Partial or complete ruptures of the tendon may also occur; however, owing to the relative ease of clinical differentiation and the importance of rapid surgical intervention, MR imaging is not routinely performed. In cases where the diagnosis is unclear, where the presence of a partial,

high-grade rupture is being considered, MR imaging will demonstrate the tendon as being irregular and frayed, with small or moderate regions of high signal on the T2-weighted sequence.[5]

In the **Achilles tendon**, which is particularly prone to rupture, these regions are usually found 4–6 cm proximal to the insertion of the tendon into the calcaneus, thought to be a less vascular region, thus rendering the tendon more susceptible to injury (Figure 7.20). They need to be differentiated from the small regions of slightly brighter signal arising from the internal architecture of the tendons, which are seen on both the T1- and T2-weighted sequences rather than the fluid-sensitive sequences alone.

The clinical presentation of a patient with an Achilles tendinosis will differ from that of a complete

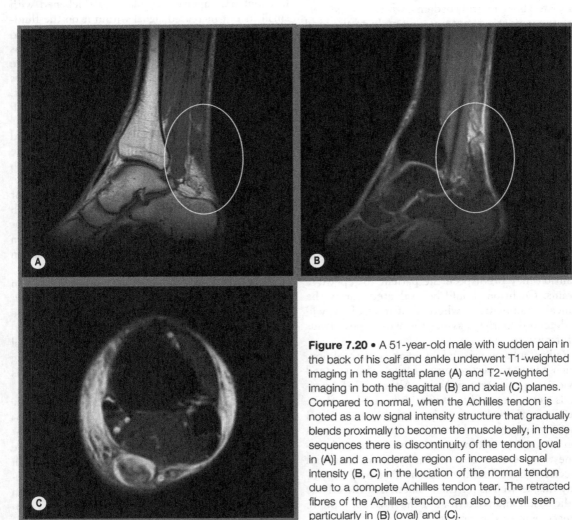

Figure 7.20 • A 51-year-old male with sudden pain in the back of his calf and ankle underwent T1-weighted imaging in the sagittal plane (A) and T2-weighted imaging in both the sagittal (B) and axial (C) planes. Compared to normal, when the Achilles tendon is noted as a low signal intensity structure that gradually blends proximally to become the muscle belly, in these sequences there is discontinuity of the tendon [oval in (A)] and a moderate region of increased signal intensity (B, C) in the location of the normal tendon due to a complete Achilles tendon tear. The retracted fibres of the Achilles tendon can also be well seen particularly in (B) (oval) and (C).

rupture of the tendon. With a patient who has tendinosis, there is, in general, local pain that worsens with activity such as running or an activity that will solicit the use of the tendon. In a patient who has a complete rupture of the tendon, the predominant complaint of the patient is a total inability to move the ankle, due to the loss of the normal function of the tendon. As a result of this, the patient will not necessarily have pain as the major symptom. In a complete rupture, MR imaging is not necessarily the technique of choice to confirm the diagnosis, the clinical history and examination usually suffice for this purpose, whereas in a tendinosis, which may be associated with micro- or small macro-tears, further imaging may be useful to determine the extent of the tear. In this case, ultrasound may be useful but not as informative as MR imaging to determine the local effect of the problem.

The **tibialis posterior** tendon is also prone to rupture, though not nearly as frequently as that of the Achilles tendon. During its course, proximal to its passage past the medial malleolus, the tendon can become irritated with a tendinopathy being created. This can be observed on the fluid-sensitive sequences as bright or high signal in the region of the tendon, which is normally found positioned deeply to its companion tendons, flexor digitorum longus and flexor hallucis longus.

As the descending tendon passes the navicular, normal variants may occur; these may, on occasion, cause irritation and tendinopathy. Such normal variants can include a large accessory navicular bone, located medial to the parent navicular. In certain populations, such as dancers and athletes, such large accessory navicular bones can produce a friction effect with the posterior tibialis tendon and also create irritation, and an inflammatory reaction with the parent bone via the partially formed synchondrosis.[39,40]

The posterior tibial artery, nerve and vein are located between flexor digitorum longus and flexor hallucis longus (Figure 7.12). Occasionally, vascular lesions such as varices can be detected on MR imaging, usually after the clinical examination. MR imaging would not be the imaging modality of choice to detect the varicosities, being detectable following the clinical examination with ultrasound; however, on occasion, large tortuous varicosities may irritate surrounding soft tissue structures such as the tendons and ligaments about the ankle, leading to the development of symptoms of pain, swelling and limitation of movement about the ankle joint.

The peronei can also develop tendinoses: the peroneus longus tendon is more prone to tendinopathy; the peroneus brevis tendon is more prone to acute tears, either partial or complete. Such tears may be associated with bony lesions, such as the *Dancer's* or *Jones' fracture*, an avulsion fracture located at the styloid process of the base of the fifth metatarsal. With such an injury, the patient will normally have focal pain, swelling and a sense of lack of stability about the lateral aspect of the midfoot (it is important to determine whether this sensation is from the ankle or, as in this case, more distally located).[31,41]

Infection

In predisposed populations, such as those with diabetes mellitus, infection of the distal lower extremity is relatively common and carries with it high morbidity and mortality; therefore, astute diagnosis and management of the patient is essential. Despite other techniques being available for the detection of infection, MR imaging remains the most cost-effective and accurate examination modality in differentiating osteomyelitis from soft tissue infection and visualizing associated complications such as abscess formation (Figure 7.21).[5]

Whilst the patient may not be fully aware of the presence or extent of infection, examination may reveal a region of focal swelling or redness, accompanied by an alteration in the general health status of the patient. Depending on the degree of sensory loss, pain and tenderness will be variable features. Close inspection of the plantar surface is particularly important, to search for portals of entry for infection; in some cases, evidence of the sinus tract will also be identifiable. Extra care is needed when palpating the foot of a diabetic, owing to the increased friability of the skin.

On routine imaging, osteomyelitis may not become visible for up to 10 days post-implantation, the *radiographic latent period*. However, it is clearly important to make the diagnosis as early as possible to instigate the appropriate management protocols, namely antibiotics and control of associated comorbidity; therefore, where clinical suspicion exists, further imaging is appropriate. This may involve a bone scan but, to best determine the presence of osteomyelitis and the effect that it has on the surrounding osseous and soft tissue architecture, MR imaging is the modality of choice, using a normal series with, if possible, the addition of gadolinium

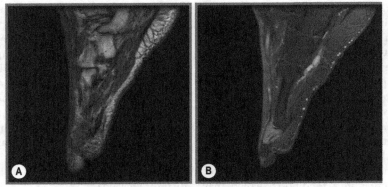

Figure 7.21 • A 79-year-old female presented with pain and swelling in her first ray. Sagittal T1-weighted (A) and STIR (B) images demonstrate a region of decreased signal intensity within the bone in (A), with an associated mass in the soft tissue surrounding the bone both superior and inferiorly. On the STIR sequence (B), the lesion is well identified in the proximal phalanx, with increased signal intensity throughout, destruction of the cortices and extension in to the surrounding soft tissues; this is an example of osteomyelitis, in this case secondary to known diabetes mellitus.

to detect subtle foci of active infection that may otherwise remain occult.[42]

Within the bone marrow, osteomyelitis will provoke a high signal intensity on the fluid-sensitive sequences; by contrast, the signal on the T1-weighted sequences will appear as hypointense compared to the normal marrow. Regions of osseous destruction will be well defined on these images. Any involvement of the surrounding soft tissue can also be demonstrated well with MR imaging: the development of a periperiosteal inflammatory response, abscess formation and eventually sinus tract development can all be evaluated, as can the response to medical management. Where surgical debridement has been employed, the results can be monitored non-invasively to confirm resolution of the osteomyelitis and the development of possible complications. This is particularly useful for patients such as diabetics, who may need to be evaluated over many years, and allows comparisons to be made with previous studies, which helps to determine subtle changes suggestive of new infective foci.[43,44]

Morton's neuroma

Most commonly occurring in between the third and fourth rays, Morton's neuroma is an enlargement of a nerve, usually at the point where the lateral plantar nerve combines with part of the medial plantar nerve. The nerve lies in subcutaneous tissue, just above the fat pad of the foot, close to an artery and vein and superficial to the deep transverse metatarsal ligament.[9,16] In patients predisposed by pes planus or by unsuitable footwear, the nerve is compressed between the contact point of a shoe and the strong, relatively inflexible ligament.[42,45]

The condition, which is not a true neuroma and is more accurately termed *Morton's metatarsalgia*, needs to be differentiated from **intermetatarsal bursitis** (Figure 7.22). It can be extremely disabling,

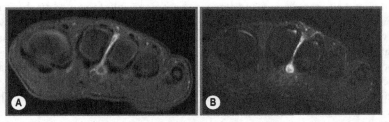

Figure 7.22 • Axial T2-weighted (A) and T1-weighted with contrast (B) MR images of the foot, demonstrating a region of high signal intensity about the inferior aspect of the intermetatarsal space between the second and third metatarsal. This region exhibits a moderate degree of enhancement with the addition of contrast (B), due to the presence of an intermetatarsal bursitis, which, clinically, can easily be confused with Morton's neuroma.

not just causing local, sometimes exquisite, pain but also altering lower limb biomechanics, limiting the choice of footwear and activities of daily living, such as shopping. Often, the patients are middle-aged women who have progressively developed pain in the second and third metatarsal spaces, either unilaterally or, at times, bilaterally.[46]

Although observation of the region does not usually reveal a great deal, palpation will often recreate the exquisite pain associated with the conditions. The standard orthopaedic test is the *squeeze test*, whereby pressure is applied in a superficial to deep direction from the first and fifth metatarsals, thereby compressing the inter-metatarsal structures and recreating pain in patients with either pathology.[47]

Routine radiography will normally provide no useful information. Ultrasonography, in the hands of an experienced operator, can be extremely helpful both in diagnosis and for guiding hydrocortisone injection into the site; however, despite the requirement in this instance for contrast, MR imaging is still widely used for evaluation of this region, partly because it is easier to interpret but also because it offers better scope for differentiating Morton's neuroma from soft tissue tumours. The lesion will be intermediate signal on T1-weighted imaging and low signal on T2-weighted imaging. If contrast is

used, the lesion is well demonstrated with intense uptake; contrast can also help with patients who redevelop symptoms after surgical resection in differentiating the development of a new neuroma from scar tissue.[42,45]

Plantar fasciitis

A potentially disabling condition, plantar fasciitis is commonest in the middle-aged patient, who typically reports the development of progressive discomfort and then pain along the proximal aspect of the plantar surface of their hind- to midfoot. On observation, there is not usually evidence of swelling, but on direct palpation over the origin of the short plantar muscles as well as of the fascia, exquisite pain may be elicited.

Whilst MR imaging is not warranted for simple cases of plantar fasciitis, for those patients with persistent pain, or where surgery is being considered, MR imaging may provide additional clinical information to determine the origin of the pain and identify which anatomical structures are involved (Figure 7.23).[48] The plantar fascia and involved muscles are well visualized on the sagittal, fluid-sensitive images, which will demonstrate regions of increased signal in and about the tendinous insertions into the

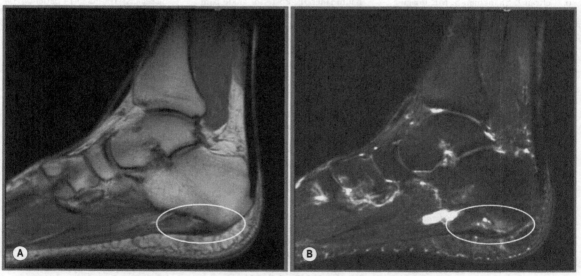

Figure 7.23 • A 54-year-old female presented with severe pain in the base of the ankle. MR imaging of the ankle has been performed in the sagittal plane using T1-weighted (A) and T2-weighted (B) sequences. On the T2-weighted image, a focal region of increased signal intensity is noted in the calcaneus at the insertion of the plantar fascia (oval). On the T1-weighted image, the same region is noted, though now with low signal intensity, with thickening of the plantar fascia noted (oval); this is an example of moderate plantar fasciitis.

calcaneus as well as thickening of the plantar fascia to more than 5 mm in thickness. MR imaging is important in those patients who are resistant to conservative management, to determine the extent of inflammation, identify the muscle origins that are the cause of the pain, provide a visual guide to any intervention for pain relief, and indicate the presence and extent of the commonly associated plantar enthesophyte, which may require surgical excision. It can also differentiate the condition from osteomyelitis in the underlying calcaneus, which can mimic the symptoms.[49]

References

1. Haukka E, Leino-Arjas P, Solovieva S, et al. Co-occurrence of musculoskeletal pain among female kitchen workers. *Int Arch Occup Environ Health*. 2006;80(2): 141–148.

2. Young MF. The physics of anatomy. In: *Essential Physics for Muscloskeletal Medicine*. Edinburgh: Elsevier; 2009.

3. Moran DS, Evans RK, Hadad E. Imaging of lower extremity stress fracture injuries. *Sports Med*. 2008; 38(4):345–356.

4. O'Connor PJ, Rankine J, Gibbon WW, et al. Interobserver variation in sonography of the painful shoulder. *J Clin Ultrasound*. 2005; 33(2):53–56.

5. Kaplan P, Helms C, Dussault R, Anderson M. Foot and ankle. In: *Musculoskeletal MRI*. Philadelphia: WB Saunders; 2001:384–430.

6. Beltran J, Shankman S. MR imaging of bone lesions of the ankle and foot. *Magn Reson Imaging Clin N Am*. 2001;9(3):553–566, xi.

7. Bergin D, Morrison WB. Postoperative imaging of the ankle and foot. *Radiol Clin North Am*. 2006;44(3):391–406.

8. Moore K. The upper limb. In: *Clinically Oriented Anatomy*. 2nd ed. Baltimore: Williams and Wilkins; 1985:626–793.

9. Standring S, ed. *Gray's Anatomy – Pelvic girdle and lower limb – foot and ankle (Section 115)*. Edinburgh: Elsevier; 2009.

10. Kaplan P, Helms C, Dussault R, Anderson M. *Musculoskeletal MRI*. Philadelphia: WB Saunders; 2001.

11. Joseph J. Muscles and fascia of the lower limb. In: Hamilton W, ed. *Textbook of Human Anatomy*. 2nd ed. London: Macmillan; 1976:179–195.

12. Lee MH, Chung CB, Cho JH, et al. Tibialis anterior tendon and extensor retinaculum: imaging in cadavers and patients with tendon tear. *Am J Roentgenol*. 2006;187(2): W161–W168.

13. Mengiardi B, Pfirrmann CW, Vienne P, et al. Anterior tibial tendon abnormalities: MR imaging findings. *Radiology*. 2005;235(3):977–984.

14. Morrison WB. Magnetic resonance imaging of sports injuries of the ankle. *Top Magn Reson Imaging*. 2003;14(2):179–197.

15. Pontell D, Hallivis R, Dollard MD. Sports injuries in the pediatric and adolescent foot and ankle: common overuse and acute presentations. *Clin Podiatr Med Surg*. 2006;23(1): 209–231, x.

16. Moore K. The lower limb. In: *Clinically Oriented Anatomy*. 2nd ed. Baltimore: Williams and Wilkins; 1985:396–564.

17. Cortes ZE, Harris AM, Baumhauer JF. Posterior ankle pain diagnosed positional MRI of the ankle: a unique case of posterior ankle impingement and osteonecrosis of the talus. *Foot Ankle Int*. 2006;27(4):293–295.

18. Messiou C, Robinson P, O'Connor PJ, Grainger A. Subacute posteromedial impingement of the ankle in athletes: MR imaging evaluation and ultrasound guided therapy. *Skeletal Radiol*. 2006;35(2):88–94.

19. Rowe L, Yochum T, eds. *Essentials of Skeletal Radiology*. 2nd ed. Baltimore: Williams and Wilkins; 2004.

20. Kaplan P, Helms C, Dussault R, Anderson M. Temporomandibular joint. In: *Musculoskeletal MRI*. Philadelphia: WB Saunders; 2001:169–173.

21. Wischer TK, Bredella MA, Genant HK, et al. Perthes lesion (a variant of the Bankart lesion): MR imaging and MR arthrographic findings with surgical correlation.

AJR Am J Roentgenol. 2002;178(1):233–237.

22. Kennedy J. What are osteochondral defects? Available from: http://www.osteochondraldefects.com Accessed 02.03.09.

23. Malfair D. Therapeutic and diagnostic joint injections. *Radiol Clin North Am*. 2008;46(3): 439–453 v.

24. Bhosale AM, Richardson JB. Articular cartilage: structure, injuries and review of management. *Br Med Bull*. 2008;87:77–95.

25. Fritz RC. MR imaging of osteochondral and articular lesions. *Magn Reson Imaging Clin N Am*. 1997;5(3):579–602.

26. De Smet AA, Fisher DR, Burnstein MI, et al. Value of MR imaging in staging osteochondral lesions of the talus (osteochondritis dissecans): results in 14 patients. *Am J Roentgenol*. 1990;154(3):555–558.

27. Sella EJ, Caminear DS, McLarney EA. Haglund's syndrome. *J Foot Ankle Surg*. 1998;37(2):110–114, discussion 73.

28. Lee JC, Calder JD, Healy JC. Posterior impingement syndromes of the ankle. *Semin Musculoskelet Radiol*. 2008;12(2):154–169.

29. Sofka CM, Adler RS, Positano R, et al. Haglund's syndrome: diagnosis and treatment using sonography. *HSS J*. 2006; 2(1):27–29.

30. Jerosch J, Schunck J, Sokkar SH. Endoscopic calcaneoplasty (ECP) as a surgical treatment of Haglund's syndrome. *Knee Surg Sports Traumatol Arthrosc*. 2007;15(7): 927–934.

31. Rowe L, Yochum T. Trauma. In: Yochum T, Rowe L, eds. *Essentials of Skeletal Radiology*. 2nd ed. Baltimore: Williams and Wilkins; 1996:653–794.

32. Leduc S, Clare MP, Laflamme GY, Walling AK. Posttraumatic avascular

necrosis of the talus. *Foot Ankle Clin.* 2008;13(4):753–765.

33. Love JN, O'Mara S. Freiberg's Disease in the Emergency Department. *J Emerg Med.* 2008;38(4):e23–5.

34. Patel CV. The foot and ankle: MR imaging of uniquely pediatric disorders. *Magn Reson Imaging Clin N Am.* 2009;17(3):539–547, vii.

35. Staser J, Karmazyn B, Lubicky J. Radiographic diagnosis of posterior facet talocalcaneal coalition. *Pediatr Radiol.* 2007;37(1):79–81.

36. Stoller D. *Magnetic Resonance Imaging in Orthopaedics and Sports Medicine.* 2nd ed. Philadelphia: Lippincott Williams and Wilkins; 1996.

37. Kavanagh EC, Zoga AC. MRI of trauma to the foot and ankle. *Semin Musculoskelet Radiol.* 2006;10(4): 308–327.

38. Chilvers M, Donahue M, Nassar L, Manoli 2nd A. Foot and ankle injuries in elite female gymnasts. *Foot Ankle Int.* 2007;28(2):214–218.

39. Fredrick LA, Beall DP, Ly JQ, Fish JR. The symptomatic accessory navicular bone: a report and discussion of the clinical presentation. *Curr Probl Diagn Radiol.* 2005;34(2):47–50.

40. Omey ML, Micheli LJ. Foot and ankle problems in the young athlete. *Med Sci Sports Exerc.* 1999;31(suppl 7): S470–S486.

41. Beers M, Berkow R. *The Merck Manual.* 17th ed. West Point, PA: Merck & Co; 1999.

42. Masala S, Fiori R, Marinetti A, et al. Imaging the ankle and foot and using magnetic resonance imaging. *Int J Low Extrem Wounds.* 2003;2(4): 217–232.

43. Stoller DW, Tirman PF, Bredella MA. *Diagnostic Imaging Orthopaedics.* Salt Lake City: Amirsys Inc; 2003.

44. Berquist T. *MRI of the Musculoskeletal System 4th ed.* Philadelphia: Lippincott Williams and Wilkins; 2000.

45. Bancroft LW, Peterson JJ, Kransdorf MJ. Imaging of soft tissue lesions of the foot and ankle. *Radiol Clin North Am.* 2008;46(6): 1093–1103, vii.

46. Hassouna H, Singh D. Morton's metatarsalgia: pathogenesis, aetiology and current management. *Acta Orthop Belg.* 2005;71(6): 646–655.

47. Eustace S, Johnston C, O'Neill P, O'Byrne J. The foot and ankle. In: *Sports Injuries: Examination, Imaging and Management.* Edinburgh: Elsevier Churchill Livingstone; 2007:19–86.

48. Osborne HR, Breidahl WH, Allison GT. Critical differences in lateral X-rays with and without a diagnosis of plantar fasciitis. *J Sci Med Sport.* 2006;9(3): 231–237.

49. Recht MP, Donley BG. Magnetic resonance imaging of the foot and ankle. *J Am Acad Orthop Surg.* 2001;9(3):187–199.

The shoulder

8

Peter J. Scordilis   Julie-Marthe Grenier
Michelle A. Wessely   Martin Young

Introduction

Upper extremity pain and, more specifically, shoulder pain is a common complaint in the general population[1,2] and is a familiar presentation to any physician in primary care.[2-4] The incidence of new episodes of shoulder pain is approximately 11 per 1000 presentations in general practice,[2] making it responsible for 16% of all musculoskeletal complaints.[1] The complex arrangements of soft tissue structures in the shoulder joint, as well as its proximity to significant neurovascular anatomy, renders it a difficult joint to assess, while the combination of the joint's instability and mobility subject it to an increased probability of injury.[5,6]

A multitude of pain generators can be responsible for shoulder pain and these are not merely limited to local structures; referred pain from spinal structures is also a common cause of shoulder pain.[7,8] This myriad of clinical factors requires the primary care physician to have an advanced understanding of shoulder joint anatomy and pathophysiology, as well as a more than cursory knowledge of appropriate physical examination and diagnostic imaging procedures to correctly diagnose an injury.

Evaluation of the shoulder joint typically includes plain film radiography; however, many common shoulder complaints involve soft tissue structures not detectable using radiographs. Magnetic resonance (MR) imaging offers unmatched anatomical detail, relative ease of assessment and high accuracy and allows multiplanar assessment.[9,10] These attributes have made MR imaging the procedure of choice for evaluation of occult fractures, articular structures and soft tissues of the shoulder including tendons, ligaments, muscles and capsulolabral structures[11] despite its relatively high cost and occasional limited availability in some regions.[12]

History and examination

In assessing the painful shoulder, it is necessary to evaluate all possible pain generators and contributing conditions. While many shoulder disorders have their signature clinical presentations, many also tend to precipitate secondary conditions or are common comorbidities; it is relatively uncommon for an isolated condition to be the sole cause of shoulder pain in a patient.[13]

Of key importance to the diagnostic process is an accurate history of both the present complaint and previous episodes; occupational- and sports-related factors; epidemiological data; injury pathomechanics; exacerbating activities; and other diagnosed conditions that may (or may not) directly affect the shoulder joint. In most cases of shoulder pain, a careful, well-directed history will lead to a correct diagnosis.[14,15]

Physical examination procedures including specific provocative tests are vital to the diagnostic picture and play a large role in directing imaging and, consequently, management decisions. Both active and passive range of motion and muscle testing will provide important information to the clinician, although many traumatic injuries may limit the ability to perform them. It is important not to mistake muscle failure resulting from the pain induced by provocation testing with muscle weakness. Palpation will help to localize

© 2011, Elsevier Ltd.
DOI: 10.1016/B978-0-443-06726-6.00008-1

the site of pain as well as identify palpable deformities related to dislocations or separations. The differential diagnosis can be further refined by conducting special tests; these tests, their associated clinical findings and significance are discussed later in conjunction with the conditions to which they pertain in order to allow the physician to correlate their imaging findings with their investigative procedures.[14]

Assessment of shoulder pain also necessitates evaluation of the cervical spine owing to the frequency of complaints coexisting in both areas.[16,17] Pain related to the majority of common shoulder conditions typically does not extend beyond the elbow; this finding should direct the clinician towards a cervical, brachial plexus or peripheral nerve lesion.[8]

Differential diagnosis

The most important differential diagnostic considerations to be given by the musculoskeletal specialist to a patient with shoulder pain are rheumatological conditions and referred pain from visceral pathology.

The most challenging aspect of these conditions is that they can often coexist with or underlie genuine musculoskeletal injury and be overlooked or only become apparent when a patient's injury starts to heal.

The range of common conditions that can mimic shoulder injury is detailed and discussed in Table 8.01.

Clinical indications for diagnostic imaging

If the history and examination are sufficiently proficient, then often the diagnosis will be self-evident and no diagnostic imaging required. However, in the event of significant trauma; if the patient's pain is uncontrolled or precludes adequate physical examination; or in the event that the patient fails to respond to conservative therapy, there is an occasionally confusing wealth of imaging possibilities available to the physician.[18]

Table 8.01 Differential diagnosis of shoulder conditions

Condition	Effect on shoulder	Clinical features
Biliary disease	Right-sided pain	Jaundice Hepatomegaly Altered stools Ascites
Blood or gas in peritoneal cavity	Referred to side of diaphragmatic irritation	Ascites Distension
Blood or gas in pleural cavity	Referred to side of diaphragmatic irritation	Cough Altered breath sounds History of trauma, smoking or tuberculosis
Subphrenic abscess	Referred to side of diaphragmatic irritation	Concomitant abdominal symptoms
Cardiac disease	Left shoulder pain	Altered heart sounds Cardiovascular findings Worsening pain on exercise
Splenic trauma	Left shoulder pain	History of abdominal trauma Ascites Anaemia
Polymyalgia rheumatica	Bilateral	Elevated ESR (>50 mm/hr) Geriatric presentation Nocturnal/morning pain Fever, weight loss

Plain radiographs are often still the first step in diagnostic imaging and can reveal fractures, dislocation and neoplastic osseous lesions; pathology in the thoracic outlet/inlet; acromioclavicular joint changes; calcification of soft tissues; and degenerative joint disease. The most common protocol for the shoulder is anteroposterior views with the shoulder in internal and then external rotation and 'baby arm' (neutral abduction); these views may be supplemented by transaxillary, scapular outlet or 'Y' (Lamy) views if indicated by the clinical findings.[19–21] The physician also must consider whether acromioclavicular, cervical spine or chest x-rays are required.

Computed tomography (CT) has, to an extent, fallen into disuse, as has arthrography; although both can have a role to play in assessment, it is rare for primary contact practitioners to order such special imaging. Advanced imaging for the most part now consists of ultrasonography and MR imaging.

Ultrasound, as a diagnostic modality, has developed markedly over recent years to the point where it can rival MR imaging in its depiction of soft tissue pathology in certain instances; these include the principal shoulder tendons. Although it is unlikely to supplant MRI as the primary means of evaluating tendon pathology and is dependent on operator skill, ultrasound plays an important role in the evaluation of the rotator cuff and offers a number of obvious advantages, including lack of ionizing radiation, portability in the office setting, high patient acceptance, low cost, and lack of medical contraindications.[22,23]

MR imaging has become the gold standard for diagnostic imaging of the shoulder, particularly with regard to injuries of the soft tissues. It is non-invasive and offers a high degree of resolution, enabling the evaluation of multiple potential pathological processes. It should be considered by the clinician whenever further evaluation of non-osseous structures is required, or as a follow-up to inconclusive plain film radiographs.[18]

Techniques and protocols

MR imaging of the shoulder should enable visualization of the anatomy surrounding the glenohumeral and acromioclavicular joints in the axial, and oblique sagittal and coronal planes. Whilst the neurovascular bundle can be visualized on typical shoulder MR images, separate MR neurography studies are required to assess the brachial plexus.[10] MR imaging

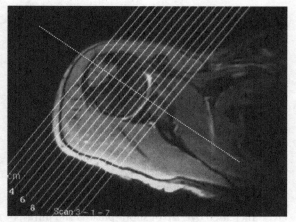

Figure 8.01 • An example of an axial scout view or 'plan scan', obtained on a 25-year-old female patient with shoulder instability. The lines demonstrate the angle of the sagittal oblique images, parallel to the glenoid fossa (approximately 30°) with 2-mm slices. The dotted line represents the plane of imaging for the coronal oblique sequences.

of the shoulder customarily includes images in all three planes with T1-weighted, T2-weighted and proton density (PD) sequences. Fat saturation techniques are usually performed only upon request and are becoming more popular during faster acquisition sequences (fast spin echo and gradient echo); their utility will be discussed later.

The localizer, or 'scout', is a single axial view through the glenohumeral joint, used to plan all the subsequent acquisitions (Figure 8.01). This view allows for the sagittal slices to be obtained parallel to the glenoid fossa; these are termed sagittal obliques, owing to their non-parallel relationship to the true anatomical plane. Based on the scout view, the coronal oblique slices are obtained perpendicular to the glenoid fossa, parallel to the supraspinatus tendon. The fibres of the supraspinatus tendon, as well as the glenohumeral joint, are slightly oblique to the true coronal plane, hence the images are orientated to reflect this, and the resultant images are termed *coronal obliques*. If true or direct coronal images were to be obtained, the supraspinatus muscle and tendon would appear discontinuous and shortened, mimicking tears.[10,24,25]

Patient placement and cooperation are critical during the procedure. The patient should lie supine with the involved arm at their side, supported by sponges, in neutral to slight external rotation. A surface coil will most likely be used to ensure greater image quality. Because the shoulder joint will be lateral to the isocentre of the magnet, the diagnostic area of the magnetic field will be inhomogeneous, which may lead to artifacts and lower-quality images without the use of a coil.[10,25]

Extreme rotation of the arm is not recommended, even if it allows good visualization of the glenoid labrum. This position is difficult to maintain for patients, causing pain, distorting the biceps tendon and increasing the chance for motion artifacts (figure motion artifact). In this position, the synovium can also become redundant and may mimic a soft tissue mass.[24,25] If the arm is placed in internal rotation, the supraspinatus tendon curves anteriorly and leaves the oblique coronal plane and the capsule will appear lax.[26] Increased overlap of supraspinatus and infraspinatus tendons, as well as signal changes at the infraspinatus insertion, may mimic tears. It is important to note that a small percentage of shoulders will demonstrate these findings when imaged in the neutral position as well,[27] making it necessary to evaluate suspected findings in all planes and with all sequences.

Some authors have also suggested image acquisition during complete abduction and external rotation of the arm, termed the ABER manoeuvre (Figure 8.02).

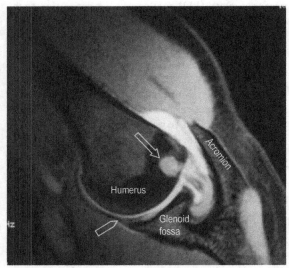

Figure 8.02 • MR imaging of the right shoulder: T2-weighted, fat-saturated sequence. This image was obtained with the patient in the ABER (abduction, external rotation) position. The patient was a 34-year-old female presenting with signs of impingement. A large, high signal area is noted in the humeral head, representing a subchondral cyst (arrow). Also noted is the close relationship between the glenoid labrum and the articular capsule (arrowhead).

Studies have shown better visualization of partial cuff tears and labrum tears utilizing this position in conjunction with arthrography than images obtained with arthrography only.[28–30] This position is, however, difficult to maintain for long periods of time, decreasing patient compliance and increasing pain level and motion artifacts.[10,24,25] Even experienced technicians require additional time for patient placement, positioning and image acquisition, adding substantial time to an already time-consuming procedure. These images will usually be obtained during MR arthrography and are typically reserved for inconclusive findings on conventional MR or arthrography.[31]

In the neutral position, both coronal oblique and axial slices allow good visualization of the rotator cuff muscles. The superior and inferior portions of the labrum as well as the subscapularis notch can be well viewed on the coronal images, whilst the anterior and posterior portions of the labrum can be well viewed on the axial slices. The supraspinatus muscle and tendon should be observed in their entire length on the coronal oblique images. Sagittal oblique projections demonstrate the coracoacromial arch, including the coracoclavicular and coracoacromial ligaments and the undersurface of the acromioclavicular joint. All of these structures are important in determining the cause and type of impingement, which will be addressed later in the chapter.

As a general guide, T1-weighted sequences have the highest level of anatomical detail. Bone marrow and peri-articular fat both display high signal intensity. On T2-weighted images, soft tissue oedema or other fluid collections, such as that seen in bursitis, are depicted as high intensity zones. These sequences are also better suited for identification of pathologies and may help in the assessment of artifacts found on T1-weighted images, such as the **'magic angle' phenomenon:** when a structure is oriented at 55° to the main magnetic field, it will appear as an area of hyperintensity on T1-weighted sequences, mimicking pathology.[32] This angle has been termed the 'magic' angle and can appear in MR imaging of various body regions, including, in the shoulder, the supraspinatus tendon, glenoid labrum and biceps tendon. Muscle, ligaments and tendons will appear as areas of low signal intensity on both sequences. Proton density-weighted sequences use a relatively long relaxation time (TR) and short echo time (TE) and have shown a high sensitivity for detection of injury to the rotator cuff and glenoid labrum and capsular complex. Fast spin echo (FSE) sequences have more recently been used to decrease imaging time and improve signal-to-noise ratio. Fat will appear brighter with this technique, which may obscure small lesions adjacent to lipid structures, including subtle defects of the rotator cuff tendons and pathological bursal fluid.[33] Fat saturation techniques can minimize these effects and help with the differentiation between fluid and fat at their interface; this can increase the sensitivity for detecting partial tears.[34]

Use of intra-articular contrast (arthrography) may enhance partial articular surface tears of the rotator cuff muscles or increase conspicuity of the capsulolabral anatomy;[35-37] however, it is usually performed only on unresponsive patients or after an inconclusive non-contrast study. To perform the procedure, a needle is inserted into the glenohumeral joint under fluoroscopy. In order to verify intra-articular positioning, a small amount of iodinated contrast is injected and an image is taken to confirm correct placement. Following this, 10 to 16 ml of dilute gadopentetate dimeglumine is injected in to the intra-articular space, avoiding both the introduction of air and overdistension of the joint.[38] An alternative procedure involves injection of saline solution followed by gentle shoulder mobilization (within patient tolerance) prior to the FSE MR imaging study.[31] The use of local anaesthetic has the advantage of not masking the area if an aberrant injection is made.[38] The procedure is typically painful to the patient and is associated with the typical risks of a mildly invasive procedure; expectations should be discussed prior to the procedure. Utilization of MR arthrography for specific conditions will be discussed individually throughout the chapter.

Normal anatomy

Osseous structures

Biomechanically, the shoulder is the most complicated articulation in the body. It comprises the glenohumeral, acromioclavicular and sternoclavicular joints, which, together with the articulation between the scapula and the true ribs, form a closed-loop kinematic chain.[39-41] The shoulder has multitudinous muscle attachments, supporting ligaments and bursae, many of which demonstrate interrelated comorbidities when the shoulder is affected by internal derangements.[5,6] The major advantage of MR imaging, as compared with plain film radiography, is the visualization of these soft tissue structures

and their pathoanatomical interrelationships, the most common source of pain when addressing shoulder complaints.[2,42]

The *sternoclavicular joint* is a synovial 'saddle' joint (sellaris) and represents the only point of contact between the pectoral girdle and axial skeleton.[6,41] The *glenohumeral joint* is a 'ball and socket' (spheroidal) synovial joint, allowing three degrees of freedom.[6,41] It occurs between the *glenoid fossa* of the scapula, which is shallow and lined with hyaline cartilage, as is the reciprocal articulating surface of the *humeral head*. Hyaline cartilage, unlike fibrocartilage, will show up as an area of intermediate signal intensity on both T1- and T2-weighted sequences. The fossa is rimmed by a fibrocartilaginous disc known as the *glenoid labrum* (Figures 8.03, 8.04), which will show up as a low intensity area on most sequences. Six labral variants have been noted, with more variability in the anterior labrum (Table 8.02).

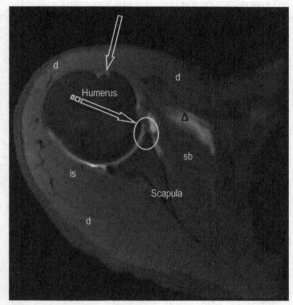

Figure 8.03 • Axial, T2-weighted, fat-suppressed MR image through the mid-portion of the glenohumeral joint, below the supraspinatus muscle. The biceps tendon is well seen, outlined by the fluid-filled synovial sheath (arrow). The subscapularis bursa is visible and identified by the delta symbol (Δ). It is of high signal intensity, or fluid-filled, due to its continuity with the articular capsule. Only the subscapularis and infraspinatus bursae should be visualized in a non-inflamed shoulder. A small cleft is visible between the glenoid labrum and the scapula, representing a normal variant, often mistaken for glenoid tears (striped arrow and oval). The key to the legend is detailed in Box 8.01.

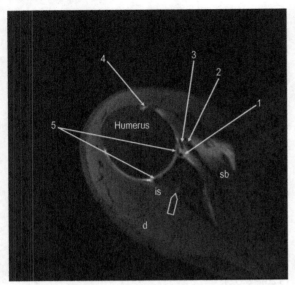

Figure 8.04 • An axial, T2-weighted, fat-suppressed MR image through the glenohumeral joint (slightly superior to Figure 8.03) through the plane of the subscapularis tendon. The suprascapular neurovascular bundle is demonstrated by the arrowhead. 1 = anterior capsular reflection; 2 = subscapularis tendon; 3 = middle glenohumeral ligament; 4 = bicipital tendon and synovial sheath; 5 = anterior and posterior glenoid labrum.

Table 8.02 The glenoid labrum: congenital variants[43]

Variant	Frequency anterior	Frequency posterior
Triangular	45%	71%
Round	19%	12%
Cleft	15%	0%
Notched	8%	0%
Flat	7%	6%
Absent	6%	8%

It is important to note these variations so as not to confuse them with pathology and to be aware of the lack of variability in the posterior labrum, where cleaved or notched patterns should raise suspicion of a tear. Of additional note is posterosuperior labral absence, which is considered a normal variant.[43] The labrum is the site of the fibrous attachment of the glenohumeral ligaments and the joint capsule to the scapula. In most patients, the hyaline cartilage of the glenoid fossa will extend beneath the labrum, creating an area of increased intensity (referred to by some as *undercutting*) that may be confused with a tear.[25,44,45] Increased signal intensity has been identified in both the posterosuperior and anteroinferior labrum without a tear, owing to the 'magic angle' phenomenon.[46] It is useful to be aware that posterosuperior labrum tears are more common in athletes involved in throwing and there should be increased clinical suspicion in the physician diagnosing this population.[47]

The articular capsule extends from the glenoid labrum to the humeral head. Three proximal capsular attachment variants have been described and can occur at the anterior labrum. Type I capsules insert at the tip or base of the labrum, whilst type II insert no more than 1 cm medial to the labrum. Both will appear with approximately the same frequency at the anterior labrum. Type III capsules occur in about 4% of shoulders, insert more than 1 cm medially and are usually indistinguishable from congenital synovial pouches or capsular stripping. If type II or III capsules are found posteriorly, this should raise clinical suspicion of injury.[43] The synovial lining of the capsule extends to form a sheath around the proximal aspect of the long head of the biceps muscle.[41]

The coracohumeral and the three glenohumeral ligaments may be difficult to evaluate separately from the capsule; indeed, they are usually regarded as capsular folds or thickenings.[10,24,48,49] Of these, the *inferior glenohumeral ligament* is the largest and most important; it forms the axillary recess of the capsule. The *superior glenohumeral ligament* is the smallest and its function is not well understood; in 3–10% of the population, it is congenitally absent.[24] In many of these instances, the *medial glenohumeral ligament* is thickened and cord-like and attaches directly to the superior labrum at the base of the biceps tendon. The combination of the two anomalies is referred to as the *Buford complex* and has been reported to occur in 1.5% of the population.[50]

Another variation of the capsular-ligamentous complex is a labrum foramen, a hole in which a small detachment of the anterosuperior corner of the labrum is present; this occurs in 12% of the population.[51] In as many as three-quarters of the population, a sublabral recess/sulcus may form between the bicipito-labral complex and the superior portion of the glenoid fossa by a synovial reflection.[52] All three of these variants can easily be mistaken for labral tears.

Anatomical variants in bone marrow may be confused with pathologies on MR. On T1-weighted MR sequences, red (haematopoietic) marrow appears as an area of **hypo**intensity, whilst yellow (fatty) marrow appears as an area of **hyper**intensity. As individuals age, red marrow is converted to yellow marrow, starting distally and moving towards the appendicular skeleton. Adult marrow patterns are typically realized by the age of 18–21 years, although residual red marrow is a common finding. It is important to note that an area of hypointensity, usually visualized as a subcortical curvilinear distribution in the medial humeral head, is a typical location for residual or reconverted marrow.[53,54] This should not be mistaken for marrow disease and will occur in the absence of soft tissue mass, cortical destruction or medullary expansion.[31] The finding will be relatively symmetrical and imaging of the contralateral shoulder may help with differentiation.

The head of the humerus has a normal anatomical flattening that occurs underneath the path of the teres minor muscle as it inserts on the lateral portion of the humeral head. It is important to differentiate this normal finding from a *Hill–Sachs impaction fracture* (Figure 8.05). Differentiation on individual axial images cannot be made with confidence by either the size of the indentation or its location in the axial plane. The most accurate way to distinguish the two entities is by their position on the long axis of the humerus. Hill–Sachs lesions will be visible within the superior 5 mm of the humeral head and typically extend up to 18 mm from the top of the humeral head. They should be visible within the first two transaxial sections. In contrast, normal flattening occurs 20 mm or more caudal to the humeral head.[55]

Whilst it may be possible for lesions to extend further caudally and overlap the normal groove, they can be differentiated by viewing the more cephalic slices. In addition, in a new or recent Hill–Sachs lesion, associated bone marrow oedema will be noted surrounding the depression of the superolateral aspect of the humeral head. Often, the Hill–Sachs lesion is associated with additional lesions, particularly the *Bankart lesion* (either cartilaginous or osteocartilaginous).[56,57]

The *acromioclavicular* joint is regarded as a 'gliding' (plane) synovial joint although in reality a number of variations exist that can affect either articular surface, though in a reciprocal manner.[41] Acromial morphology was first categorized by Bigliani[58] into three shapes:

- Type I acromion is characterized by a flat undersurface.
- Type II is characterized by a curved undersurface.
- Type III is characterized by a hooked undersurface (Figure 8.06).

The last two, non-planar variations are associated with a higher predisposition to degenerative change.[59] A fourth acromial configuration, with a convex undersurface, has since been identified[60] but it is considered uncommon and no correlation has been made between this shape and impingement.[31] The prevalence of each acromial type in the general population and in subjects with painful shoulders remains uncertain.[58,61,62]

Both joint surfaces are covered by fibrocartilage, sometimes mixed with the hyaline cartilage more typically associated with synovial articulations.[41,63] The joint contains a disc, which is highly variable: true discs are relatively rare but, when present, can divide the joint in two; more commonly, the disc is a meniscus, whose fibrocartilage structure can be difficult to differentiate from the articular surfaces of the joint. The disc is frequently degenerate and can be congenitally absent.[63,64]

When viewing the acromion in the coronal oblique plane, a common finding is an area of hypointensity projecting inferolaterally from the lateral aspect of the acromion, termed a 'pseudospur'; this is the normal inferior tendon slip of the deltoid insertion on the acromion and should not be confused with a spur.[45] If any doubt exists, correlation with findings on other imaging planes or plain film radiography will be helpful (Figure 8.07).

Muscles

MR imaging also allows for a good assessment of the major muscle groups of the shoulder and their tendons, in particular the rotator cuff group, the biceps and deltoid muscles. Muscle and tendon should appear hypointense on T1- and T2-weighted sequences (Figures 8.03, 8.04, 8.08–8.12; Box 8.01). When observing the supraspinatus tendon on T1-weighted sequences, any areas of increased signal intensity must be correlated with T2-weighted images to avoid misdiagnosis due to the magic angle phenomenon (Figure 8.13).[30] This most commonly occurs at the critical zone, where the tendon angles anteriorly and where tendon pathology is most commonly located.[45]

On axial slices, the biceps tendon is well visualized within the bicipital groove; it is maintained there in part by the transverse ligament of the humerus, an

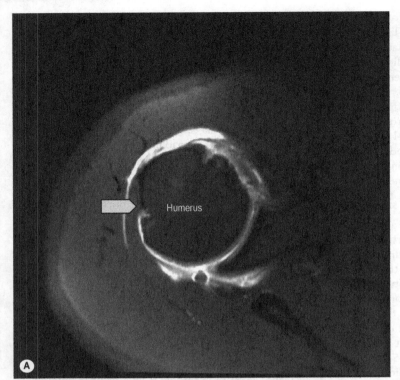

Humerus

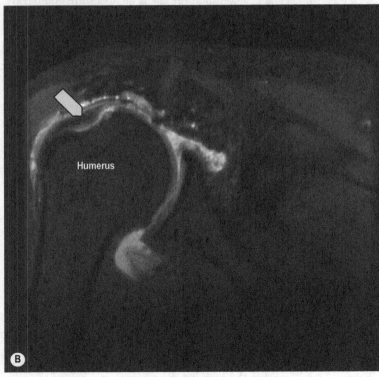

Humerus

Figure 8.05 • T2-weighted axial (A) and coronal oblique (B) MR images demonstrate a Hill–Sachs deformity in the classic location, superior posterolateral aspect of the humeral head (arrowhead).

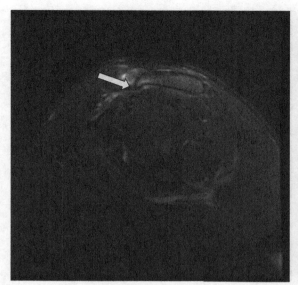

Figure 8.06 • Sagittal oblique MR image demonstrating a 'hooked' or type III acromion (arrow). This acromial type has been most clearly linked with impingement.

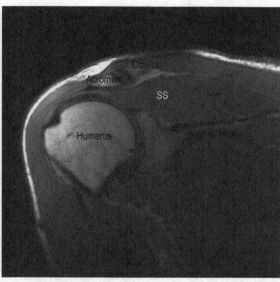

Figure 8.08 • Coronal oblique, T1-weighted MR image. Note the hyperintensity of fat and the increased intensity of bone as compared to the T2-weighted images.

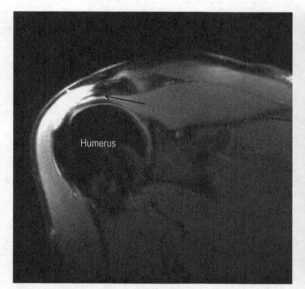

Figure 8.07 • Coronal oblique, T2-weighted MR image demonstrating a low signal intensity structure projecting inferiorly from the lateral border of the acromion (arrow). This 'pseudospur' can be further evaluated through plain film imaging or on alternate imaging planes for confirmation.

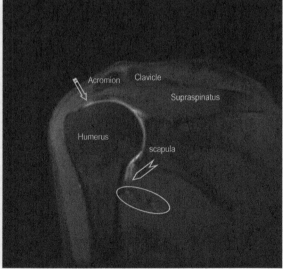

Figure 8.09 • Coronal oblique, T2-weighted, fat-suppressed image through the supraspinatus muscle and tendon. Note the variability in the signal of the supraspinatus tendon. The focal, high intensity region is called the 'critical zone' (striped arrow). This image also allows for good visualization of the acromioclavicular joint and capsule. The axillary recess is identified by the arrowhead. The neurovascular bundle is visible just below as circular areas of variable signal intensities (oval).

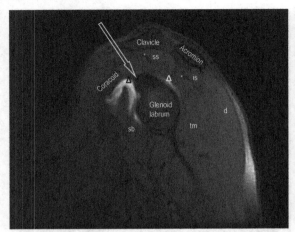

Figure 8.10 • Sagittal oblique, T2-weighted, fat-suppressed MR image through the glenohumeral joint. The main muscle groups are identified. The supraspinatus and infraspinatus tendons respectively are visualized as intramuscular, low intensity zones (*). The root of the biceps tendon is indicated by the arrow. The subscapularis and infraspinatus bursae are seen as high intensity zones (Δ).

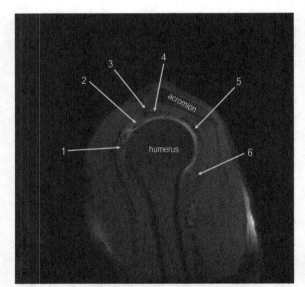

Figure 8.11 • Sagittal oblique, T2-weighted, fat-suppressed MR image through the middle of the humerus, several slices lateral to Figure 8.10. This slice allows for visualization of the tendons of the main muscle groups. These structures are most at risk for impingement, owing to their proximity to the undersurface of the coracoacromial arch. 1 = subscapularis tendon and muscle; 2 = long head of the biceps; 3 = coracoacromial ligament; 4 = supraspinatus tendon; 5 = infraspinatus tendon; 6 = teres minor muscle and tendon.

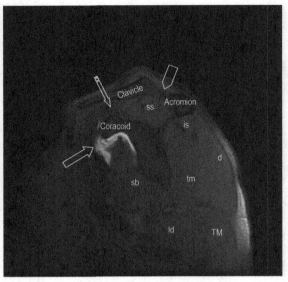

Figure 8.12 • Sagittal oblique, T2-weighted, fat-suppressed MR image though the medial scapula demonstrating the coracoacromial arch and main muscle groups. This image is slightly medial to Figure 8.05. The high intensity zone adjacent to the coracoid process represents the subscapularis bursa (arrow). Note the position of the supraspinatus muscle and tendon, occupying the entire space between the clavicle and scapula. The coracoclavicular ligament is shown by the striped arrow and the acromioclavicular ligament by the arrowhead.

Box 8.01

Key to legend for figures

ss:	Supraspinatus muscle
is:	Infraspinatus muscle
sb:	Subscapularis muscle
d:	Deltoid muscle
tm:	Teres minor muscle
TM:	Teres major muscle
ld:	Latissimus dorsi muscle
MTJ:	Musculotendinous junction

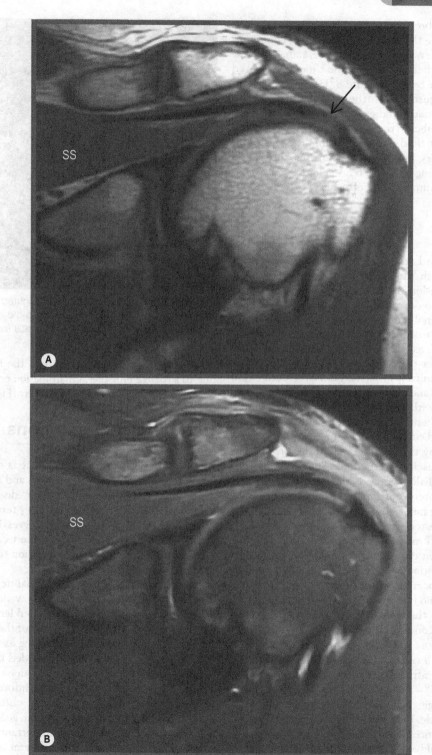

Figure 8.13 • Coronal oblique, T1-weighted MR image (A) showing a hyperintense region (arrow) in the supraspinatus tendon region that does not increase in intensity on the T2-weighted image (B); this is the 'magic angle' phenomenon.

expansion of fibres contributed by the subscapularis tendon. Because the biceps tendon sheath communicates with the glenohumeral joint space, a small amount of fluid in the sheath is normal and should be located posterior to the tendon (Figure 8.03). A round, focal fluid collection just lateral to the biceps tendon may also be noted; anatomical studies have identified this as the anterolateral branch of the anterior circumflex humeral vessels, and not fluid collection within the sheath. In normal shoulders, fluid should not encircle the tendon and such a finding indicates tendon injury, inflammation or a glenohumeral joint effusion.[45]

Bursae

The subscapular bursa is the only bursa communicating directly with the glenohumeral joint and represents an extension of the capsular synovial sheath. Communication occurs mainly between the superior and middle glenohumeral ligaments. It is considered that the purpose of this bursa is to protect the subscapularis tendon as it travels beneath the coracoid process and over the scapular neck.[65]

The most clinically important bursal structures are the subdeltoid and subacromial bursae. They do not communicate with the joint; however, in most individuals, they are contiguous structures although are variable in size and configuration. Superiorly, the bursae are bordered by the acromion and inferiorly by the rotator cuff muscles and tendons. The medial border stretches medially beyond the acromioclavicular joint, and the lateral portion to the greater tuberosity. Anteriorly, the bursa covers portions of the bicipital groove and posteriorly it lies between the deltoid and rotator cuff muscles. This ensures proper gliding motion between the rotator cuff and coracoacromial arch. Inflammation of these bursae can be related to impingement or rotator cuff diseases.[65,66]

A subcoracoid bursa is common and does not communicate with the glenohumeral joint but has been reported to communicate with the subdeltoid–subacromial bursa in anywhere from 11% to 55% of subjects.[67] Both calcific and non-calcific subcoracoid bursitis is an infrequent cause of isolated anterior shoulder pain.[68]

The MR imaging appearance of all bursae should be isointense to muscle. If increased signal is observed on T2-weighted sequences, it should be considered a sign of effusion. Fluid should only be observed in the joint space as a fine line between the two articular surfaces, in communicating bursae or surrounding the long head of the biceps

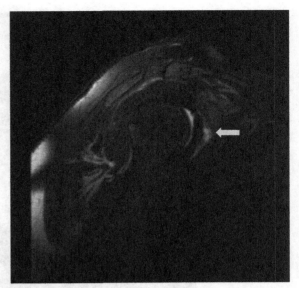

Figure 8.14 • Sagittal oblique, T2-weighted MR image; note the hyperintense area posterior to the coracoid process indicative of subcoracoid bursitis (arrow).

tendon. Increased signal intensity in the bursa can be due to a rotator cuff tear, inflammation or inadvertent injection into the bursa on arthrography (Figure 8.14).[66]

Pathological conditions

In assessing the painful shoulder, it is necessary to evaluate all possible pain generators and contributing conditions. While many shoulder disorders have their own clinical presentations, they tend to precipitate or follow each other in the progression of shoulder dysfunction, yielding concomitant conditions. It is uncommon for an isolated condition to be the sole cause of shoulder pain in a patient.

The multitude of imaging modalities, tests and physical examination procedures available further compound the complexity of shoulder evaluation. In addition, clinicians need be aware of the normal variants and diagnostic pitfalls appearing as normal with MR imaging. The information provided by MR imaging should never be solely relied upon but should instead be integrated with clinical information so as to improve diagnosis and treatment outcomes.

When identifying the primary pain generator in the shoulder, two entities are very important to consider: rotator cuff disease and glenohumeral instability, as they are typically involved as either precipitating factors for or consequences of shoulder injuries.

Rotator cuff disease

The term *rotator cuff disease* covers a wide range of conditions involving the muscles and tendons of the rotator cuff and associated structures. The rotator cuff is responsible for shoulder movement, dynamic stabilization and muscular balance about the glenohumeral joint. Two important actions of the group are depression of the humeral head by counteracting the force of the deltoid and compression of the humeral head into the glenoid fossa, reinforcing the joint capsule.[6] Controversy still exists regarding the pathophysiology of rotator cuff disease, although several mechanisms have been described. An understanding of the anatomy of the region as well as the kinematics of the joints is necessary to determine which mechanism is responsible for the cuff pathology.[69–71]

Impingement syndromes

Subacromial impingement syndrome (SIS) is a frequent cause of rotator cuff disease and occurs most commonly when the rotator cuff tendons, long head of the biceps brachialis or subacromial bursa are compressed and inflamed.[72] Put more simply, any structure travelling through the subacromial space that is subject to inflammation or injury can be affected by any number of obstructions in the space.

Primary, extrinsic impingement involves the anatomical structures of the coracoacromial arch. This has been attributed to forward elevation of the shoulder[73] as well as to variant acromial morphology, as discussed earlier.[58–60] Type I acromion has the least correlation to impingement syndrome (3%) while the type III acromion (Figure 8.06) has the highest correlation (70%–80%). Variable frequencies of each of the three types of acromion have been reported in the population. It is important to note that symmetrical morphology is frequent (70%) and that type III acromion is more common in males.[62] Acromial slope and position have also been implicated in impingement syndrome[74] as they can alter the shape and size of the outlet, although this remains controversial.[75–77] A low-lying acromion has been correlated to degenerative changes[74] and may be due to instability of the acromioclavicular joint.

Osteophytes of the acromioclavicular joint and the undersurface of the acromion have both been implicated in impingement (Figure 8.15).[31] An *os acromiale*, the unfused apophysis of one or more of the three ossification centres of the acromion, has been reported to occur in 1%–15% of the population (Figure 8.16).

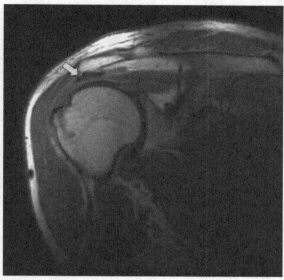

Figure 8.15 • Coronal oblique, T1-weighted MR image with a subacromial degenerative spur pointing inferior (arrow).

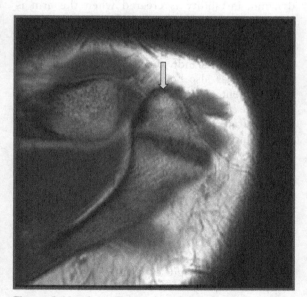

Figure 8.16 • Axial, T1-weighted MR image through the superior portion of the joint. Note the unfused ossification centre of the acromion, termed an os acromiale (arrow).

The presence of osteophytic spurring or instability of the os acromiale may lead to supraspinatus impingement.[78] The subacromial space may also be narrowed by a thickened coracoacromial ligament.[79]

Secondary, extrinsic impingement usually occurs without any abnormalities of the coracoacromial arch.

Table 8.03 Classification factors in glenohumeral instability

Factor	Range
Frequency	Acute
	Chronic
	Recurrent
Degree	Subluxation
	Dislocation
Aetiology	Traumatic
	Microtraumatic
	Atraumatic
Direction	Anterior
	Posterior
	Inferior
	Multidirectional

Instead, the impingement syndrome is related to glenohumeral instability (Table 8.03). This dynamic instability is created when the arm is abducted and externally rotated, causing impingement against the acromion and coracoacromial ligament; rotator cuff pathology is typically less advanced in these individuals.[80,81] Scapulothoracic instability has also been implicated in secondary impingement, where abnormal scapular motion can create a narrowed subacromial space.[82,83] Clinically, differentiation between these two causes of impingement is vital to allow treatment to address the underlying instability.[84]

Primary impingement generally occurs in the post-35-year-old population and presents with positive impingement tests without shoulder instability. Secondary impingement is due to anterior instability from repetitive trauma or the excessive demands of throwing and overhead activities. It generally affects a younger, athletic population, under the age of 35 years, and presents with positive impingement and stability tests. Neer and Hawkins tests (Figure 8.17) have demonstrated high sensitivities and positive predictive values for subacromial impingement only, which is useful considering this is the most common location.[72]

More recently described lesions involve the articular side of the cuff tendon. Impingement between the posterosuperior glenoid rim and the humeral head is termed *posterior internal impingement* and presents with posterior shoulder pain that occurs when placing the shoulder in 90° of abduction and external rotation.[85,86] *Anterior internal impingement* can occur when the articular side of the tendon contacts the anterosuperior labrum. Patients will present with anterior shoulder pain with positive impingement signs in the absence of instability (Figure 8.18).[87]

Subcoracoid impingement is a rare yet clinically important entity as patients may present following surgical intervention without resolution of their pain. It occurs when the interval between the coracoid process and the humerus is decreased, placing the subscapularis tendon, the tendon of the long head of the biceps, and the middle glenohumeral ligament at risk of impingement.[88] Clinically, patients present with isolated anterior shoulder pain that can be reproduced by assuming a position of adduction, internal rotation and flexion. While the subcoracoid–humeral interval can be evaluated by MR imaging, findings are of poor predictive value, making the diagnosis mostly clinical.[89]

Another consideration, especially in athletes, is muscle hypertrophy or overdevelopment.[10,24] This can be seen as an indentation of the muscle or tendon adjacent to the acromioclavicular joint on the coronal or sagittal slices. Patients typically present with the same symptoms as primary subacromial impingement syndrome, exacerbated by shoulder abduction. This will typically occur without changes in coracoacromial outlet size.

As well as extrinsic causes of rotator cuff disease, intrinsic cuff degeneration must also be considered as an aetiology. The distal supraspinatus tendon has an area of decreased vascularity 1 cm medial to its insertion; this is termed the 'critical zone'.[42,90] It is known to be a key component of rotator cuff disease as the majority of cuff tears begin on the *articular* side of the tendon; if extrinsic bony impingement was the cause, the tears should occur on the *bursal* surface.[42,91]

In order to explain the degenerative processes that accompany rotator cuff disease, the following theory has been proposed: following tendinopathy and failure of the supraspinatus muscle, superior migration of the humeral head causes the degenerative spurring that is seen in these patients. This can be shown by the lack of degenerative spurring in patients with rotator cuff tendinopathy.[92] Proponents of this theory feel that for rotator cuff disease caused by an intrinsic mechanism treatment should focus on debridement of the supraspinatus tendon and avoidance of an unnecessary acromioplasty.

Whilst dispute still exists among experts as to the cause of rotator cuff pathology, it is likely that a

Figure 8.17 • *Hawkins* (A) and *Neer* (B) are both tests for impingement of the rotator cuff against the coracoacromial arch and are considered positive when the patient's pain is reproduced. In the former, an overpressure is exerted by the examiner, without resistance by the patient. The Neer test can be performed seated or standing with the examiner stabilizing the mid-thoracic spine. The shoulder is flexed by the examiner, noting both patient response and joint end feel.

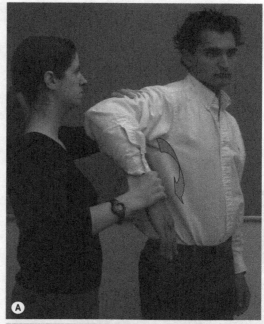

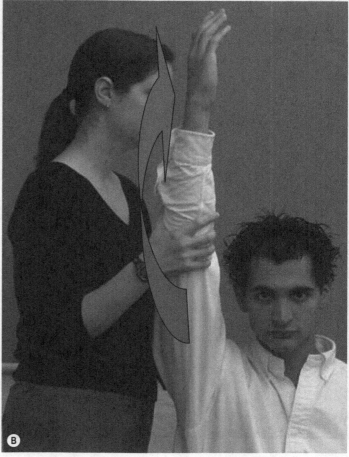

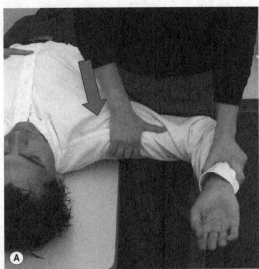

Figure 8.18 • The *subluxation/relocation test* (A) is used to determine subtle anterior impingement. Facing the patient's head, the examiner grasps the forearm and the most proximal portion of the humerus. Gentle anterior pressure is applied, noting any pain. Relief of pain following a gentle posterolateral force is a positive sign. The *load and shift test* (B) is for directional anteroposterior instability. Whilst grasping the humerus slightly lateral to the head, medial pressure is applied; this is followed by anteromedial and posterolateral translations. A unilateral increase in laxity compared to the uninjured shoulder indicates corresponding directional instability.

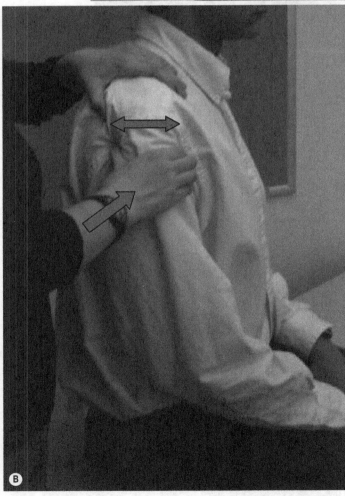

combination of the above factors plays a role in the aetiology. Careful evaluation of the mechanisms and clinical correlation will allow proper diagnosis and thus proper management. Treatment should be directed at the primary cause of the cuff disease to avoid unnecessary invasive procedures.

Extrinsic impingement may present with several bone changes, including acromial joint osteophytes, subacromial spurs, and sclerosis and cysts of the humeral head. The subacromial bursa may appear thickened and compressed by the anterior acromion. An area of increased signal intensity will be seen in the supraspinatus tendon without tendon retraction. This is indicative of tendinopathy or cuff disruption without tendon retraction. Intensity approaching fluid may be evident in the subdeltoid bursa, representing inflammation.[93] Coracoacromial ligament thickening may contribute to a decrease in supraspinatus outlet size and can best be viewed on sagittal oblique images.[94]

Trauma

Trauma can play either a primary or secondary role in the development of rotator cuff tears. Severe trauma such as a car accident or a fall may result in an anterior dislocation with a tear of the supraspinatus muscle. More commonly, trauma can worsen an already torn or degenerated tendon. In an older population, history of minor trauma may often be elicited; in these patients, the trauma probably plays a secondary role in an ongoing degenerative process.[95] Typically, there will be tears of more than one tendon. Younger patients tend to present without a history of trauma but instead a history of pain related to athletics.[31]

Tears will typically involve one tendon and are related to instability and impingement with a final episode of traumatic symptomatology. True traumatic tendon rupture is uncommon and occurs in the absence of tendon degeneration.[96] The patient is typically younger and has no symptoms prior to the injury[48]; the injury will be substantial, such as a fall on an outstretched hand (FOOSH).[96,97] In these traumatic tears, two entities should be investigated using MR imaging: greater tuberosity fractures in patients under 40 years of age and subscapularis tears in patients over the age of 40.[96]

Tendon tears

Rotator cuff tears have been classified by a number of different systems including the size or shape of the tear, the number of involved tendons, the location of the tear, the age of the injury or the aetiology, as described above.[31,98] Most of these classification systems are important only when determining the efficacy of surgical intervention or the appropriateness of specific surgical approaches. Of importance to the physician is the differentiation between complete and partial tears, which tendons are involved and the location of the tear (bursal or articular) as these factors alter the clinical picture.

A complete, or full thickness, tear is one that extends from the bursal to the articular surface and allows direct communication between the subdeltoid bursa and the joint cavity (Figure 8.19).[48] Partial thickness tears involve either the bursal or the articular side of the tendon (Figure 8.20).

The typical presentation of rotator cuff tears is the complaint of pain with overhead activity and weakness on lifting the arm. Partial thickness tears usually present with pain, less severe weakness and posterior capsule tightness[99]; full thickness tears are likely to present with weakness on resisted isometric contraction with the shoulder in the 'full can' testing position (Figure 8.21).[48,99]

Superior glenohumeral instability has been described in conjunction with supraspinatus tears; in these instances, it is usually unclear if the tear is a result of instability and secondary impingement or the chronic rotator cuff dysfunction was the cause of the instability as described above.[99] Differentiation requires a complete understanding of the mechanism of injury and its temporal progression. Another presentation of a supraspinatus lesion is a subacromial abrasion, which presents with crepitus as the humerus rotates under the acromion in the absence of pain or weakness.[99]

These orthopaedic tests are generally good at either ruling out tendinopathies (high sensitivity) or confirming tendinopathies (high specificity) but never both. The 'empty can' and 'full can' tests are better at ruling out pathology and are more accurate for complete rupture (positive is weakness) as opposed to tendinopathy (positive is pain).[100] The *Codman's drop arm* or, more simply, drop arm test is highly specific for full thickness tears but has a low sensitivity.[99] No conclusive evidence exists for the decisive diagnostic ability of one test over another.[101]

Subscapularis tendon tears can occur following anterior shoulder dislocation in an older patient or following trauma with external rotation of the arm at the side or extension of the humerus.[102] Patients will usually report a traumatic injury, suffer from

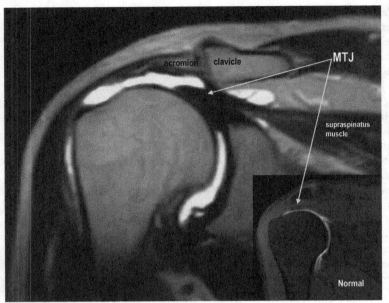

Figure 8.19 • Coronal oblique, T1-weighted MR imaging sequence with contrast showing a full-thickness supraspinatus tear with retraction of the musculotendinous junction (MTJ) and prominent fluid accumulation in the subacromial bursa. The normal position of the MTJ is lateral to the acromioclavicular articulation.

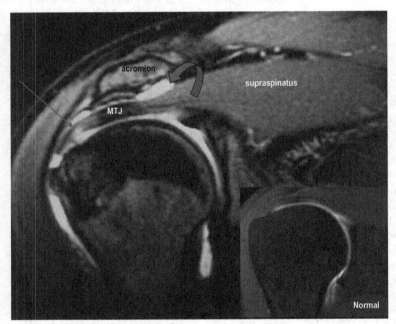

Figure 8.20 • Coronal oblique, T2-weighted MR image with fat suppression. A focal defect or partial tear of the supraspinatus is present on the articular surface of the tendon. The fibres on the bursal aspect of the tendon are continuous. Fluid in the subacromial bursa (curved arrow) is noted as a secondary sign. The signal intensity of the muscle and musculotendinous junction is normal.

recurrent anterior instability and are generally younger than those who present with degenerative supraspinatus tears.[48] Anterior shoulder pain, night pain due to anatomical location in relation to sleep position and weakness are common presentations.[102] Clinicians should be aware of limitations in activities of daily living (ADLs), such as the inability to tuck in the back of a shirt, fasten a brassiere or place a wallet in the back pocket, which could point to a tear.[102] Physical examination reveals weakness on internal rotation and increased external rotation. If the patient has full range of motion, the *Gerber*[99] and *Modified Gerber* tests[103] should be performed. Lack of abduction or internal rotation could create a false positive and necessitates use of the Napoleon sign (Figure 8.22).[99,102]

Figure 8.21 • The *empty can* (full internal rotation) and *full can* (full external rotation) positions should both be tested in the scapular plane (30° anterior to coronal). Utilizing a consistent hand placement and pressure, the examiner instructs the patient to resist movement from the starting position. Pain or muscle weakness (4/5 or less) is considered positive for pathology of the supraspinatus.

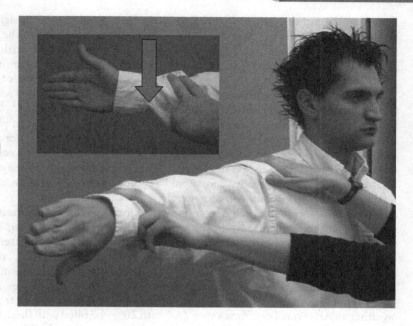

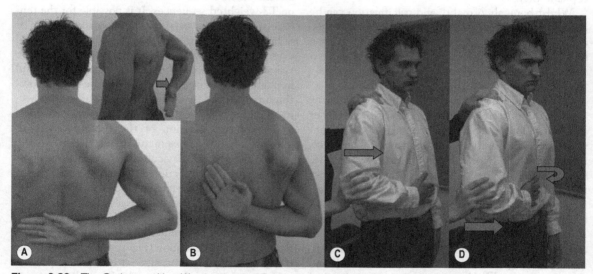

Figure 8.22 • The *Gerber position* (A) and *Modified Gerber position* (B) (maximal internal rotation) are used to isolate the subscapularis muscle. The inability to lift the hand away from the back indicates severe subscapularis weakness, most probably from a tear. Before asking the patient to lift the hand, it is important to verify that the patient is actually able to achieve the position. The *Napoleon sign* is elicited by asking the patient to press on their belly whilst attempting to avoid wrist flexion, and keeping the elbow in the coronal plane (C, D).

Both the teres minor and infraspinatus are frequently overlooked when evaluating the rotator cuff. Because most tears of these tendons occur in the presence of other rotator cuff tears, suspicion of any tear necessitates their assessment. Infraspinatus tears present with severe weakness, impairment and a positive *dropping sign*. Teres minor tears present with an inability to externally rotate the shoulder, and full thickness tears present with positive Hornblower's sign, in which the shoulder is externally rotated with 90° of abduction with the examiner supporting the arm in the scapular plane. The elbow is flexed to 90° and the patient is asked to rotate the arm externally against the resistance; a positive sign is the inability to maintain the externally rotated position with the arm dropping back to a neutral position.[104]

When indicated by the history and physical examination, plain radiographs should be taken to assess bony abnormality or soft tissue calcification. Signs such as a sclerotic greater tuberosity or acromion or a decreased acromiohumeral interval may point to advanced rotator cuff disease or a large unbalanced rotator cuff tear, respectively, and should prompt further studies. Glenohumeral degenerative joint disease can be seen on both the anteroposterior (AP) view and the axillary view. Supraspinatus calcification (CPPD) can be detected on external and internal rotation views. Acromial morphology can be viewed utilizing the Rockwood view (coronal AP with 30° caudal tilt) or the supraspinatus outlet view. Acromioclavicular degeneration can be viewed on either an AP coronal or a Zanca view (AP with 20° cephalic tilt).

Whilst bony abnormality and calcification can be observed with conventional radiography, only inferences as to the state of the soft tissue structures can be made. Radiographs can help to guide clinical decisions but do not have absolute information regarding the soft tissue pathologies.

Once clinical suspicion is established, MR imaging is often the procedure most appropriate for further evaluation. This modality has demonstrated high sensitivity and specificity of approximately 90% in multiple studies.[105–107] Although MR arthrography has shown higher figures, it is not routinely employed, being reserved for difficult patients or when aggressive management options are considered.[24,108] MR imaging can show the size, orientation and degree of retraction of the tears as well as the quality of the torn edges, with good correlation on surgical evaluation; it can also demonstrate associated muscle and osseous changes.[109–112] Even with the high level of confidence that these imaging modalities provide, it is important to note that patients still may suffer from rotator cuff tears with a negative study; clinical correlation is always key.[113]

The normal signal pattern for the rotator cuff tendon is low to intermediate intensity on most common sequences, including T1-weighted, T2-weighted and fat-suppressed.[10,24,48,114] Variations in the signal intensity can be attributed to pathological changes such as tears or degeneration but also to technical factors.[10,24,30] The magic angle phenomenon, the focal change in signal intensity when a structure is oriented 55° to the main magnetic field, occurs only on sequences with short echo time (T1 and spin density). If a tear is suspected, one should look for secondary signs of tears and for correlation with the T2-weighted sequences, where this phenomenon does not occur.[10,24,30] A full thickness tear is present when there is complete disruption of the fibres in the superior to inferior direction, creating an area of communication between the capsule and the bursa, however small it may be. Some tendon fibres may, however, still be intact, especially at the posterior aspect.

Tears occur most commonly at the anterior, distal portion of the supraspinatus tendon near the insertion of the greater tuberosity. They also occur at the *critical zone*, an area of the tendon located 1 cm proximal to the insertion.[10,11,115] Discontinuity of the tendon fibres is the best evidence to indicate the presence of a tear. The gap between the fibres will be filled with fluid, which will appear as high intensity zones on the T1-weighted sequence with contrast and on T2-weighted sequences. It is possible for the tendon gap to be obscured by granulomatous tissue or debris, making the tear difficult to identify. If clinical evidence points to a tear but the defect cannot be visualized, there are secondary signs that can be useful in establishing a diagnosis.[10,24,111] These include focal thinning, blurred tendon margins or tendon displacement and may all be indicative of a tear.

The normal position of the musculotendinous junction of the supraspinatus is just lateral to the level of the acromioclavicular joint. Medial displacement, indicating retraction, is a useful sign. High signal intensity on T2-weighted sequences (fluid) in the subacromial/subdeltoid bursa is always abnormal and is another sign of a tear. The fluid indicates communication between the bursa and the articular capsule due to a tear in the tendon (Figure 8.12). This finding is not specific, however, since it can also be present with partial tear or bursitis. The last indirect sign is muscle atrophy, seen as loss of muscle bulk, change of shape and streaks of increased T1 signal, associated with fatty infiltration.[10,24] The presence of these signs is useful not only for detection of tears but also for evaluation of the patient's prognosis. With severe atrophy and fatty infiltration, a surgical repair will likely not be undertaken, owing to the poor chances of success; the muscle would likely not be able to perform its function even if reattached.[116]

Partial or incomplete tears are more frequent but slightly more difficult to detect. An area in the tendon of increased signal intensity on T2-weighted images, with or without fat suppression, is the best sign, but in many cases will not be present. Often, the defect will appear as isointense to muscle, or an area of intermediate signal surrounded by the normal low signal intensity of the rest of the tendon. The edges of the defect may also be smooth and regular, making the tendon appear thinned, as opposed to torn. The location will indicate whether the damage involves the articular surface (most common), the bursal surface or is intratendinous (Figure 8.20).

On T1-weighted images, the involved area will be of low to intermediate signal intensity.[10,24] Tendinosis or degenerative changes usually demonstrate similar signal on both types of sequences, allowing some differentiation between the two conditions.[10]

Evaluation of subscapularis tears is best achieved on axial or sagittal oblique images, in which the tendon can be visualized in its entirety.[117,118] Discontinuity of the fibres or intrasubstance signal change, as with the supraspinatus, is the best evidence of tears (Figure 8.23). The tears will be areas of bright signal on T1-weighting with contrast and on T2-weighted sequences. Fatty infiltration of the muscle belly, abnormal tendon position or shape, and fluid leak under the tendon insertion on the lesser tuberosity (subscapularis recess) are all supporting or secondary signs of tears.

Anomalies of the long head of the biceps are usually associated with subscapularis tears. Tears in both tendons are frequently missed, making assessment of secondary signs exceedingly important. Seventy per cent of patients also have a concurrent supraspinatus tear, glenoid labral tear or subcoracoid bursitis.[117,118] The imaging findings for complete or partial tears of the infraspinatus and teres minor are similar to the other rotator cuff pathologies. Intrasubstance signal change and displacement are the most obvious signs.

Glenohumeral instability

Owing to the mobile nature of the shoulder joint and the range of motion that it allows, instability is a common entity in the shoulder. Instability is clinically defined as only occurring in the presence of pain, as the humeral head may move beyond the boundaries of the glenoid in the absence of symptoms.[119] It is important to differentiate generalized joint laxity from glenohumeral instability, although laxity may be a predisposing factor and the two may, therefore, coexist. Classification systems of instability involve several factors; authors tend to utilize different systems depending on whether their focus is clinical or surgical.[31,48,49]

Figure 8.23 • Axial, T2-weighted image with fat suppression. Note the high signal intensity and change in shape of the subscapularis tendon near its insertion. The inset image demonstrates the appearance of a normal subscapularis tendon.

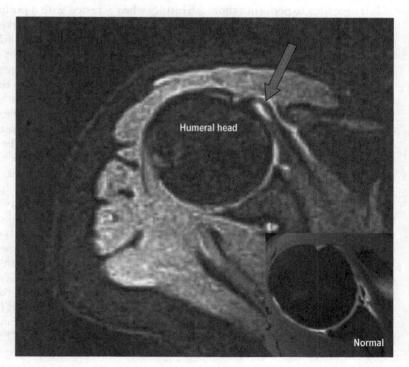

Humeral head

Normal

The acronyms TUBS and AMBRI encompass the ends of a spectrum of instability. TUBS stands for traumatic instability, unidirectional in nature, Bankart lesion present, responds to surgery. AMBRI stands for atraumatic aetiology, multidirectional bilateral involvement, responds to rehabilitation and rarely requires an inferior capsule shift (although this may become necessary if conservative measures fail). A third group has recently been added to include persons with microtraumatic instability; AIOS stands for acquired instability related to overstress of the joint and responds to surgery. This group consists mainly of athletes involved in overhead activities.[120]

Glenohumeral stability is provided by a combination of static and dynamic mechanisms, failure of which may produce instability. Static factors include the labrum, the glenohumeral ligaments, the long head of the biceps, the posterior capsule and the negative intra-articular pressure in the joint. Dynamic stability is accomplished in coordination with the static stabilizers. Balanced function of the rotator cuff, biceps and scapulothoracic musculature provides compression of the humerus into the glenoid as well as positioning the glenoid for optimal articular contact.[119] Disruption of static or dynamic shoulder stabilizers may lead to instability and it is important to assess these structures in determining the aetiology of the instability.

It is necessary to perform a thorough history when assessing a patient for instability. As noted above, the multifactorial nature of instability requires detailed information about any previous trauma, including arm position and severity of the event. A force applied to an abducted, externally rotated and extended arm will point towards anterior instability, while forward flexion adduction and internal rotation are more likely in posterior instability (Figure 8.09).[31] Anterior instability is the most common and can occur with or without a history of trauma. Posterior instability is infrequent and is typically associated with severe trauma, seizures or electrical shock. Atraumatic posterior instability can be attributed to athletic activities that repeatedly require the arm to be placed in flexion, adduction and internal rotation. Severe traumatic dislocation in the young has a high incidence of recurrence, whilst the same event in the elderly is associated with rotator cuff tears.[31] Physician-assisted relocation of traumatic dislocation will typically have a higher incidence of labral pathology. Pain localization is harder in patients with instability owing to its dynamic nature and should be correlated with specific movements.

Anterior shoulder pain associated with abduction and external rotation, such as the cocking phase of a throw, indicates anterior instability. Superior pain is generally related to rotator cuff pathology or osteoarthritis. Posterior pain experienced in adduction and internal rotation, such as punching, can be related to posterior instability. Pain while lifting with the arm at the side is identified in inferior instability.[121] An important clinical entity is the voluntary dislocator. This individual will typically dislocate at will for social approval and will typically not be forthcoming with information regarding history of dislocation.

When assessing the patient, it is important to evaluate for generalized joint laxity; this is most commonly assessed using the Beighton scale.[121] Shoulder hypermobility comprising laxity without pain is not instability. Shoulder range of motion in patients with instability is typically normal to increased. Apprehension or discomfort in any range of motion may point to instability. Increases in external rotation are associated with laxity of the inferior glenohumeral ligamentous complex or a tear of the subscapularis, as discussed previously. An increase in internal rotation points to stretching of the posterior capsule. Abnormal scapulothoracic motion will affect dynamic stabilization of the glenohumeral joint. Tests to identify altered biomechanics of the scapula include 'winging', tested with a pushup against a wall, which indicates long thoracic nerve palsy.[83]

Specific tests for instability are used to assess the static stabilizers by passive end range motion.[122] Each test should be performed bilaterally with specific attention paid to the degree of humeral head translation and pain provocation.[123] The 'sulcus test' is used to evaluate inferior instability: inferior-directed traction is placed on the arm while it is at the side. The force must be applied superior to the elbow so as not to involve the biceps. A positive sulcus sign will usually point to multidirectional instability.[122] Numerous tests have been identified for clinically addressing unidirectional anterior or posterior instability, including the apprehension tests, drawer tests, load and shift tests and the posterior stress test.[101,102] What the examiner is identifying with any of these tests is movement beyond the glenoid accompanied by pain. Instability alone is not diagnostic and pain alone may point to another involved structure, such as the rotator cuff (Figure 8.18).[120,121] The compression rotation, clunk, crank and anterior slide tests as well as the O'Brien sign have been extensively studied and have relatively strong predictive value

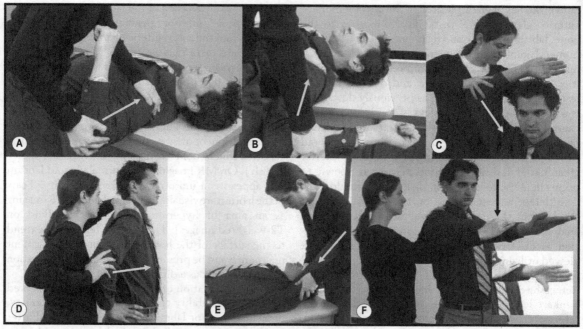

Figure 8.24 • Orthopaedic manoeuvres to assess glenoid labrum integrity. (A, B) The *compression rotation test* in the starting and rotating phases. The humerus is compressed in the glenoid fossa during different degrees of rotation of the arm. Reproduction of pain, or catching, may indicate a SLAP (Superior Labrum from Anterior to Posterior) lesion. (C) The *crank test*. The arm is in an overhead position and compression is applied with different levels of humeral rotation. Pain, particularly during external rotation, or reproduction of the pain and catching, constitutes a positive test. (D) An example of the *anterior slide test*. Anterior and slightly superior pressure is applied to the patient's elbow. Anterior pain and clicking are considered positive findings. (E) The *labral clunk test*, in which the patient's shoulder is flexed. Compression is applied caudally at first, followed by compression and circumduction. Pain, clunking and locking indicate a positive test. (F) The *O'Brien's sign*. The patient resists downward pressure with the arm in flexion, mild adduction and maximal internal rotation (insert). The manoeuvre is repeated with the arm in maximal external rotation. Pain with internal rotation that disappears with external rotation is considered a positive test.

(Figure 8.24). Reproduction of pain, clicking and clunking during the manoeuvres are good indicators of tears.[99] Combinations of these tests have been found to have greater sensitivity than MRI without contrast for detecting glenoid labrum tear.[4,124,125]

Initial evaluation of shoulder instability should include plain radiography, although bony defects associated with instability are difficult to identify and appear in a minority of instability patients.[122] Specialized views such as the apical oblique view will help to identify osseous Bankart injuries of the glenoid, whilst the Stryker notch view and AP internal rotation can help identify a Hill–Sachs deformity. Plain radiography will typically be normal, as the above-listed lesions only occur with traumatic or repetitive dislocations. A very specific finding on the anteroposterior film with a humeral avulsion of the glenohumeral ligaments (HAGL lesion) is scalloping of the medial side of the neck of the humerus and/or a small bone fragment medial to it; this is discussed in more detail later. While these findings are very specific to the lesion, they occur in a minority of cases.[126]

Anterior instability is the most common form and presents following one or multiple episodes of dislocation or subluxation. Dislocations may occur posteriorly, inferiorly or anteriorly, with the last-mentioned occurring up to 98% of the time.[127] The mechanism for anterior dislocation is abduction, extension and external rotation of the shoulder. Recurrent subluxation or dislocation is very common in those under the age of 30, occurring in up to 90% of patients, and is more common in men. Recurrence rates drop as low as 15% or less after the age of 40. Anterior subluxation does not require a history of dislocation or injury to occur; repetitive microtrauma or overuse has been implicated in the development of anterior glenohumeral instability.[31] Injuries to the bone, labrum, capsule and ligaments about the glenohumeral joint have all been implicated in anterior instability. The two most common bone abnormalities identified are Hill–Sachs and osseous Bankart lesions. A Hill–Sachs lesion, as previously described, is a posterolateral notch defect of the humeral head caused by contact between the posterolateral portion of the humeral head and the anteroinferior glenoid rim. This finding is specific to a prior anterior inferior glenohumeral dislocation and has been shown to occur in 47% to 100% of dislocated shoulders.[62] The defect is best viewed on transverse images at the level of the coracoid; remember that a normal anatomical groove will be found caudal to this location. Acute cases with marrow oedema can best be viewed utilizing fat-suppressed T2-weighted or STIR sequences. The accuracy of MR diagnosis of this defect has been placed as high as 94%.[128] A bony Bankart lesion involves the avulsion of the anteroinferior capsulolabral complex – a Bankart lesion, with a fracture of the adjacent glenoid rim.[129] Fragment size will affect treatment course, as larger defects can give rise to recurrent instability even following surgical soft tissue repair. These defects will require fragment refixation or bone grafting. Smaller defects may be overlooked on MR and may necessitate CT with or without contrast. Larger defects are well demonstrated on MR imaging and may alter glenoid geometry, creating an inverse pear shape.[62] Look to sagittal oblique images to evaluate glenoid shape as well as cystic changes, sclerosis and the marrow changes associated with osseous Bankart lesions.[31]

Injuries to the labrum, capsule and glenohumeral ligaments have been correlated with recurrent anterior subluxation and dislocation. Soft tissue lesions associated with anterior instability have recently come under the term avulsion/injury of the anteroinferior labroligamentous complex.[130] This complex and, most notably, the anterior band of the inferior glenohumeral ligament will most frequently fail at its glenoid insertion, causing an avulsion of the labrum resulting in variations of the Bankart lesion. Failure less frequently occurs at the humeral insertion site or intrasubstance.[122]

The **Bankart lesion** has been found in a large majority (87%–100%) of traumatic anterior instability cases.[131] It has also been reported in microtraumatic and atraumatic instability,[130] although labral fraying and degeneration is more common in the latter.[119]

The lesion is an avulsion of the labroligamentous complex (capsule, inferior glenohumeral ligament and labrum) from the anteroinferior portion of the glenoid, termed the 3 to 6 o'clock position.[31] The lesion and the displaced fragment may also extend superiorly, beyond the typically described location. Disruption of the scapular periosteum occurs in all Bankart variants. When attempting to identify this lesion, variants and pitfalls need to be ruled out. The labrum is a common site of the magic angle phenomenon, undercutting and anatomical variation which could resemble a tear (as discussed previously). On MR imaging, the normal glenoid labrum will appear as a uniform signal hypointensity. Tears of the labrum are visualized on unenhanced MR imaging as an area of hyperintensity (less than fluid on T2-weighted images). The Bankart lesion will extend to the surface of the lesion and a detached fragment may or may not be present, while internal degeneration will appear only as a diffuse area of hyperintensity.[57]

One presentation of the Bankart lesion, observed in chronic instability cases, is a thick, low intensity, detached anterior labral fragment. It is named after its description on MR: glenoid labrum ovoid mass (GLOM).[132] Unenhanced MR has a high specificity and sensitivity for anterior labral tears, similar to that of MR arthrography.[133] The sensitivity and specificity for unenhanced MR imaging decreases when evaluating superior and posterior tears.[31] When arthrography is employed, contrast will extend into the labral defect and will highlight labral fraying better than will MR imaging. Identification of these injuries will be enhanced with ABER position as well, but this painful position should be employed only following equivocal MR arthrography.[28,29]

Bankart variants are typically identified utilizing MR arthrograms and specialized positions. The Perthes lesion has been defined as a non-displaced Bankart, whereby the periosteum remains intact but is stripped.[31,57] In these cases, the labrum can rest in its normal position and heal, leaving only the redundant periosteum.[31] During traditional MR arthrography, contrast may not extend into a healed fragment, making diagnosis difficult.[119] Even with arthrography, these lesions can be hard to identify, particularly without prior knowledge of the lesion.[134] The ABER position may help to separate the labrum from the glenoid, allowing better visualization.[57,119,134]

The **anterior labroligamentous periosteal sleeve avulsion** (ALPSA) is a medially displaced avulsion of the anterior labrum.[135] In this lesion, the periosteum will remain intact, like the Perthes variant. The labroligamentous complex will strip down the scapular neck, resembling the rolling up of a shirt-sleeve, and will cause incompetence of the inferior glenohumeral ligament. Common terms to describe the lesion are 'peel back lesion' and 'medialized Bankart' lesion. This lesion is more common in recurrent dislocation than in first-time traumatic dislocation.[136]

It is important not to mistake a slightly displaced labrum with a congenital labral variant.[136] The typical finding on MR arthrography is a cleft between the glenoid and the nodular-shaped fibrous tissue.[137] There is some doubt as to the value of unenhanced MR in detecting Bankart and variant lesions; most of these lesions have only been described utilizing contrast-enhanced MR.[137] It is important for the clinician to remember that a negative test does not indicate the absence of a lesion, which should be investigated fully if clinical suspicion remains.

A second classification of anterior instability lesion does not involve the labroligamentous complex at its glenoid insertion. The humeral avulsion of the glenohumeral ligaments (HAGL) lesion is an isolated tear of the inferior glenohumeral ligament at its humeral insertion and has been correlated with instability. The typical presentation is an older, male patient suffering a violent dislocation. In the absence of a Bankart lesion in a patient with anterior instability, the incidence of a HAGL lesion is 27%.[126] Overall, in cases of anterior instability, the incidence of such lesions has been reported as being between 7% and 9%. The majority of patients with a HAGL lesion will have associated injuries such as labral tears, Bankart lesions, Hill–Sachs lesions or rotator cuff tears.[120] Whilst identification on conventional MR is possible, it requires joint effusion to be present. On coronal oblique T2-weighted images, the lesion can be identified by the conversion of the inferior glenohumeral ligament from a U-shaped, fluid-distended structure to a J-shaped structure with fluid extravasation beyond the humeral attachment of the ligament.[120] HAGL lesions have been missed on arthroscopic Bankart repair and have been identified as the cause of continued complaints post surgery[96,109]; this makes presurgical identification important for appropriate management.[120,126]

In approximately 20% of HAGL cases, a bony avulsion from the humeral attachment will occur (BHAGL). This can typically be seen on plain film radiography and may resemble a fragment from an osseous Bankart. Medial scalloping of the humeral neck is very specific to the BHAGL and can help differentiate the two lesions.[126]

A final Bankart variation is the 'floating' anterior band of the inferior glenohumeral ligament (AIGHL). This lesion occurs when there is a classic Bankart lesion in conjunction with a humeral avulsion. It is a rare occurrence and will be treated surgically.[57]

'SLAP' lesions are injuries to the glenoid labrum involving the insertion of the tendon of the long head of the biceps muscle. When the arm is bent inward forcefully at the shoulder, the superior portion of the glenoid labrum is torn away from the cavity in an anterior to posterior direction.[4,124] The acronym 'SLAP' refers to the location and direction of the tear: **Superior Labrum, Anterior to Posterior lesion**. Patients with labral tears usually present with painful locking of the shoulder through specific movement patterns and signs of anterior shoulder instability. The latter may include pain, apprehension, loss of function and aggravation of symptoms in overhead and abduction/external rotation positions.[4,138]

SLAP lesions were originally classified by Snyder into four types: type I, fraying of the free edge of the superior labrum (11%); type II, avulsion of the labrum and the biceps tendon anchor (41%); type III, bucket-handle tear without involvement of the biceps tendon anchor (33%); type IV, bucket-handle tears with extension into the biceps anchor (15%).[139] More recent delineation of the above classifications have been made and more categories have been added to further classify the lesions. On conventional MR, identification of SLAP lesions can be difficult. Cartland et al have identified the following findings in their study. Type I lesions exhibit minimal irregularity of the articulating labral contours. Type II lesions exhibit globular high signal interposed between the superior part of the glenoid labrum and the superior part of the glenoid fossa. Type III lesions exhibit areas of high signal intensity within the superior section of the labrum separate from the normal superior part of the labral recess. Type IV lesions exhibit diffuse high signal intensity within the glenoid labrum with marked abnormal high signal intensity extending into the proximal biceps tendons.[140] In more difficult cases, arthrography may be necessary to visualize a SLAP lesion.

Posterior instability is a very rare entity, accounting for only 2%–4% of all cases of shoulder instability[56,141]; however, the majority of these cases can be treated conservatively with strengthening exercises, and surgical intervention is rare.[142] Despite its infrequency, posterior instability can present a clinical challenge due to the inconsistency of its aetiology and lack of distinct signs. Bilateral posterior dislocation is nearly always caused by electric shock or epileptic convulsion and does not commonly recur. Unilateral traumatic posterior dislocation will usually occur after a violent force is applied to an adducted internally rotated arm, and is prone to recurrence, especially in the presence of large bony defects. The most common clinical lesion involves repeated posterior subluxation due to repetitive microtrauma in the adducted flexed and internally rotated position.

There are no definitive lesions of posterior instability. Prior violent dislocation may result in an osseous impaction of the anteromedial humeral head on the posterior glenoid rim: a reverse Hill–Sachs lesion. Abnormalities of the bony glenoid include fractures in traumatic dislocation and marrow oedema, sclerosis or cystic lesions with repetitive impaction.[31] In cases of atraumatic posterior instability, glenoid rim insufficiency and retroversion and humeral retroversion have been implicated.[141] Posterior labral tears are less indicative of posterior instability than anterior tears are of anterior instability; in fact, tears of the posterior labrum have been found in cases of anterior instability – a consequence of repetitive dislocation – and in cases of clinically stable shoulders.[141,143]

The **posterior labrocapsular periosteal sleeve lesion (POLPSA)** can occur when the capsule strips the labrum from the scapular periosteum. Isolated labral tears are uncommon and may be due to trauma or unidirectional or multidirectional instability. Posterior labral tears have been identified in contact-sport athletes, such as offensive linemen in American football, who engage their opponents with their arms in front of

the body.[144] MR studies will exhibit high signal outlining the lesions, which will brighten on T2-weighting and become more defined with fat suppression. Arthrography will allow contrast material to extravasate beneath lesions, allowing improved delineation.

A very specific injury to the posterior labrum in overhead throwers has been termed the *Bennett lesion*. Traction placed on the inferior glenohumeral ligament, caused by the deceleration and follow-through phases of pitching, can create an avulsion injury of the posterior capsule.[145] These forces create enthesophytes, which, when mineralized, can be seen using conventional radiographs, CT or MR imaging as a crescent shape at the posterior inferior glenoid rim. The associated soft tissue injuries to the rotator cuff, labrum and capsule can be identified on MR imaging.

Biceps tendinopathy

Biceps tendinopathies consist of tendinosis, instability and rupture and typically affect young or middle-aged individuals with a history of overhead arm activity.[2] Imaging findings for bicipital tendon tears will be similar to those for other tendon tears, with increased intrasubstance high-signal changes and alteration in the course of the tendon. Tears unrelated to impingement occur distal to the musculoskeletal junction. The 'empty bicipital groove sign' or 'naked humerus sign' occurs when there is distal retraction of the tendon and muscle and can be seen in both types of tear (Figure 8.25).[52]

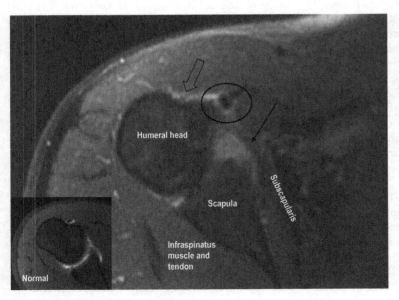

Figure 8.25 • Axial, T2-weighted sequence showing a biceps tendon dislocation (oval region). The bicipital groove is empty (thick arrow). There is also displacement of the subscapularis tendon (thin arrow).

It is, however, important to scrutinize both the axial and the parasagittal oblique slices, since the findings can be subtle.[55]

Primary tendinopathy is caused by eccentric overload, hypovascularity or bicipital groove abnormalities, which lead to tendon attrition. Tendinopathy can also occur secondary to glenohumeral joint instability or rotator cuff impingement. Approximately 95%–98% of patients diagnosed with biceps tendinopathy have impingement primarily, with the secondary tendinopathy as the pain generator.[58] Pain is typically present in the proximal, anterior aspect of the shoulder, sometimes extending into the biceps muscle belly and rarely radiating into the neck or beyond the biceps.[2] Instability of the tendon, although a common diagnosis, occurs infrequently and has been attributed to tears of the transverse humeral ligament[60]; however, even with complete transection of this ligament, subluxation of the tendon is nearly impossible with an intact rotator cuff.[61]

When instability is suspected, the rotator cuff should be examined for incompetence to determine whether there is a primary problem therein (in cases where the rotator cuff is incompetent or dysfunctional, the 'subluxation' of the tendon is a secondary phenomenon). Patients with instability typically present with the same pattern as those with tendinopathy, although a palpable snap is evident on motion.[2] Isolated biceps tendon rupture can be due to acute trauma or the end result of any of the above-listed tendon disorders. Most ruptures are associated with rotator cuff tears and necessitate evaluation of these tendons. Ruptures present with acute pain and may have a palpable snap. Because of its attachment, the biceps anchor can be injured along with the glenoid labrum, which can cause a click or snap.

References

1. Urwin M, Symmons D, Allison T, et al. Estimating the burden of musculoskeletal disorders in the community: the comparative prevalence of symptoms at different anatomical sites, and the relation to social deprivation. *Ann Rheum Dis*. 1998;57(11): 649–655.

2. van der Windt DA, Koes BW, de Jong BA, Bouter LM. Shoulder disorders in general practice: incidence, patient characteristics, and management. *Ann Rheum Dis*. 1995;54(12):959–964.

3. Berkow R. Neck, shoulder and upper limb pain. In: *The Merck Manual*. 16th ed. West Point, PA: Merck & Co; 1992:1362.

4. Souza T. *Differential Diagnosis and Management for the Chiropractor*. 2nd ed. Riverwoods, IL: Aspen; 2000.

5. Moore K. The upper limb. In: *Clinically Oriented Anatomy*. 2nd ed. Baltimore: Williams and Wilkins; 1985:626–793.

6. Palastanga N, Field D, Soames R. The upper limb. In: *Anatomy and Human Movement: Structure and Function*. 5th ed. Edinburgh: Elsevier Butterworth Heinemann; 2006: 43–234.

7. Travell J, Simons D. *Myofascial Pain and Dysfunction*. Baltimore: Williams and Wilkins; 1992.

8. Lindsay K, Bone I, Callander R. Localised neurological disease and its management. In: *Neurology and Neurosurgery Illustrated*. Edinburgh: Elsevier; 1991:213–466.

9. Stoller D. *Magnetic Resonance Imaging in Orthopaedics and Sports Medicine*. 2nd ed. Philadelphia: Lippincott Williams and Wilkins; 2006.

10. Berquist T. *MRI of the Musculoskeletal System*. 4th ed. Philadelphia, PA: Lippincott Williams and Wilkins; 2000.

11. Shahabpour M, Kichouh M, Laridon E, et al. The effectiveness of diagnostic imaging methods for the assessment of soft tissue and articular disorders of the shoulder and elbow. *Eur J Radiol*. 2008; 65(2):194–200.

12. Fotiadou AN, Vlychou M, Papadopoulos P, et al. Ultrasonography of symptomatic rotator cuff tears compared with MR imaging and surgery. *Eur J Radiol*. 2008;68(1): 174–179.

13. Harryman 2nd DT, Hettrich CM, Smith KL, et al. A prospective multipractice investigation of patients with full-thickness rotator cuff tears: the importance of comorbidities, practice, and other covariables on self-assessed shoulder function and health status. *J Bone Joint Surg Am*. 2003;85-A(4):690–696.

14. Bates B. The musculoskeletal system. In: Bates B, ed. *A Guide to Physical Examination*. 3rd ed. Philadelphia: JB Lippincott; 1983:324–370.

15. Bates B, Hoekelman R. Interviewing and the health history. In: Bates B, ed. *A Guide to Physical Examination*. 3rd ed. Philadelphia: JB Lippincott; 1983:1–27.

16. Ndetan HT, Rupert RL, Bae S, Singh KP. Prevalence of musculoskeletal injuries sustained by students while attending a chiropractic college. *J Manipulative Physiol Ther*. 2009;32(2):140–148.

17. Abbassian A, Giddins GE. Subacromial impingement in patients with whiplash injury to the cervical spine. *J Orthop Surg*. 2008;3:25.

18. Stevenson JH, Trojian T. Evaluation of shoulder pain. *J Fam Pract*. 2002;51(7):605–611.

19. Rowe L, Yochum T. Radiographic positioning and normal anatomy. In: Yochum T, Rowe L, eds. *Essentials of Skeletal Radiology*. Baltimore: Williams and Wilkins; 1987:1–93.

20. Bianchi S, Prato N, Martinoli L, Derchi E. Shoulder radiography. In: Davies M, Hodler J, eds. *Imaging of the Shoulder: Techniques and Applications*. London: Springer; 2003:3–20.

21. Blum A, Carrillon Y, Railhac J-J, et al. Instability. In: Davies M, Hodler J, eds. *Imaging of the Shoulder: Techniques and Applications*. London: Springer; 2003:161–190.

22. Parker BJ, Zlatkin MB, Newman JS, Rathur SK. Imaging of shoulder injuries in sports medicine: current protocols and concepts. *Clin Sports Med*. 2008;27(4):579–606.

23. Prickett WD, Teefey SA, Galatz LM, et al. Accuracy of ultrasound imaging of the rotator cuff in shoulders that are painful postoperatively. *J Bone Joint Surg Am*. 2003; 85-A(6): 1084–1089.

24. Stoller D. *Magnetic Resonance Imaging in Orthopaedics and Sports Medicine*. 1st ed. Philadelphia: Lippincott Williams and Wilkins; 1996.

25. Mirowitz S. *Pitfalls, Variants and Artifacts in Body MR Imaging*. St Louis: Mosby; 1996.

26. Bloem J, Sartoris D. *MRI and CT of the Musculoskeletal System: A Text-Atlas*. Baltimore: Williams and Wilkins; 1992.

27. Davis SJ, Teresi LM, Bradley WG, et al. Effect of arm rotation on MR imaging of the rotator cuff. *Radiology*. 1991;181(1):265–268.

28. Cvitanic O, Tirman PF, Feller JF, et al. Using abduction and external rotation of the shoulder to increase the sensitivity of MR arthrography in revealing tears of the anterior glenoid labrum. *Am J Roentgenol*. 1997;169(3):837–844.

29. Choi JA, Suh SI, Kim BH, et al. Comparison between conventional MR arthrography and abduction and external rotation MR arthrography in revealing tears of the antero-inferior glenoid labrum. *Korean J Radiol*. 2001; 2(4):216–221.

30. Tirman PF, Bost FW, Garvin GJ, et al. Posterosuperior glenoid impingement of the shoulder: findings at MR imaging and MR arthrography with arthroscopic correlation. *Radiology*. 1994; 193(2):431–436.

31. Zlatkin MB. MRI of the postoperative shoulder. *Skeletal Radiol*. 2002;31(2):63–80.

32. Timins ME, Erickson SJ, Estkowski LD, et al. Increased signal in the normal supraspinatus tendon on MR imaging: diagnostic pitfall caused by the magic-angle effect. *Am J Roentgenol*. 1995; 165(1): 109–114.

33. Kijowski R, Farber JM, Medina J, et al. Comparison of fat-suppressed T2-weighted fast spin-echo sequence and modified STIR sequence in the evaluation of the rotator cuff tendon. *Am J Roentgenol*. 2005;185(2):371–378.

34. Reinus WR, Shady KL, Mirowitz SA, Totty WG. MR diagnosis of rotator cuff tears of the shoulder: value of using T2-weighted fat-saturated images. *Am J Roentgenol*. 1995;164(6): 1451–1455.

35. Palmer WE, Brown JH, Rosenthal DI. Rotator cuff: evaluation with fat-suppressed MR arthrography. *Radiology*. 1993; 188(3):683–687.

36. Palmer WE, Caslowitz PL, Chew FS. MR arthrography of the shoulder: normal intraarticular structures and common abnormalities. *Am J Roentgenol*. 1995;164(1):141–146.

37. Chandnani VP, Yeager TD, DeBerardino T, et al. Glenoid labral tears: prospective evaluation with MRI imaging, MR arthrography, and CT arthrography. *Am J Roentgenol*. 1993;161(6): 1229–1235.

38. Jacobson JA, Lin J, Jamadar DA, Hayes CW. Aids to successful shoulder arthrography performed with a fluoroscopically guided anterior approach. *Radiographics*. 2003;23(2):373–378; discussion 9.

39. Young MF. The physics of anatomy. In: *Essential Physics for Muscloskeletal Medicine*. Edinburgh: Elsevier; 2009.

40. Standring S, ed. *Gray's Anatomy - Pectoral girdle and upper limb:* *General organization and surface anatomy of the upper limb (Section 48)*. Edinburgh: Elsevier; 2009.

41. Standring S, ed. *Gray's Anatomy – Pectoral girdle and upper limb: Pectoral girdle, shoulder region and axilla (Section 49)*. Edinburgh: Elsevier; 2009.

42. Uhthoff HK, Sarkar K. An algorithm for shoulder pain caused by soft-tissue disorders. *Clin Orthop Relat Res*. 1990;(254): 121–127.

43. Neumann CH, Petersen SA, Jahnke Jr AH, et al. MRI in the evaluation of patients with suspected instability of the shoulder joint including a comparison with CT-arthrography. *Rofo*. 1991;154(6):593–600.

44. Liou JT, Wilson AJ, Totty WG, Brown JJ. The normal shoulder: common variations that simulate pathologic conditions at MR imaging. *Radiology*. 1993; 186(2):435–441.

45. Kaplan PA, Bryans KC, Davick JP, et al. MR imaging of the normal shoulder: variants and pitfalls. *Radiology*. 1992;184(2): 519–524.

46. Sasaki T, Yodono H, Prado GL, et al. Increased signal intensity in the normal glenoid labrum in MR imaging: diagnostic pitfalls caused by the magic-angle effect. *Magn Reson Med Sci*. 2002; 1(5):149–156.

47. Roger B, Skaf A, Hooper AW, et al. Imaging findings in the dominant shoulder of throwing athletes: comparison of radiography, arthrography, CT arthrography, and MR arthrography with arthroscopic correlation. *Am J Roentgenol*. 1999;172(5):1371–1380.

48. Rockwood C, Matsen 3rd FA. *The Shoulder*. 2nd ed. Philadelphia: WB Saunders; 1998.

49. Ianotti J, Williams G. *Disorders of the Shoulder: Diagnosis and Management*. Baltimore: Lippincott: Williams and Wilkins; 1999.

50. Williams MM, Snyder SJ, Buford Jr D. The Buford complex—the "cord-like" middle glenohumeral ligament and absent anterosuperior labrum complex: a normal anatomic capsulolabral variant. *Arthroscopy*. 1994; 10(3):241–247.

51. Kwak SM, Brown RR, Resnick D, et al. Anatomy, anatomic variations, and pathology of the 11- to 3-o'clock position of the glenoid labrum: findings on MR arthrography and anatomic sections. *Am J Roentgenol.* 1998; 171(1):235–238.

52. Smith DK, Chopp TM, Aufdemorte TB, et al. Sublabral recess of the superior glenoid labrum: study of cadavers with conventional nonenhanced MR imaging, MR arthrography, anatomic dissection, and limited histologic examination. *Radiology.* 1996;201(1):251–256.

53. Richardson ML, Patten RM. Age-related changes in marrow distribution in the shoulder: MR imaging findings. *Radiology.* 1994;192(1):209–215.

54. Mirowitz SA. Hematopoietic bone marrow within the proximal humeral epiphysis in normal adults: investigation with MR imaging. *Radiology.* 1993;188(3):689–693.

55. Richards RD, Sartoris DJ, Pathria MN, Resnick D. Hill-Sachs lesion and normal humeral groove: MR imaging features allowing their differentiation. *Radiology.* 1994; 190(3):665–668.

56. Bui-Mansfield LT, Taylor DC, Uhorchak JM, Tenuta JJ. Humeral avulsions of the glenohumeral ligament: imaging features and a review of the literature. *Am J Roentgenol.* 2002;179(3): 649–655.

57. Takase K, Yamamoto K. Intraarticular lesions in traumatic anterior shoulder instability: a study based on the results of diagnostic imaging. *Acta Orthop.* 2005; 76(6):854–857.

58. Bigliani L, Morrison D, April E. The morphology of the acromion and its relationship to rotator cuff tears. *Orthop Trans.* 1986;10:216.

59. Shah NN, Bayliss NC, Malcolm A. Shape of the acromion: congenital or acquired—a macroscopic, radiographic, and microscopic study of acromion. *J Shoulder Elbow Surg.* 2001;10(4):309–316.

60. Vanarthos WJ, Monu JU. Type 4 acromion: a new classification. *Contemp Orthop.* 1995; 30(3):227–229.

61. Epstein RE, Schweitzer ME, Frieman BG, et al. Hooked acromion: prevalence on MR images of painful shoulders. *Radiology.* 1993;187(2):479–481.

62. Getz JD, Recht MP, Piraino DW, et al. Acromial morphology: relation to sex, age, symmetry, and subacromial enthesophytes. *Radiology.* 1996;199(3): 737–742.

63. Heers G, Gotz J, Schubert T, et al. MR imaging of the intraarticular disk of the acromioclavicular joint: a comparison with anatomical, histological and in-vivo findings. *Skeletal Radiol.* 2007; 36(1):23–28.

64. Salter Jr EG, Nasca RJ, Shelley BS. Anatomical observations on the acromioclavicular joint and supporting ligaments. *Am J Sports Med.* 1987;15(3):199–206.

65. Duranthon LD, Gagey OJ. Anatomy and function of the subdeltoid bursa. *Surg Radiol Anat.* 2001;23(1):23–25.

66. White EA, Schweitzer ME, Haims AH. Range of normal and abnormal subacromial/subdeltoid bursa fluid. *J Comput Assist Tomogr.* 2006;30(2):316–320.

67. Grainger AJ, Tirman PF, Elliott JM, et al. MR anatomy of the subcoracoid bursa and the association of subcoracoid effusion with tears of the anterior rotator cuff and the rotator interval. *Am J Roentgenol.* 2000;174(5): 1377–1380.

68. Schraner AB, Major NM. MR imaging of the subcoracoid bursa. *Am J Roentgenol.* 1999; 172(6):1567–1571.

69. Nho SJ, Yadav H, Shindle MK, Macgillivray JD. Rotator cuff degeneration: etiology and pathogenesis. *Am J Sports Med.* 2008;36(5):987–993.

70. Budoff JE, Nirschl RP, Ilahi OA, Rodin DM. Internal impingement in the etiology of rotator cuff tendinosis revisited. *Arthroscopy.* 2003;19(8):810–814.

71. Tang KL, Habermeryer P, Li QH, et al. Etiology, classification and clinical evaluation of partial-thickness tears of rotator cuff. *Chin J Traumatol.* 2003; 6(5):309–317.

72. Calis M, Akgun K, Birtane M, et al. Diagnostic values of clinical diagnostic tests in subacromial impingement syndrome. *Ann Rheum Dis.* 2000;59(1):44–47.

73. Neer 2nd CS. Rotator cuff tears associated with os acromiale. *J Bone Joint Surg Am.* 1984;66(8): 1320–1321.

74. Edelson JG, Taitz C. Anatomy of the coraco-acromial arch. Relation to degeneration of the acromion. *J Bone Joint Surg Br.* 1992;74(4): 589–594.

75. Moses DA, Chang EY, Schweitzer ME. The scapuloacromial angle: a 3D analysis of acromial slope and its relationship with shoulder impingement. *J Magn Reson Imaging.* 2006;24(6):1371–1377.

76. Yao L, Lee HY, Gentili A, Shapiro MM. Lateral down-sloping of the acromion: a useful MR sign? *Clin Radiol.* 1996; 51(12):869–872.

77. Chang EY, Moses DA, Babb JS, Schweitzer ME. Shoulder impingement: objective 3D shape analysis of acromial morphologic features. *Radiology.* 2006; 239(2):497–505.

78. Park JG, Lee JK, Phelps CT. Os acromiale associated with rotator cuff impingement: MR imaging of the shoulder. *Radiology.* 1994; 193(1):255–257.

79. Gallino M, Battiston B, Annaratone G, Terragnoli F. Coracoacromial ligament: a comparative arthroscopic and anatomic study. *Arthroscopy.* 1995;11(5):564–567.

80. Ticker JB, Fealy S, Fu FH. Instability and impingement in the athlete's shoulder. *Sports Med.* 1995;19(6):418–426.

81. Jobe FW, Kvitne RS, Giangarra CE. Shoulder pain in the overhand or throwing athlete. The relationship of anterior instability and rotator cuff impingement. *Orthop Rev.* 1989;18(9): 963–975.

82. Michener LA, McClure PW, Karduna AR. Anatomical and biomechanical mechanisms of subacromial impingement syndrome. *Clin Biomech (Bristol, Avon).* 2003;18(5):369–379.

83. Voight ML, Thomson BC. The role of the scapula in the rehabilitation of shoulder injuries. *J Athl Train.* 2000;35(3):364–372.

84. Hebert LJ, Moffet H, McFadyen BJ, Dionne CE. Scapular behavior in shoulder impingement syndrome. *Arch Phys Med Rehabil.* 2002;83(1):60–69.

85. Jobe CM. Posterior superior glenoid impingement: expanded spectrum. *Arthroscopy.* 1995; 11(5):530–536.

86. Edelson G, Teitz C. Internal impingement in the shoulder. *J Shoulder Elbow Surg.* 2000; 9(4):308–315.

87. Struhl S. Anterior internal impingement: An arthroscopic observation. *Arthroscopy.* 2002;18(1):2–7.

88. Dines DM, Warren RF, Inglis AE, Pavlov H. The coracoid impingement syndrome. *J Bone Joint Surg Br.* 1990;72(2):314–316.

89. Giaroli EL, Major NM, Lemley DE, Lee J. Coracohumeral interval imaging in subcoracoid impingement syndrome on MRI. *Am J Roentgenol.* 2006; 186(1):242–246.

90. Fuduka H. Shoulder impingement and rotator cuff disease. *Curr Orthop.* 1990;4:225–232.

91. Ozaki J, Fujimoto S, Nakagawa Y, et al. Tears of the rotator cuff of the shoulder associated with pathological changes in the acromion. A study in cadavers. *J Bone Joint Surg Am.* 1988; 70(8):1224–1230.

92. Budoff JE, Nirschl RP, Guidi EJ. Debridement of partial-thickness tears of the rotator cuff without acromioplasty. Long-term follow-up and review of the literature. *J Bone Joint Surg Am.* 1998; 80(5):733–748.

93. Seeger LL, Gold RH, Bassett LW, Ellman H. Shoulder impingement syndrome: MR findings in 53 shoulders. *Am J Roentgenol.* 1988;150(2):343–347.

94. Brossmann J, Preidler KW, Pedowitz RA, et al. Shoulder impingement syndrome: influence of shoulder position on rotator cuff impingement—an anatomic study. *Am J Roentgenol.* 1996; 167(6):1511–1515.

95. Norwood LA, Barrack R, Jacobson KE. Clinical presentation of complete tears of the rotator cuff. *J Bone Joint Surg Am.* 1989;71(4):499–505.

96. Zanetti M, Weishaupt D, Jost B, et al. MR imaging for traumatic tears of the rotator cuff: high prevalence of greater tuberosity fractures and subscapularis tendon tears. *Am J Roentgenol.* 1999;172(2):463–467.

97. Quillen DM, Wuchner M, Hatch RL. Acute shoulder injuries. *Am Fam Physician.* 2004;70(10):1947–1954.

98. Morag Y, Jacobson JA, Miller B, et al. MR imaging of rotator cuff injury: what the clinician needs to know. *Radiographics.* 2006; 26(4):1045–1065.

99. Ellenbecker T. *Clinical Examination of the Shoulder.* Philadelphia: Elsevier WB Saunders; 2004.

100. Itoi E, Kido T, Sano A, et al. Which is more useful, the "full can test" or the "empty can test", in detecting the torn supraspinatus tendon? *Am J Sports Med.* 1999;27(1): 65–68.

101. Dinnes J, Loveman E, McIntyre L, Waugh N. The effectiveness of diagnostic tests for the assessment of shoulder pain due to soft tissue disorders: a systematic review. *Health Technol Assess.* 2003;7(29): iii, 1–166.

102. Kelly J. Shoulder pain and weakness. *Physician Sportsmed.* 2004;32:11.

103. Stefko JM, Jobe FW, VanderWilde RS, et al. Electromyographic and nerve block analysis of the subscapularis liftoff test. *J Shoulder Elbow Surg.* 1997;6(4):347–355.

104. Walch G, Boulahia A, Calderone S, Robinson AH. The 'dropping' and 'hornblower's' signs in evaluation of rotator-cuff tears. *J Bone Joint Surg Br.* 1998;80(4):624–628.

105. Sahin-Akyar G, Miller TT, Staron RB, et al. Gradient-echo versus fat-suppressed fast spin-echo MR imaging of rotator cuff tears. *Am J Roentgenol.* 1998; 171(1):223–227.

106. Schibany N, Zehetgruber H, Kainberger F, et al. Rotator cuff tears in asymptomatic individuals: a clinical and ultrasonographic screening study. *Eur J Radiol.* 2004;51(3):263–268.

107. Martin-Hervas C, Romero J, Navas-Acien A, et al. Ultrasonographic and magnetic resonance images of rotator

cuff lesions compared with arthroscopy or open surgery findings. *J Shoulder Elbow Surg.* 2001;10(5):410–415.

108. Magee T, Williams D, Mani N. Shoulder MR arthrography: which patient group benefits most? *Am J Roentgenol.* 2004; 183(4):969–974.

109. Bryant L, Shnier R, Bryant C, Murrell GA. A comparison of clinical estimation, ultrasonography, magnetic resonance imaging, and arthroscopy in determining the size of rotator cuff tears. *J Shoulder Elbow Surg.* 2002;11(3):219–224.

110. Motamedi AR, Urrea LH, Hancock RE, et al. Accuracy of magnetic resonance imaging in determining the presence and size of recurrent rotator cuff tears. *J Shoulder Elbow Surg.* 2002;11(1):6–10.

111. Rafii M, Firooznia H, Sherman O, et al. Rotator cuff lesions: signal patterns at MR imaging. *Radiology.* 1990;177(3):817–823.

112. Teefey SA, Rubin DA, Middleton WD, et al. Detection and quantification of rotator cuff tears. Comparison of ultrasonographic, magnetic resonance imaging, and arthroscopic findings in seventy-one consecutive cases. *J Bone Joint Surg Am.* 2004;86-A(4):708–716.

113. Nakatani T, Fujita K, Iwasaki Y, et al. MRI-negative rotator cuff tears. *Magn Reson Imaging.* 2003;21(1):41–45.

114. Mirowitz SA. Normal rotator cuff: MR imaging with conventional and fat-suppression techniques. *Radiology.* 1991;180(3):735–740.

115. Tuite MJ, Turnbull JR, Orwin JF. Anterior versus posterior, and rim-rent rotator cuff tears: prevalence and MR sensitivity. *Skeletal Radiol.* 1998; 27(5):237–243.

116. Lam F, Mok D. Open repair of massive rotator cuff tears in patients aged sixty-five years or over: is it worthwhile? *J Shoulder Elbow Surg.* 2004; 13(5):517–521.

117. Tung GA, Yoo DC, Levine SM, et al. Subscapularis tendon tear: primary and associated signs on MRI. *J Comput Assist Tomogr.* 2001;25(3):417–424.

118. Li XX, Schweitzer ME, Bifano JA, et al. MR evaluation of subscapularis tears. *J Comput Assist Tomogr*. 1999;23(5):713–717.

119. McCluskey GM, Getz BA. Pathophysiology of anterior shoulder instability. *J Athl Train*. 2000;35(3):268–272.

120. Woertler K, Waldt S. MR imaging in sports-related glenohumeral instability. *Eur Radiol*. 2006;16(12):2622–2636.

121. Cordasco FA. Understanding multidirectional instability of the shoulder. *J Athl Train*. 2000;35(3): 278–285.

122. Gerber C, Ganz R. Clinical assessment of instability of the shoulder. With special reference to anterior and posterior drawer tests. *J Bone Joint Surg Br*. 1984;66(4): 551–556.

123. Ellenbecker TS. Rehabilitation of shoulder and elbow injuries in tennis players. *Clin Sports Med*. 1995;14(1):87–110.

124. Liu SH, Henry MH, Nuccion S, et al. Diagnosis of glenoid labral tears: a comparison between magnetic imaging and clinical examinations. *Am J Sports Med*. 1996;24:149–154.

125. O'Brien SJ, Pagnani MJ, Fealy S, et al. The active compression test: a new and effective test for diagnosing labral tears and acromion-clavicular joint abnormality. *Am J Sports Med*. 1998;26:610–613.

126. Palmer WE, Caslowitz PL. Anterior shoulder instability: diagnostic criteria determined from prospective analysis of 121 MR arthrograms. *Radiology*. 1995; 197(3):819–825.

127. Bokor DJ, Conboy VB, Olson C. Anterior instability of the glenohumeral joint with humeral avulsion of the glenohumeral ligament. A review of 41 cases. *J Bone Joint Surg Br*. 1999; 81(1):93–96.

128. Chalidis B, Sachinis N, Dimitriou C, et al. Has the management of shoulder dislocation changed over time? *Int Orthop*. 2007;31(3):385–389.

129. Workman TL, Burkhard TK, Resnick D, et al. Hill-Sachs lesion: comparison of detection with MR imaging, radiography, and arthroscopy. *Radiology*. 1992; 185(3):847–852.

130. Itoi E, Lee SB, Berglund LJ, et al. The effect of a glenoid defect on anteroinferior stability of the shoulder after Bankart repair: a cadaveric study. *J Bone Joint Surg Am*. 2000;82(1):35–46.

131. Massengill AD, Seeger LL, Yao L, et al. Labrocapsular ligamentous complex of the shoulder: normal anatomy, anatomic variation, and pitfalls of MR imaging and MR arthrography. *Radiographics*. 1994;14(6):1211–1223.

132. Ly JQ, Beall DP, Sanders TG. MR imaging of glenohumeral instability. *Am J Roentgenol*. 2003; 181(1):203–213.

133. Legan JM, Burkhard TK, Goff 2nd WB, et al. Tears of the glenoid labrum: MR imaging of 88 arthroscopically confirmed cases. *Radiology*. 1991;179(1):241–246.

134. Gusmer PB, Potter HG, Schatz JA, et al. Labral injuries: accuracy of detection with unenhanced MR imaging of the shoulder. *Radiology*. 1996;200(2):519–524.

135. Wischer TK, Bredella MA, Genant HK, et al. Perthes lesion (a variant of the Bankart lesion): MR imaging and MR arthrographic findings with surgical correlation. *Am J Roentgenol*. 2002;178(1): 233–237.

136. Waldt S, Burkart A, Imhoff AB, et al. Anterior shoulder instability: accuracy of MR arthrography in the classification of anteroinferior labroligamentous injuries.

137. Radiology. 2005;237(2): 578–583.

138. Neviaser TJ. The GLAD lesion: another cause of anterior shoulder pain. *Arthroscopy*. 1993;9(1):22–23.

138. Warren RF, Craig EV, Altchek DW. *The Unstable Shoulder*. Philadelphia: Lippincott Raven; 1999.

139. Snyder SJ, Karzel RP, Delpizzo W, et al. SLAP lesions of the shoulder. *Arthroscopy*. 1990;6:274–279.

140. Cartland JP, Crues 3rd JV, Stauffer A, et al. MR imaging in the evaluation of SLAP injuries of the shoulder: findings in 10 patients. *Am J Roentgenol*. 1992;159(4): 787–792.

141. Hottya GA, Tirman PF, Bost FW, et al. Tear of the posterior shoulder stabilizers after posterior dislocation: MR imaging and MR arthrographic findings with arthroscopic correlation. *Am J Roentgenol*. 1998;171(3): 763–768.

142. Tung GA, Hou DD. MR arthrography of the posterior labrocapsular complex: relationship with glenohumeral joint alignment and clinical posterior instability. *Am J Roentgenol*. 2003;180(2): 369–375.

143. Shin RD, Polatsch DB, Rokito AS, Zuckerman JD. Posterior capsulorrhaphy for treatment of recurrent posterior glenohumeral instability. *Bull Hosp Jt Dis*. 2005;63(1–2):9–12.

144. Minkoff J, Cavaliere G. Glenohumeral instabilities and the role of magnetic resonance imaging techniques. The orthopedic surgeon's perspective. *Magn Reson Imaging Clin N Am*. 1993;1(1): 105–123.

145. Escobedo EM, Richardson ML, Schulz YB, et al. Increased risk of posterior glenoid labrum tears in football players. *Am J Roentgenol*. 2007;188(1):193–197.

The elbow

9

Julie-Marthe Grenier   Michelle A. Wessely
Kristin L. Hurtgen-Grace

Introduction

There is little doubt that magnetic resonance (MR) imaging of the elbow fails to attract the same level of interest as the same investigations in the lumbar spine and larger peripheral articulations, yet, for those involved in treating elbow pain and functional impairment in daily practice, it is a useful modality to consider. This is particularly true in those cases where other forms of imaging have failed to provide a definitive diagnosis and where an in-depth visualization of the articulation and surrounding neuromuscular, musculotendinous and vascular tissue is necessary.

The elbow is a complex articulation in both structure and function[1] and this demands from the clinician a detailed knowledge of the normal anatomical relationships, whether treating clinically or interpreting diagnostic imaging. It is worth reviewing these before proceeding further; this can be done by studying Figures 9.01 and 9.02.

A variety of injury and pathology may affect the elbow, involving both the soft tissue and the osseous components. Therefore, a complete familiarity with the fundamentals of the normal MR imaging appearance of the principal structures of the elbow is an essential prerequisite for the practitioner if they are to be able to correctly assess the anatomical relationships and identify the presence or absence of pathology.

However, diagnosis of elbow conditions does not begin with MR imaging. As with any other area of the body, an appropriate history and physical examination cannot be replaced by any diagnostic imaging modality. Not only do these establish a differential diagnosis that determines the necessity for and type of imaging required, but also it allows for clinical correlation of any pertinent findings.[2]

History and examination

Whenever the clinician is assessing a patient presenting with pain in or around the elbow, their evaluation should include the whole of the associated kinematic chain: hand, forearm, arm, shoulder and cervicothoracic spine. The contralateral elbow should also be considered for both comparison and evidence of compensation, which as well as indicating the level of disability can also determine the onset of adaptive injury.[3]

When taking the patient's history, in addition to the customary questions, there are some key points that will help direct the physician to the most appropriate differential diagnoses. These are detailed in Box 9.01.

Differential diagnosis

Mentally dividing the elbow into four regions is a valuable exercise, and assists both in constructing an initial differential diagnosis and in determining the imaging appearance. Each of the quadrants can be associated with specific pain-generators, pathologies and, to a certain extent, mechanisms of injury (Table 9.01); of course, disorders such as loose body formation or significant trauma may cause pain in any location.

Correlating the localization of the pain to the timing of the complaint may help to further refine

DOI: 10.1016/B978-0-443-06726-6.00009-3

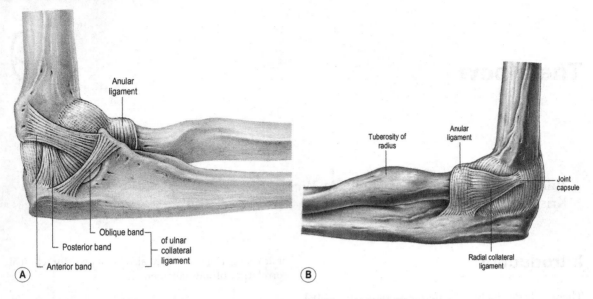

Figure 9.01 • Ligamentous structures of the left elbow: medial (A) and lateral (B) aspects.

the diagnostic list. For example, pain at the anterior aspect of the elbow during the early cocking phase of a throw may be consistent with biceps tendonitis.[4,5] Likewise, a tendinopathy involving the flexors and pronator teres will most likely manifest as anterior-medial pain during the late acceleration phase of a throw where forearm pronation and wrist flexion are maximal.[6]

These examples are specific to sports such as baseball, rounders or cricket, which involve throwing. The structures of the elbow are also specifically solicited during sports such as tennis,[7–12] badminton,[12–14] golf,[12,15–18] squash/racquetball[12,19,20] and basketball.[21,22] Occupational injuries at the elbow are also frequent: ask any construction worker, musician or computer enthusiast![23–28] In addition, the forearm also becomes very active in compensation for shoulder or core deficiencies.[15,29,30]

Clinical indications for diagnostic imaging

MR imaging of the elbow is useful in the evaluation of an array of neuromusculoskeletal disorders. These commonly involve acute trauma or the chronic repetitive application of mechanical stress to the elbow, leading to pain and restriction of the patient's normal activity.

The initial imaging modality for the elbow remains plain film radiography: it is useful, widely available and inexpensive. Many projections are available and demonstrate the osseous anatomy well. The standard examination protocol involves an antero-posterior (AP) view with the forearm in supination and a lateral view, taken with the elbow in 90° of flexion and the forearm in neutral (i.e. without pronation or supination).[31,32] A medial oblique view with the forearm in pronation is the most common supplementary view. Depending on the clinical question, projections specifically designed for the olecranon and the radial head are also commonly taken and can be very useful.[31,32]

Ultrasonographic evaluation of the elbow is becoming more and more popular. There is minimal bony interference in the elbow area, allowing for a good acoustic window. The tissues evaluated are also relatively superficial.[33,34] Ultrasound examination can also be performed in real time and in a dynamic fashion with immediate patient feedback and localization of the region of complaint.[35] The evaluation of the ulnar nerve in a patient with cubital tunnel syndrome, chronic epicondylitis or bursitis may be much more convenient and cost-effective with this modality than with MR imaging.[36–42]

Ultrasonography is also quite popular for the evaluation of the paediatric patient, since the use of MR imaging in young children can be quite problematic.

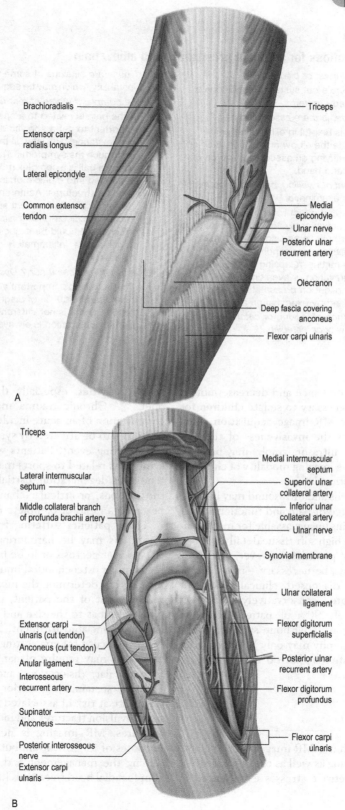

Figure 9.02 • The posterior left elbow: superficial (**A**) and deep (**B**) structures.

Box 9.01

Historical considerations for a patient presenting with elbow pain

- *Is the complaint unilateral or bilateral?*
  - This may help to rule out systemic conditions or occupation-related problems.
- *Does the pain radiate; is there associated pain?*
  - This information is helpful in eliminating pain-generators outside the elbow articulation itself or, alternatively, identifying an associated source of pain in the wrist and hand.
- *Is there any complaint of swelling, bruising or oedema?* (to be confirmed on examination)
  - Acute conditions and direct trauma may of course lead to swelling; however, systemic diseases, such as rheumatoid arthritis, may also be responsible. On occasion, inflammatory conditions can demonstrate a remitting–relapsing pattern in response to aggravation or even time of day, such that swelling is absent on presentation and so cannot be identified by examination alone.
- *Is there any experience of locking or catching; any sensation of giving way or instability?*

- These are all signs of some form of ligamentous instability, which may be sequelae to previous injury.
- *Is the complaint worse at rest or following activity?*
  - If the pain is related to a specific action, it is important to get a specific description of the circumstances and later, in the examination, to try to reproduce the symptoms. The action of throwing or hitting a ball is a complex movement, which may be separated into multiple phases, each engaging specific structures. Acute onset of pain is often related to a specific event such as a fall or direct impact. Insidious-onset pain may also be related to trauma, but could be associated with chronic degenerative, inflammatory or synovially-based disorders.
- *Exactly where does it hurt? Describe the pain.*
  - This is the most important area of questioning. It is often said that 90% of diagnoses comes from the history, and it is not different in the elbow region! Careful localization is always very useful.

In order to ensure compliance and decrease motion artifacts, it is often necessary to sedate children for the relatively lengthy MR image acquisition time. This process increases the invasiveness of the MR technique, and is why ultrasonography may be preferentially chosen as the imaging modality of choice in the paediatric population.[43,44]

Although radiographs and ultrasound may be used to determine the source of pain and functional deficit, MR imaging remains unsurpassable for many conditions because of the high soft tissue detail and bone marrow information it provides; however, this information may not always be necessary – many elbow conditions may be diagnosed clinically without any imaging and treated conservatively with great success. Approximately 90% of patients with an epicondylitis recover well without surgery.[45] MR imaging or ultrasonography may only be appropriate for the remaining patients that do not respond to conservative care.[46]

Trauma

Trauma often necessitates MR imaging of the elbow in both the acute setting as well as the chronic situation such as the repetitive stresses experienced in

sports activities, especially those involving a racquet.[46,47] Chronic trauma may also arise from a complication of an acute incident where the patient continues to be affected by symptoms long after the precipitating event. Patients with persistent elbow symptoms related to sports may develop scar tissue, tendinous degeneration, partial or complete tears of the tendons, or articular changes, all of which can preclude a rapid or complete recovery.[19,46]

Those patients suffering from persistent elbow symptoms may be harbouring complications such as avascular necrosis or loose body formation resulting from an osteochondral injury. In such cases, MR imaging can determine the most appropriate clinical management of the patient, providing a wealth of information as to the size and position of the lesion and any associated fragment.[48–51]

In the acute trauma setting, there are also situations that may require planar imaging such as MR; in particular, dislocations and complex fractures. Patients sustaining posterior dislocations of the elbow are at risk of associated ligament and capsular tears, avulsion fractures and instability. In the case of fractures, MR imaging is not always needed for purposes of identification, but can be vital in determining the management and prognosis.[52] When a simple radial head fracture is identified on plain film,

Table 9.01 Structures and pathologies associated with different quadrants of the elbow

Structures	Pathologies
Lateral quadrant	
Radius Capitellum Lateral epicondyle Lateral collateral ligament & capsule Common extensor tendon Radial nerve Posterior interosseous nerve	Osteochondral defects (especially at the capitellum) Radiocapitellar chondromalacia Degenerative changes Radial head fractures Lateral epicondylitis Radial nerve entrapment Posterolateral instability Muscular pathology
Medial quadrant	
Ulna Trochlea Medial epicondyle Medial collateral ligament & capsule Common flexor tendon Cubital tunnel Ulnar nerve	
Anterior quadrant	
Coronoid process of the ulna Anterior capsule and synovial recess Brachialis and biceps muscles Distal biceps tendon Brachial artery Median nerve Radial nerve	Musculotendinous strains Degenerative processes affecting the trochlea-ulna articulation
Posterior quadrant	
Olecranon process of the ulna Triceps and anconeus muscles/tendon Posterior capsule and synovial recess Olecranon bursae	Avulsion or tendinosis/tendinopathy of triceps tendon Stress fractures Osteophytes at the olecranon causing impingement Extension overload syndromes

the treatment plan is usually straightforward: initial immobilization and early rehabilitation to avoid capsular restriction, particularly into extension. No advanced imaging is normally performed; however, the management and prognosis of comminuted fractures is often based on the associated injuries as opposed to the fracture itself. In these instances, cross-sectional imaging becomes indicated.

MR imaging of the elbow may also provide important information regarding the neural elements that pass by the articulation during their course into the forearm and hand. The radial, median and ulnar nerves follow complicated pathways and are prone to entrapment in multiple locations by a wide variety of causes such as injury, mass compression or developmental variants.[53-56] Surgery may also provoke scar tissue formation about the nerves, leading to adhesions, irritation, entrapment and, eventually, chronic denervation.[57,58] In such syndromes, the use of MR imaging can be useful in determining the extent of any neuropathy and associated denervation and evaluating the potential for recovery. Clinical examination, electromyography and nerve conduction tests are also essential parts of the work-up, allowing for both the structure and function of the involved neural structures.

Techniques and protocols

Imaging of the elbow has benefited greatly from technological developments; in particular, high field strength magnets (1–3 T) and better surface coils have improved the speed and quality of the images.[59] MR imaging of the elbow involves the patient lying in the supine position with the arm resting against the body. A surface coil, wrapped around the patient's elbow, is used to improve the final image quality. With the patient in this position, motion artifacts are minimized.[60]

If there is clinical suspicion of a lesion to the distal biceps tendon or median nerve, the 'FABS' position (flexed elbow, **ab**ducted shoulder, supinated forearm) may be utilized to obtain a longitudinal view of the tendon and nerve. In this instance, the patient lies prone on the MR table with the involved arm overhead, the elbow flexed to 90° and the forearm supinated with the thumb pointing upwards. MR imaging can also be performed on a patient wearing a cast but, since the arm is sometimes fixated in an odd flexion position, it may cause difficulties in patient positioning. The cast also adds bulk, making the use of a standard elbow coil difficult.[61]

When possible, the three planes of interest are all included: axial, sagittal and coronal, maximizing the three-dimensional visualization of anatomical structures. The images are usually obtained with 4-mm slices and a 10% (0.4-mm) gap to prevent cross-talk (Figure 9.03). Since not all the aforementioned

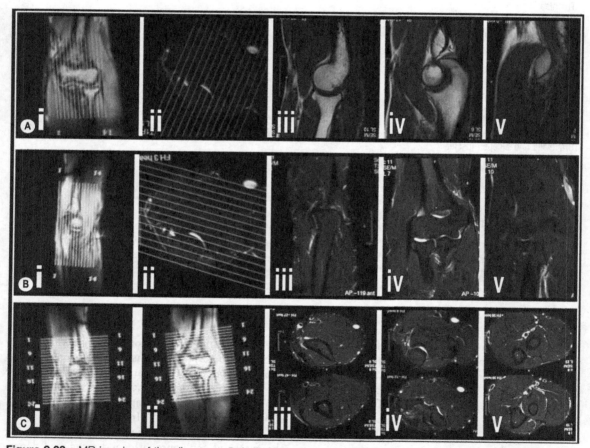

Figure 9.03 • MR imaging of the elbow usually includes imaging sequences in all three orthogonal planes: sagittal, coronal and axial. This figure demonstrates the scout views (Ai/ii, Bi/ii and Ci/ii), the initial imaging views that assist in the planning of each sequence. Note particularly on Figure Ci/ii the numbers, which correspond to the individual slices that have been performed. The remaining images correspond to the resulting sequences. Aiii–v are sagittal, T1-weighted views; Biii–v are coronal plane, short tau inversion recovery (STIR) sequences; Ciii–v are again STIR sequences, this time in the axial plane.

sequences are necessarily performed on a routine scan, it is always helpful to provide the radiographer and radiologist with the clinical findings and diagnostic suspicions, so that the appropriate parameters can be applied.[62] Another useful trick that may be utilized when looking for a specific problem is to tape a capsule of vitamin E on the skin of the patient, adjacent to the area of complaint. This will serve as a marker to indicate the problematic region on the images and can be seen on the final image as a round, or oval, area of high signal focus lying on the patient's skin (Figure 9.04).[63]

On occasion, intravenous contrast may be added, particularly if the clinical question involves the identification of a mass or the evaluation of an active, synovial-based disorder. MR arthrography is limited to assessing undersurface collateral tears or finding intra-articular loose fragments. The use of contrast carries risks and increases the invasiveness of the technique. The decision as to whether contrast is appropriate and, indeed, the most appropriate investigative protocol is based largely on the nature of the structure(s) under investigation (Table 9.02).[64,65]

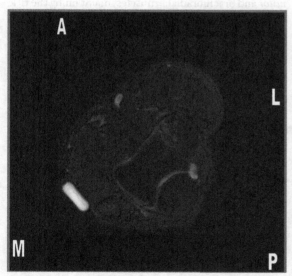

Figure 9.04 • On the axial slices of this STIR sequence of the elbow, note the bright, high signal lozenge-shaped region superficial to the subcutaneous tissues along the medial elbow, which represents a vitamin E capsule, placed by the radiographer alongside the clinically relevant region so as to indicate to the radiologist the area of clinical complaint when reading the imaging (M = medial, L = lateral, A = anterior, P = posterior).

Table 9.02 Optimum sequences for the visualization of different structures

Bone and marrow	STIR in all three planes
Articular cartilage	STIR and gradient echo, Proton Density Fat Saturated coronal/sagittal planes
Ligaments	STIR in the coronal plane
Tendons	T1-weighted and STIR in all planes
Nerves	T1-weighted and STIR in the axial plane

Normal imaging anatomy

Osseous anatomy (Figures 9.05–9.07, Box 9.02)

The elbow is a compound, hinge-type synovial joint (ginglymus) composed of the distal humerus, proximal ulna and proximal radius (Figures 9.01, 9.02).[66]

On the distal **humerus**, there are two prominent processes, the *medial* and *lateral epicondyles*. The distal articular surface of the humerus is wide and flat. The lateral third, the *capitellum*, articulates with the head of the **radius**, which has a disc-shaped articular surface. The medial third, the *trochlea*, articulates with the *trochlear notch* of the **ulna**.[67]

This notch, which is large and C-shaped, is also sometimes termed the *semilunar notch*. The projection forming its upper border is called the *olecranon process*. It articulates with the posteriorly situated *olecranon fossa* of the humerus and may be palpated as the angular 'point' of the elbow. The projection that forms the inferior border of the trochlear notch, the *coronoid process*, enters the *coronoid fossa* of the humerus when the elbow is flexed. This fossa is separated from the *cubital fossa* anteriorly by only a thin layer of bone.[68]

The lateral side of the coronoid process has a small, shallow notch or groove, called the *radial notch*. This articulates with the head of the radius, forming a synovial *pivot* (trochoid) joint, which allows supination and pronation of the forearm.[69] On the medial aspect of the coronoid process, approximately 2 cm posterior to the coronoid tip, is the *sublime tubercle*, the site of insertion for the ulnar collateral ligament.[70]

Nerves

Nerves are distinguishable on MR imaging owing to their surrounding layer of fatty myelin. The median, radial and ulnar nerves are usually obvious on axial images of the elbow (Figure 9.05E); however, they can be difficult to identify owing to their size, variable anatomical relationships and low signal intensity. They have complex courses, running through multiple compartments.

Ulnar nerve

Of the three, the **ulnar nerve** is the most vulnerable to injury, probably because of the superficial position that the nerve takes as it passes through the joint. The elbow is also the most common site for traumatic injury to the ulnar nerve, particularly where it passes through the *cubital tunnel*.[53,69] The tunnel floor is made from the posterior and transverse portion of the *ulnar collateral ligament* (or *medial collateral ligament of the elbow*) as well as the articular capsule. The aponeurosis of the *flexor carpi ulnaris muscle* and the *cubital tunnel retinaculum* create the roof of the tunnel. This retinaculum, sometimes called the *arcuate ligament*, runs from the olecranon to the medial epicondyle and is not present in everyone.[1] In some individuals, it is replaced by an accessory muscle, the *anconeus epitrochlearis*, which offers an additional site of potential entrapment and compression of the ulnar nerve.[71,72]

Median nerve

The **median nerve** may be better identified if the patient's forearm is placed in pronation during imaging.[73] If there is a clinical question regarding this nerve, it is thus wise to impart this information to the radiologist.

In the region of the elbow, the median nerve travels between the *bicipital aponeurosis* and the *brachialis muscle*, through the cubital fossa. The median nerve gives off its *anterior interosseous* branch just after passing between the two origins of the pronator teres muscle, as they arise from the medial epicondyle and coronoid process, offering a potential site of entrapment. If this pathology occurs before the separation of the nerve into its distal branches, it is termed **pronator syndrome**. If the entrapment occurs after the separation, it is referred to as **anterior interosseous nerve syndrome**.[69,74,75]

Radial nerve

The **radial nerve** can be found in the anterolateral portion of the elbow region, between the *brachialis* and *brachioradialis* muscles. It divides into two branches: the superficial sensory branch passes between the *supinator* and brachioradialis muscles, maintaining the title of the radial nerve, while the purely motor *posterior interosseous nerve* forms at the level of the capitellum and courses between the heads of the supinator muscle, in a fibrous tunnel named the *arcade of Frohse*.[66,69,75]

Box 9.02

Key to anatomical features marked on subsequent MR images

H humerus	14. Anterior fat pad
R radius	15. Common extensor tendon
U ulna	16. Anconeus muscle
1. Brachial artery	17. Flexor carpi ulnaris muscle
2. Cephalic vein	18. Flexor digitorum (superficialis and profundus) muscle
3. Radial nerve	19. Extensor digitorum muscle
4. Ulnar nerve	20. Extensor carpi ulnaris muscle
5. Median nerve	21. Supinator muscle
6. Basilic vein	22. Palmaris longus muscle
7. Brachioradialis muscle	23. Flexor carpi radialis muscle
8. Brachialis muscle	24. Radial collateral ligament
9. Extensor carpi radialis longus muscle	25. Olecranon fossa
10. Triceps muscle	26. Biceps tendon
11. Pronator teres muscle	27. Posterior fat pad
12. Common flexor tendon	28. Ulnar collateral ligament
13. Biceps muscle	29. Articular cartilage

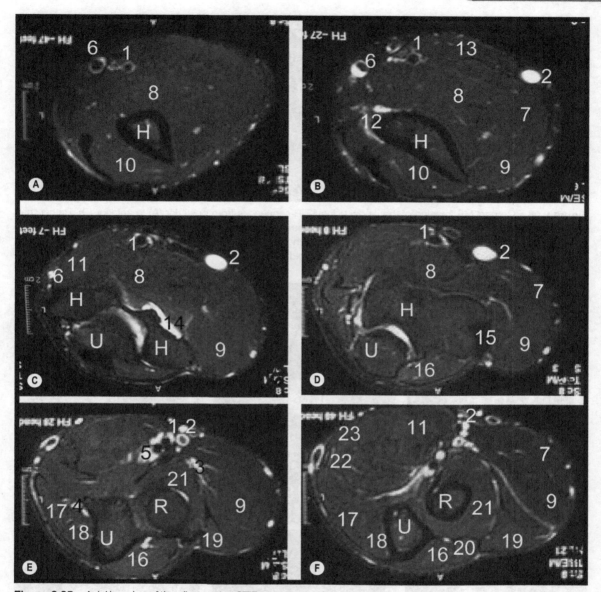

Figure 9.05 • Axial imaging of the elbow using STIR sequences, demonstrating the full spectrum of the intricate anatomical structures revealed by MR imaging. The radial (3), ulnar (4) and median (5) nerves are all clearly visualized (E). A method for reviewing the anatomy is to select an individual anatomical structure and to trace it from proximal (A) to distal (F). Although time-consuming, this allows accuracy in identification of the structure and determination of any lesion affecting it.

Muscles and bursae

Anterior

The group of muscles that contribute to the soft tissue structures anteriorly comprise the biceps brachii and brachialis. The two proximal heads of the biceps brachii unite to form a common tendon above the elbow that inserts on the *radial tuberosity*. The tendon anchors into the *bicipital aponeurosis* (or *lacertus fibrosus*). The brachialis muscle lies deep to the biceps brachii. It originates from the distal half of the anterior humerus and inserts onto the coronoid process.[66,68] Both muscles are best seen on axial and sagittal images (Figures 9.05 and 9.07 respectively).

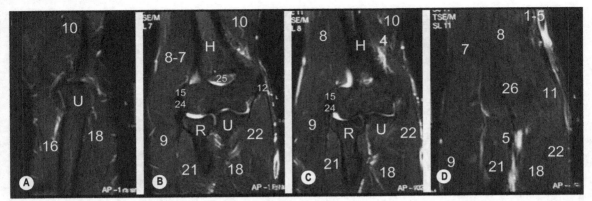

Figure 9.06 • Coronal MR imaging of the elbow using STIR sequences from posterior (A) to anterior (D). Rather than be overwhelmed by the number of structures to identify, it is useful for the clinician to choose those structures that commonly present in practice with pathology, for example the common extensor tendon (structure 15) and appreciate the normal appearance in this set of images of a 24-year-old student.

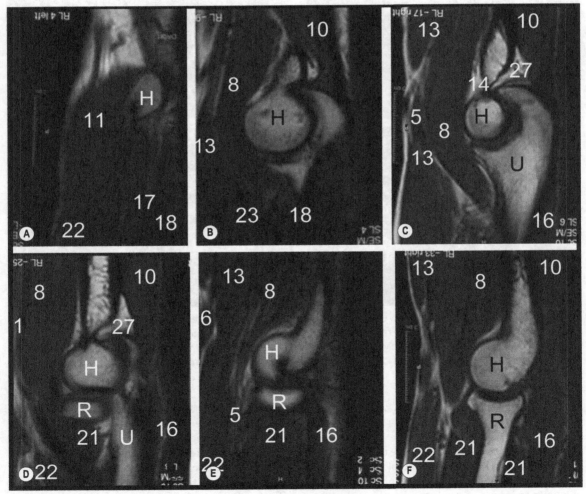

Figure 9.07 • Sagittal T1-weighted MR imaging of the elbow sequences demonstrating the normal anatomical relationships about the articulation from medial (A) to lateral (F).

The *bicipitoradial* and *interosseous bursae* separate the extrasynovial, paratenon-wrapped distal tendon of the biceps from the anterior aspect of the radial tuberosity.[68] The bursae are not normally visible on MR images, unless they have become inflamed and/or distended.

Posterior

The muscles contributing to the posterior elbow group are the *anconeus* and *triceps muscles*.[76] The axial and sagittal sequences are the most useful to assess both these muscles (Figures 9.05 and 9.07 respectively). The anconeus is a small, triangular muscle that originates on the posterior aspect of the lateral epicondyle and inserts on the posterior superior surface of the ulna.[76] Although it assists the (*postero-*) *lateral ulnar collateral ligament* (LUCL) in resisting varus stress, since it blends with the triceps distally, it is often considered as functionally part of this muscle.[68] The triceps attaches to the posterior surface of the olecranon process and it is at this site that the tendon's fibres become intertwined with fibrofatty slips that may be radiologically mistaken for a partial tear. This phenomenon will appear as an increased signal on both T1- and T2-weighted images. The *olecranon bursa* lies between the triceps tendon and the olecranon.[69]

Medial

The medial group of muscles consists of the pronator teres, the palmaris longus (when present) and the flexors of the hand (flexor digitorum superficialis and profundus; flexor carpi radialis, flexor carpi ulnaris and flexor pollicus longus).[1] The pronator teres muscle is the most superficial of the group. It has two origins: from the medial condyle (the humeral head) and from the coronoid process of the ulna (the ulnar head). The pronator inserts onto the lateral surface of the mid-third of the radius. The remaining muscles unite in the common flexor tendon, which inserts into the medial epicondyle of the humerus.[76] The ulnar (or medial) collateral ligament may also be identifiable along its course. It offers supports to the common flexor tendon in resisting valgus stresses. For best visualization, one should assess the axial and coronal images (Figures 9.05 and 9.06 respectively). Normal ligaments and tendons will be demonstrated as homogeneously low signal structures inserting onto the medial epicondyle.[77]

Lateral

The supinator and brachioradialis muscles, along with the extensor muscles of the hand, form the lateral group of elbow muscles.[1] The supinator muscle is the deepest muscle, originating on the lateral epicondyle of the humerus and inserting onto the proximal third of the radius. It contributes to the floor of the cubital fossa whilst the brachioradialis serves as the lateral boundary of the cubital fossa.[68] Originating at the supracondylar ridge of the humerus, the brachioradialis inserts onto the lateral surface of the distal radius.[76] The extensor muscle group originates as the common extensor tendon from the lateral epicondyle. The tendon is common to *extensor carpi radialis brevis* and *carpi ulnaris* and to *extensor digitorum* and *digiti minimi*. The *extensor carpi radialis longus* is part of the lateral group but originates slightly more proximally on the lateral condyle of the humerus.[69] The axial and coronal images are again the best to visualize the lateral compartment muscles (Figures 9.05 and 9.06 respectively).

Ligaments and capsule

The *articular capsule* of the elbow extends from the humerus, covering all the articular surfaces down to the radial neck and inferior aspect of the coronoid process of the ulna. It is weaker on its anterior and posterior aspects, the medial and lateral aspects being strengthened by the medial and lateral collateral ligament complexes.[68] The anterior and posterior fat pads may be seen on lateral radiographs of the elbow joint as well as on MR imaging. Normally, with the elbow in a flexed position, the anterior fat pad is visible on radiographs as a relatively linear lucency in contact with the anterior aspect of the distal humerus. The posterior fat pad is not normally visible as it is hidden deep within the olecranon fossa. Articular oedema from effusion, haemarthrosis or synovitis will cause these fat pads to be displaced away from the humerus, resulting in radiographic visualization of the posterior fat pad and anterosuperior elevation of the anterior fat pad which adopts a curvilinear configuration.[78] The fat pads are visible on MR imaging, particularly on T1-weighted or fat-sensitive sagittal sequences (Figure 9.08).

The ulnar collateral ligament (UCL) complex contributes to medial elbow stability (Figure 9.01A). It comprises three distinct bundles: the anterior, posterior and transverse portions.[69] The anterior bundle extends from the medial epicondyle to the coronoid process and is best seen on coronal images

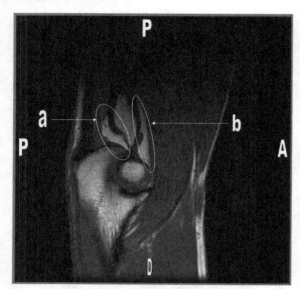

Figure 9.08 • Sagittal T1-weighted MR imaging of the elbow demonstrating the normal appearance of the posterior (a) and anterior (b) fat pads which surround the articular capsule of the elbow. Note that the anterior fat pad is seen as being flush with the anterior humerus, the normal appearance which is reproduced on the lateral radiograph as a thin radiolucent line.

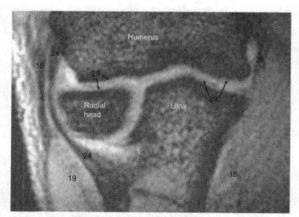

Figure 9.09 • Coronal T2-weighted MR imaging sequence of the elbow with an exquisite depiction of the lateral or radial collateral ligament (structure 24). This ligament should appear as a low signal intensity band coursing its way in an arc-like fashion laterally, as demonstrated in this image. The medial or ulnar collateral ligament can also be clearly seen in the proximal aspect (28).

(Figure 9.09).[65,68] Its proximal aspect is flared and tapers distally; it is the principal restraint against valgus stress.[79,80] The posterior fibres extend from the medial epicondyle to the olecranon. The transverse (or oblique) portion extends from the olecranon to the

coronoid process and does not really contribute to stability of the joint. The posterior and transverse portions are not always present, but this is rarely an issue from a biomechanical or clinical standpoint.[68] They are difficult to see on MR images; however, their presence is inferred as they form the floor of the cubital tunnel.[81]

The radial collateral ligament complex includes the lateral collateral ligament (LCL), the *annular* and *accessory collateral ligaments* and the LUCL (Figure 9.01B).[68] It contributes to the lateral stability of the elbow and resists varus stress.[82,83]

The LCL extends from the anterior aspect of the lateral epicondyle and inserts into the annular ligament and supinator fascia. The posterior bundle, the LUCL, extends from the lateral epicondyle and inserts into the ulna (hence the name) at the crista supinatoris.[68] The LUCL is the prime restraint against varus stress and its disruption will severely diminish the stability, leading to posterolateral rotatory instability of the elbow.[83,84] This ligament is best seen on coronal images. The better-known annular ligament is the prime stabilizer for the proximal radioulnar joint[69] and is best assessed on axial slices (Figure 9.05).[65]

Normal variants and diagnostic pitfalls

Unlike some other areas in the body, few variations from normal anatomy are to be found in the elbow. This section will focus on the supracondylar process, followed by the accessory muscles and ossicles that may, on occasion, be found. Paediatric considerations in the developmental anatomy of the elbow will then be discussed.

Osseous variants

Most commonly asymptomatic, the *supracondylar spur* (or *process*) and its associated ligament are found in approximately 1% of the population. The spur, which is located on the anteromedial surface of the humerus, 5–6 cm above the epicondyle, can be rudimentary and tubercle-like or quite large.[85] The *ligament of Struthers* connects the bony outgrowth to the medial epicondyle, forming the *supracondylar foramen* or *arcade of Struthers*. The median nerve and branches of the brachial artery run through the foramen (Figure 9.10). In some cases, the arcade can be the site of an anomalous origin of the pronator teres muscle.[86–88] These close anatomical relationships can account for the symptoms that may be

The patella cubiti is a rare sesamoid bone found in the tendon of the triceps, mimicking the patella in the quadriceps tendon. It may also be asymptomatic or cause restriction in the extension range of motion.[91]

Muscular variants

The other major elbow variants consist of accessory muscles or additional muscular bundles. Again, they may be incidental findings, although their size may cause impingement on neurovascular bundles. Clinically, this would present as any other proximal impingement syndrome with nerve-specific muscle weakness and paraesthesia in the forearm and hand.

Many types of aberrant muscles have been described, such as additional origins that may be fused or partially fused with neighbouring muscles. Variations in the location of the insertions may also be present. These variants are not at all rare and have been described for many years; it is therefore somewhat surprising that their existence is not generally appreciated by clinicians and often overlooked by them when formulating a differential diagnosis.

The biceps brachii provides a good example of this. Although the name of the muscle suggests the unvarying presence of two heads, the biceps can in fact possess anywhere between one and five heads. A third head is found in some 10%–20% of the population,[92,93] so is not in any way a rarity. As long ago as 1875, the anatomist Macalister published a review of 48 different variations for the morphology of the biceps,[94] and more have been reported since.[95–99] Another example of relatively frequent variation is the brachioradialis muscle, which may be conjoined with the supinator. Alternatively, its tendon may be split into different slips and cause entrapment if the radial nerve passes between them.[75]

Although accessory muscles or muscle bundles may not cause overt symptoms in the patient, they can be quite puzzling to the practitioner examining the MR images. The goal is not to be familiar with each and every variation (unless one is in search of a new life-long hobby), but to acknowledge that they are not rare occurrences and to be sufficiently familiar with the 'normal' muscles to identify a variant.

Paediatric considerations

The elbow region undergoes a significant transformation during the process of bony maturation. The multiple apophyses and epiphyses ossify at different

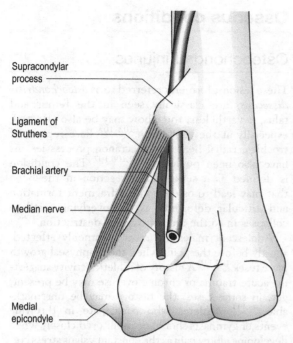

Supracondylar process

Ligament of Struthers

Brachial artery

Median nerve

Medial epicondyle

Figure 9.10 • The anomalous ligament of Struthers runs from the supracondylar spur, an anatomical variant, to the medial epicondyle. It forms the arcade of Struthers, which contains the brachial artery and the median nerve and can be a site of entrapment.

experienced by some patients and will be addressed along with the other causes of median nerve entrapment.

This variant is easy to visualize on plain film radiographs, especially if the arm is in a slightly oblique position. The spur will point towards the elbow joint, as opposed to its principal differential diagnosis, the osteochondroma, which points away from the joint. Although location and appearance are key to distinguishing the two, MR imaging demonstrates the cartilaginous cap in a developing osteochondroma.[86]

Two accessory ossicles are known to occur about the elbow joint: the *os supratrochleare* and the *patella cubiti*. The os supratrochleare is a developmental ossicle believed to originate from an accessory ossification centre of the olecranon. When present, it is located within the joint capsule in the olecranon fossa. It may restrict extension or can be asymptomatic. Because of its intra-articular position, it may benefit from synovial nutrition and increase in size. Its shape may be altered by the battering received from the adjacent olecranon. It is most common in the dominant arm of males.[89,90]

times, making the evaluation of images of the growing child quite challenging and potentially confusing.

Until recently, it was customary to obtain radiographs of the uninvolved arm; however, the increased exposure to ionizing radiation of developing tissue is no longer considered acceptable on a routine basis. On plain film, it is difficult on occasion to differentiate between a newly ossified centre and a fracture fragment. Fortunately, the ossification process follows a predictable order, for which the acronym *CRITOE* or *CRITOL* may be used in order to remember its sequence (Table 9.03).

The capitellum is the first such centre to become ossified and therefore radiologically visible; this happens towards the end of the first year of life. This is followed at approximately 2-yearly intervals by the radial head, medial (or, for acronymic purposes, internal) epicondyle, trochlea, olecranon process and, lastly, the lateral (external) epicondyle. These centres are usually completely fused by 16 years of age.[100,101]

This knowledge aids the practitioner quite considerably in their diagnosis: if, for example, an osseous fragment is noted in the region of the lateral epicondyle and the olecranon process centre is not yet visible, it would be appropriate to suspect a fracture. Understanding the process of maturation may, therefore, eliminate the need for cross-sectional imaging. Nonetheless, there are cases in which MR may be required to assess any cartilaginous injuries that may have been sustained; these will be discussed later. Ossification centres may also be multicentric and appear fragmented. On MR images, normal developing centres will demonstrate high signal intensity on T1-weighted images, corresponding to their higher fatty marrow content.

Table 9.03 Ossification centres for the elbow in order of appearance: the CRITOE acronym

Structure	Approximate age of appearance
Capitellum	1 year
Radial head	3 years
Internal (medial) epicondyle	5 years
Trochlea	7 years
Olecranon process	9 years
External (lateral) epicondyle	11 years

Osseous conditions

Osteochondral injuries

These lesions, formerly referred to as *osteochondritis dissecans*, are classically seen in the femur and talus; nevertheless, the elbow may be also affected, especially at the capitellum.[102–105] Rare reports of trochlea, radial head and olecranon process lesions have also been published.[102,106,107] The condition is defined as a subchondral reaction in the bone that may lead to osteochondral fragment formation and articular deformity as the overlying cartilage collapses in to the area of osseous destruction.[108]

Adolescent males are most commonly affected, shortly before the point when the epiphyseal growth plate fuses.[109,110] A history of athletic activity suggesting acute trauma or chronic overuse may be present; yet, in some cases, the history may be unremarkable.[109,111] Athletes who participate in throwing events or gymnasts should be monitored closely when developing elbow pain as the constant valgus stress created by impaction accentuates the stress on the lateral aspect of the elbow.[107,112] Patients may present with pain, tenderness and swelling, particularly in the lateral soft tissues surrounding the joint. Catching or locking sensations are suggestive of the presence of a loose fragment.[109,113]

It is important to clarify the terminology before moving on. There is much confusion between the terms 'osteochondritis dissecans', 'Panner's disease' and 'osteochondrosis of the capitellum'. Some authors utilize the terms interchangeably; some others establish them as different entities, although the evolution and pathophysiology of the processes are not well understood. Regardless of these semantic differences, most authors agree on this: the term 'osteochondritis' is undesirable owing to the inconsistency of inflammatory markers in this condition.[109,113,114] When considered as separate entities, Panner's disease is described as a condition affecting younger children (aged 5 to 11 years) which does not lead to loose body formation or residual deformity. For others, the conditions are linked and part of the continuum of osteochondrosis, wherein Panner's disease would represent an early phase of the spectrum.[115–118] Here, the terms 'osteochondrosis' (to identify the condition) and 'osteochondral defect' (to define the sequelae) will be used.

Although radiographs remain the initial evaluation method of choice for osteochondrosis, the use of MR imaging is increasing owing to its sensitivity and the aid that it provides in determining the prognosis and, thereby, patient management. MR imaging is definitely superior to plain film radiography in detecting early osteochondral defects (Figure 9.11).[64,104,119,120]

In the early stages, plain film radiology may appear normal or show only subtle density changes. Flattening of the articular surface and fragmentation of the subchondral bone may be observed as the condition progresses. Free fragments may be observed in the later stages, often lodged in the coronoid or olecranon fossae.[109]

MR imaging can demonstrate significant abnormalities, even when radiographs are normal. Signal changes can be observed on most sequences. Fat-suppressed T2-weighted images will demonstrate a focal increase in signal intensity in the subchondral region of the capitellum. On the T1-weighted sequences, focal areas of either low signal intensity surrounding a more intermediate signal area or of homogeneous low signal intensity correspond to the involved area (Figure 9.12). If fragments are present, these will be of the same intensity as the native bone, and are easier to locate if surrounded by joint effusion. MR imaging is also superior in assessing the size, location, displacement, stability and viability of any fragment, all of which are factors in treatment and prognosis determination.[63,64]

A high intensity zone surrounding the fragment on both T2-weighted and post-contrast T1-weighted images is a sign of instability of the fragment, suggesting that surgical intervention may be required. Imaging enhancement of the fragment with contrast is considered a positive sign suggesting adequate blood supply and viability. Timely detection may therefore determine the most appropriate management protocol, providing a better outcome for the patient.[64,110,121]

Early or stable lesions respond well to conservative treatment, mainly the discontinuation of the aggravating activity. The cessation or serious limitation

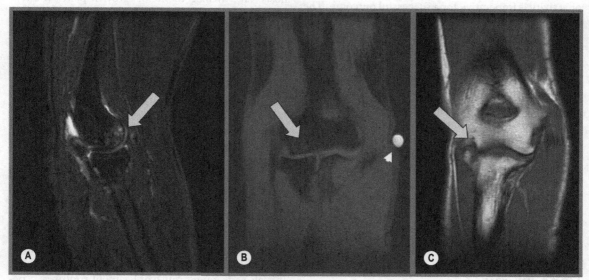

Figure 9.11 • Fat-suppressed T2-weighted MR imaging of the elbow in the sagittal (A) and coronal (B) planes together with T1-weighted imaging in the coronal plane (C). A region of increased signal intensity is noted in the subarticular area of the capitellum, most notably anteriorly (arrow in A). A mild joint effusion is also present with a collection of fluid posterior to the distal humerus. In figure B, a small region of increased signal is again noted in the region of the capitellum (arrow) with the suggestion of slight flattening of the subchondral bone. Note the small, round high signal region adjacent to the medial aspect of the elbow on the skin (arrowhead), which is a vitamin E tablet placed to indicate where the patient is symptomatic to assist the interpreter in localizing the region of complaint. In figure C, a focal defect is suggested in the capitellum. The imaging features are consistent with an osteochondral injury with an associated joint effusion, with no evidence of displacement of a fragment. These multiple images demonstrate changes consistent with early stages of osteochondrosis/osteochondral injury. Heterogeneous signal changes are noted in the anterior aspect of the capitellum on the sagittal (A) and coronal (B) fat-suppressed images. Subtle changes are also noted on the coronal T1-weighted image (C), which was obtained slightly more posteriorly than that of image B.

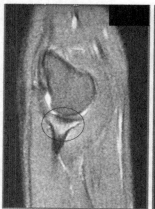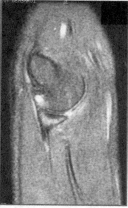

Figure 9.12 • Sagittal T2-weighted MR imaging sequence of the elbow demonstrating focal high signal in the trochlea adjacent to the articular surface (oval). This represents bone marrow contusion/infarction of the bone secondary to avulsion of the medial collateral ligament (not visualized in current study).

of activity is imperative for a successful outcome. The prognosis for the condition also depends on the age of the patient and the severity of the original lesion. Unstable lesions, where an isolated fragment is present, usually necessitate surgical management. The principal long-term complication in osteochondrosis is degenerative joint disease.[122]

A normal variant may mimic the presentation of osteochondral defects in the elbow. Occasionally, the junction of smooth articular cartilage of the capitellum and the rough, non-articular cartilage on the posterior aspect of the lateral epicondyle may form a groove and simulate a bony defect. This appearance is referred to as the 'pseudodefect of the capitellum'. The location on the posterior side is the key to recognition along with recognition of the continuity of the cartilage interface and lack of underlying osseous change.[110,123]

Bone injuries

MR imaging is not usually necessary to initially detect the majority of elbow fractures; however, MR imaging is superior to radiography in the evaluation of occult fractures, stress injuries and bone contusions, which may significantly affect both prognosis and management.[78,123] Fat-suppressed T2-weighted images are considered the most sensitive but least specific images for their detection of these often subtle osseous conditions.[64]

Fractures are demonstrated as a linear pattern of increased T2-weighted and decreased T1-weighted signal intensities. Signal changes associated with bone bruises are typically more diffuse, visible as a large region of increased signal intensity on fluid-sensitive sequences, affecting the subchondral bone and bony marrow about the site of the injury (Figure 9.12).[64]

MR imaging is also the best modality to evaluate the inevitable soft tissue injuries associated with fractures and determine their effect on both the clinical management and the prognosis of the trauma. For example, radial head fractures are often associated with disruption of the lateral and medial collateral ligaments. The damage to the soft tissues and the small fragments cannot be seen on plain film radiographs.[124,125]

Assessing damage to the growth plate and developing articular cartilage can also be performed using MR imaging. This makes the modality particularly useful for assessing traumatic injuries in the paediatric patient, notwithstanding the difficulties in imaging younger patients discussed above. The prognosis and management of growth-plate (Salter–Harris) injuries is greatly influenced by the location of the damage, making an accurate description of the injury a high priority. MR imaging offers an important advantage since the ossification centres of the distal humerus are not well seen on plain film radiographs. However, this benefit has to be clinically weighed against the risks of sedation in this population, often necessary to ensure image quality.[64,110,123]

Certain sites within the elbow are more prone to fractures than others; the most common location of fracture in adults is the radial head.[78] The mechanism of injury always involves some form of axial overloading, such as falling on an outstretched hand (*FOOSH*).[126] The '*FOOSH*' mechanism may also be responsible for injuries throughout the upper extremity: fractures at the distal radius (Colles' fracture), capitellum or the scaphoid as well as dislocations of the wrist, elbow or even glenohumeral joint. It is also a frequent cause of ligament ruptures, especially of the ulnar collateral ligament.[78,127]

When examining a patient with a suspected radial head fracture, it is therefore of the utmost importance to assess the rest of the upper extremity to explore the possibility of comorbid damage.[3] With conventional radiographic evaluation of radial head fractures, it is imperative to look for the anterior fat pad 'sail sign' or the elevated capsular fat plane posteriorly, both of which indicate capsular oedema and are very closely associated with radial head fractures, even in the absence of overt findings.[128] If the fracture is radiographically occult on plain films, MR imaging can confirm the presence of a fracture by demonstrating effusion, marrow oedema and the actual fracture line.

In adults, the anterolateral aspect of the radial head is especially vulnerable to injury because it lacks subchondral bone.[129] By contrast, in children, fracture of the radial neck is more common, though the morphological appearance is similar.[130] The degree of comminution is important to assess in all fractures of the proximal radius as it is one of the most important factors in the long-term prognosis. When the fracture is not well visualized on plain film radiography, MR imaging may be indicated.[131]

Fractures of the coronoid process of the ulna are distraction injuries caused by the avulsion of the brachialis muscle from dislocation or hyperextension. They can occur in conjunction with or independently from fractures of the radial head. If seen together, they are likely the result of a posterior dislocation caused by a *FOOSH*.[132] When associated with a sprain of the ulnar collateral ligament, they form the 'terrible triad of the elbow', invariably challenging from a management standpoint.[133,134]

Fractures of the medial and lateral epicondyles are both most commonly avulsion injuries caused by contraction of the flexor or extensor/supinator muscle groups respectively. Direct impact, creating varus or valgus stress, may also be a cause. MR imaging is helpful once again to determine the degree of comminution and damage to the adjacent articular cartilage. Complex fractures will most likely be managed surgically.[135,136]

Dislocations

The elbow joint is the second most commonly dislocated joint in adults (following the shoulder). In children, it is the commonest site of such injuries and the mechanism of injury is usually traction.[78,123,137] This is referred to technically as radial head subluxation, and colloquially as 'pulled elbow' or 'nursemaid's elbow' referring to the frequent presentation whereby a parent (or nursemaid) has jerked or pulled a small child's arm whilst holding hands; the injury is usually inadvertent. It may be reduced successfully in most cases without any requirement for imaging. In adults, a *FOOSH* or forced hyperextension is the typical cause of this injury and the situation is usually rather more complex.[138–141]

The ulna and radius can dislocate together or individually. Because of the requirement for pronation and supination, they are closely approximated in all movements. This nature of this closed kinematic chain means that when significant trauma is detected in one area of the chain, the remaining components should be carefully scrutinized to eliminate collateral injury.[29,142] Classical examples of this phenomenon include the Monteggia fracture-dislocation (radial head dislocation associated with an ulnar fracture) and the Essex-Lopresti injury (a comminuted, displaced fracture of the radial head with dislocation of the distal radioulnar joint).[78]

These injuries are usually quite evident both clinically and with conventional radiography. The utility of MR imaging mainly resides in the assessment of the adjacent soft tissue damage, underlying osseous complications and surgical planning (Figures 9.13–9.16). In particular, small fractures and capsular disruptions missed on plain film may be linked to residual instability.[125] Other injuries associated with dislocation are contusions at the anterior coronoid process, radial head and posterior capitellum; musculotendinous strains involving the brachialis muscle; ligamentous and capsule sprains; and neurovascular damage.[143]

Ligamentous trauma

The ulnar and radial collateral ligament complexes, as well as the capsule, can all be well evaluated with MR imaging. Damage to the collateral ligaments is a common, sports-related, chronic stress injury. It may, however, also occur following acute events such as dislocation.[136,143]

On plain film radiographs, subtle soft tissue densities corresponding to avulsed fragments adjacent to the involved epicondyle and gapping of the joint may be the only sign of injury. Any gapping may be accentuated on stress radiographs.[78] By contrast, MR images may demonstrate signs of acute or chronic ligamentous sprain: increased signal in or surrounding the ligament on T2-weighted images, representing oedema or haemorrhage; thickening or thinning of the ligament and waviness, laxity or discontinuity of the fibres (Figure 9.17). Ligamentous ruptures will be demonstrated by discontinuous fibres and abnormalities of the surrounding signal.[143–145]

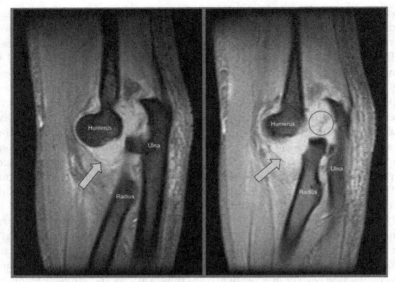

Figure 9.13 • Sagittal, fat-suppressed, T2-weighted MR imaging sequences of the elbow. A dramatic example of a posterior dislocation of the ulna and radius demonstrating the complete loss of articular apposition and also the extent of joint effusion and disruption of the soft tissue anatomy with massive oedema (arrows). Such information may be important prior to surgical intervention to guide the approach used. As well as the joint effusion, regions of low signal intensity also are noted within, which are likely to correspond to areas of intra-articular haemorrhage and/or cartilage lesions resulting from the trauma (circle).

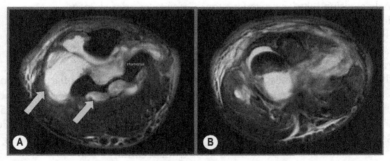

Figure 9.14 • Axial, fat-saturated, T2-weighted MR imaging sequences of the elbow performed through the distal humerus (A) and proximal forearm (B) in a patient with an acute posterior dislocation of the elbow. The images show massive soft tissue oedema (arrows) with fluid present in the olecranon and radial head fossa. There is also complete loss of apposition of the articular surface of humerus and ulna. In such a case, MR imaging may be performed to determine the extent of soft tissue involvement including the neurovascular damage. Also note the extent of the posterior subcutaneous oedema.

Ulnar collateral ligament

Ruptures of the UCL are usually an acute occurrence, whereby the patient experiences sudden pain, which may be associated with a popping sensation. They most often occur during sports involving throwing.[145] For most ordinary beings, the treatment will be conservative – the flexor-pronator muscle group will be sufficient to stabilize the elbow. In elite athletes, surgical reconstruction may be attempted in order to allow further pursuit of the sport of choice.[80,146]

The aetiology of the injury may, however, be chronic, arising from repetitive valgus force – typically from throwing activities – placing a high amount of stress on the UCL. Over time, these stresses lead

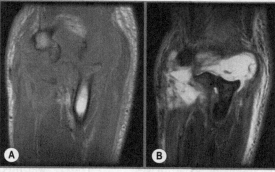

Figure 9.15 • Coronal T1-weighted (A) and fat-suppressed T2-weighted (B) MR imaging sequences of the elbow. The images demonstrate the complete loss of articular apposition between the distal humerus and the radius/ulna in a case of an acute traumatic posterior elbow dislocation. Note the extent of the synovial effusion with total disruption of normal anatomic integrity in both images.

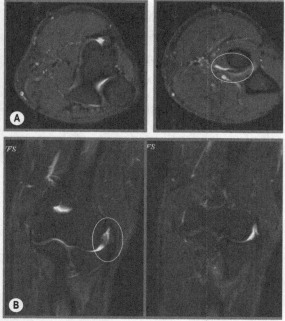

Figure 9.17 • Axial, T2-weighted, fat-suppressed MR imaging of the elbow (row A) and coronal, T2-weighted, fat-suppressed images (row B) demonstrating a partial lateral collateral ligament avulsion injury. In row A, a region of low signal intensity surrounded by high signal is noted about the radial head consistent with oedema about the lateral collateral ligament (oval). In row B, the region of abnormality is noted about the lateral aspect of the distal humerus, with an area of decreased signal intensity and enlargement of the lateral collateral ligament (oval) as well as a slightly wavy appearance. A mild joint effusion is also noted on both coronal images, which may be associated with such injuries.

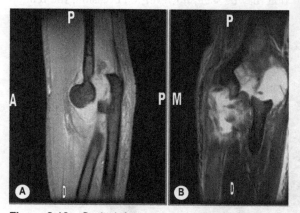

Figure 9.16 • Sagittal, fat-suppressed, T2-weighted MR imaging (A) of the elbow following severe trauma showing joint distension with posterior dislocation of the ulna. Surprisingly, the triceps insertion is still intact despite the degree of force necessary to dislocate the articulation. The same protocols in the coronal plane (B) also demonstrate the extensive joint effusion as well as the subcutaneous oedema. On closer inspection of the osseous components, note how the proximal radius, in particular the head and neck, demonstrate high signal owing to the bone marrow oedema associated with a fracture. Lateral dislocation of the radial head and an intra-articular fragment are also noted.

to repeated microtrauma, inflammatory changes, weakening and eventually rupturing of the ligament. Clinically, this may present as medial elbow instability. By far the most common site for tears of the UCL

is the mid-substance of the anterior bundle of the ligament.[80] Avulsions of the proximal attachment (3% of cases) or distal attachment (10% of cases) site have also been reported.[147,148] Chronic degeneration with thickening of the ligaments over time may lead to radiographically visible calcific changes or heterotopic bone formation, similar to that found in Pellegrini–Stieda disease in the medial collateral ligament of the knee. In patients who have undergone repetitive valgus stress, a characteristic osteophyte may be present at the insertion of the UCL on the coronoid process.[80]

With acute tears of the UCL, bone contusions may also be present in the lateral compartment. These will be demonstrated as high signal intensity on

T2-weighted sequences. Partial tears may occur as well, but detection with MR imaging is much less reliable unless intra-articular contrast is used.

Radial collateral ligament

Injuries to the radial collateral ligament may occur in acute traumatic events such as a *FOOSH*, causing hyperextension along with a varus stress, or as a result of chronic epicondylitis, causing lateral epicondylar soft tissue degeneration and tearing of the common extensor tendon.[48] Rotational instability may be present but difficult to elicit if the patient is guarding.[82] On MR images, as with other ligament tears, there will be discontinuous fibres with adjacent signal irregularities (Figure 9.18). Posterolateral rotatory instability, as seen with lateral ulnar collateral ligament (LUCL) incompetence, will result in a rotary subluxation of the humeroulnar joint and subluxation or dislocation of the radiohumeral joint. This pattern of instability may also be secondary to a surgical lateral extensor release.[149]

Tendinous injuries

Although uncommon injuries, biceps and triceps tendon tears can be assessed with MR imaging, which can confirm the rupture and distinguish between complete and partial tears as well as excluding differential diagnoses.[123,149] Rupture of the biceps tendon typically occurs acutely in middle-aged men. If it occurs distally, it will arise near or at the insertion site on the radial tuberosity.[144,150,151] On MR imaging, the low signal intensity of the tendon will be absent on axial images.[123,143] The T2-weighted images will show high signal intensity corresponding to oedema in the antecubital fossa (Figure 9.19). Retraction of the tendon fibres may be observed on the sagittal images. The amount of retraction is usually linked to a concomitant injury to the bicipital aponeurosis (lacertus fibrosus).

Tendinopathy and partial tears are also common. In both chronic and acute injury, thinning of the tendon may be seen; however, on occasion, the tendon

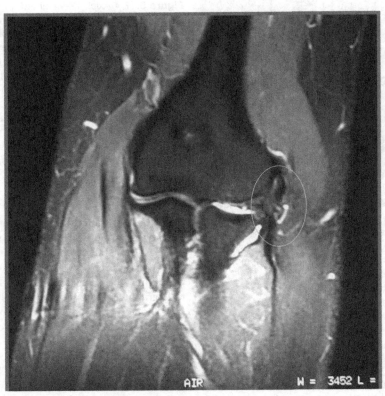

Figure 9.18 • Coronal STIR MR imaging of the elbow demonstrating the ruptured radial collateral ligament which is continuous, 'bunched-up' and disorganized (oval). However, remember that it would be necessary to review all slices in the planes available to confirm the presence and full extent of the lesion.

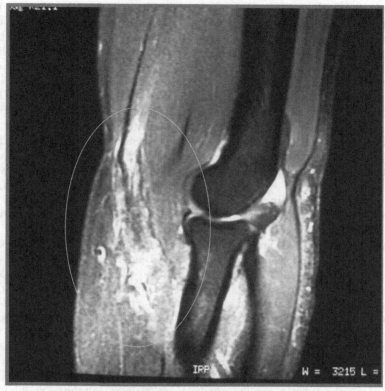

Figure 9.19 • Sagittal STIR MR imaging of the elbow demonstrating a region of diffuse increase in signal intensity in the anterior compartment of the elbow, running along the biceps muscle and tendon (oval). This represents disruption of the muscle/tendinous fibres due to a partial rupture of the lower portion of the biceps tendon.

may also appear thickened. In the acute scenario, this is due to the oedema associated with the intrasubstance damage. By contrast, the thickening seen in chronic injury is caused by accumulated fibrosis, which will have a less intense signal on the fluid-sensitive images. Partial ruptures are also characterized by the presence of high T2-weighted signal intensity, indicating bone marrow oedema in the radial tuberosity; and presence of fluid (high T2 signal intensity) in the interosseous fossa, corresponding to associated bursitis.[64,152] Low signal intensity on both T1-weighted and T2-weighted images represents osseous proliferation at the radial tuberosity, which may result from such an injury.[151] Differentiation of partial tears from bicipital tendinopathy is difficult as one may predispose to the other. It is important to consider and correlate the clinical presentation to inform the differential diagnosis.

Tears of the triceps tendon, whether complete or partial, are even rarer injuries. Tears may be seen after acute incidents (such as a *FOOSH* injury) or from chronic, repetitive events related to sports. The MR imaging findings will be similar to those described in the biceps tendon, but will be present in or surrounding the olecranon process, with associated bone marrow changes observed on both axial and sagittal images. Small avulsion fractures may be visualized at the olecranon on MR imaging and also on the lateral plain film views.[63,141]

Epicondylitis

Epicondylitis of the elbow is a common clinical disorder. It involves partial avulsion of the tendons attaching to the epicondyles of the humerus.[150–152] The diagnosis can be made clinically without imaging.[3,44] Radiographs are classically normal but may show dystrophic calcification adjacent to the involved epicondyle, particularly if the disorder is chronic. This finding represents calcific changes or heterotopic bone formation in the adjacent tendons.[153] MR imaging may, however, demonstrate characteristic findings when the study is performed to rule out concomitant or mimicking injuries, especially in the case where there is inadequate resolution of symptoms despite appropriate care. MR imaging may also assist in surgical planning to evaluate the presence of associated tendinous tears.[141,150,151]

MR imaging findings will be similar in both medial and lateral epicondylitis and pathology is usually seen best on coronal images, which can demonstrate a range of changes, from a mild thickening of a tendon through to a partial interstitial tendon tear or complete avulsion with tears of the adjacent collateral ligament.[142,150,152]

The signal intensity within and about the involved epicondyle may be increased on T2-weighted, fat-saturated T2-weighted and inversion recovery sequences, consistent with localized bone and soft tissue oedema (Figure 9.19). Tendons normally display homogeneous low signal intensity on all sequences. In epicondylitis, thickening and increased signal intensity will be seen in the substance of the tendon on T1- and T2-weighted images, most often 1–2 cm below the attachment. Complete tears will be demonstrated by a lack of continuity of the tendon fibres. Paratendinous oedema (on high T2-weighted signal) is also commonly seen.[141,151] It is important to be aware of recent therapeutic corticosteroid injections, as they may also cause this appearance. Signal changes in the tendon also seem to be chronic and persist after the regression of the symptoms. Associated abnormalities in signal intensity may be visualized in the surrounding ligaments and muscles, as pathology in the collateral ligaments have common mechanisms of injuries.[154]

In **lateral epicondylitis**, the primarily involved structure is the extensor carpi radialis brevis. The signal changes will be more apparent 1–2 cm below the attachment point, in the hypovascular area of the tendon.[153,154] The origins of the extensor carpi radialis longus, extensor digitorum and extensor carpi ulnaris may also demonstrate changes.[141,155] This condition is also commonly referred to as 'tennis elbow'; however, most sufferers do not actually play tennis. Any sport requiring the use of a racquet may of course be predisposing, but, realistically, anyone using a hand tool repetitively is at risk (construction workers, tailors, drummers, computer users, etc.). The condition is caused by chronic varus stress where the wrist extensor and supinator muscles are overutilized.[27,28,154]

Patients will classically experience lateral elbow pain, particularly with resisted wrist extension (Cozen's sign). Pain may also be present with passive wrist flexion when the elbow is in full extension. Tenderness will likely be elicited upon palpation of the conjoined tendon distal to the lateral epicondyle. If tenderness is present more distally, it may be more indicative of a radial nerve syndrome.[155] Chronic, long-standing and severe lateral epicondylitis may lead to strains or tears of the LUCL and, in turn, radial collateral ligament instability.[79,134,156]

Medially, in 'golfer's elbow' or 'pitcher's elbow', the pronator teres and common flexor tendon are affected.[155,157] As opposed to those with its lateral counterpart, **medial epicondylitis** patients usually participate in sports: golf, baseball, bowling, archery or weightlifting.[17–19,143,158] They experience pain primarily on the medial aspect of the elbow and demonstrate symptoms aggravated by wrist flexion and forearm pronation. Elbow extension may also be limited. Tenderness will be elicited distally and anteriorly to the medial epicondyle around the origin of the pronator teres and the flexor carpi ulnaris.[3,155] Medial epicondylitis or partial tendon tears may occur after chronic, repetitive valgus stress or acute overload. During a valgus motion, the medial aspect of the elbow is stretched and the lateral aspect is compacted; consequently, in acute cases, it is important to assess the ulnar collateral ligament for signs of tears/strain as well the capitellum for osteochondral injuries and bone contusion.[141,151] In the skeletally immature patient, the stress may even lead to complete avulsion of the epicondyle ('Little-leaguer's' elbow).[113,121,159]

Nerve entrapment

All three major nerves of the upper extremity can be trapped as they pass through the elbow and present clinically as neuropathies that need to be differentiated from more proximal and distal entrapment syndromes. Consideration will also need to be made as to the possibility of 'double crush' injuries; positive findings in the elbow do not remove the requirement for a full analysis of the kinematic chain as a whole.[54,85,160]

Compression of the ulnar nerve in the cubital tunnel (**cubital tunnel syndrome**) is the second most common neuropathy in the adult population (after carpal tunnel syndrome with median nerve neuropathy).[28,52,54,161] Pronator (median nerve) and radial tunnel syndrome are also quite regular clinical presentations.[54,55,141] The aetiology is often varied but is mostly associated with chronic overuse processes.[4,120]

The symptoms are variable and may be similar to those of tendinous injuries, particularly in patients with radial entrapment, which may present as a lateral epicondylitis that has been unresponsive to treatment. Long-term medial epicondylitis may also be associated with median nerve entrapments.[54,141]

The median, radial and especially the ulnar nerve are surrounded by a layer of fat, which permits good visualization of each nerve on axial sequences.[143] Inflammatory changes will be shown as heterogeneous or homogeneous increased signal intensity on T2-weighted sequences within the contours of the nerve. The diameter of the nerve may be increased around the compression site and there may be blurring of the individual fascicles (Figures 9.20–9.22).[63,142]

The surrounding muscular structures may demonstrate changes as well. It is important to assess the surrounding muscles for the presence of associated morphological changes such as muscle denervation or oedema (increased T2-weighted, fat-saturated T2-weighted and inversion recovery sequences), muscle atrophy and fatty degeneration (reduction in overall muscle belly size and increased T1-weighted signal). Early diagnosis and treatment offer the best prognosis, as these trophic changes may be irreversible after 6 months.[63,141,142]

With neuropathies, the location and aetiology of compression may be determined at the same time. The radiologist and clinician need to identify and clinically correlate normal variations; muscular hypertrophy; soft tissue masses relating to tumours or infection; trauma-induced neuropathies; or scar tissue formation. The presence of any of these findings does not automatically constitute a diagnosis unless there is evidence of entrapment *that explains the patient's clinical* presentation; no clinician wants to treat a radiological finding that was, in fact, benign!

Cubital tunnel syndrome or neuropathy is compression of the ulnar nerve in the area of the cubital tunnel retinaculum.[69,156] A wide variety of causes

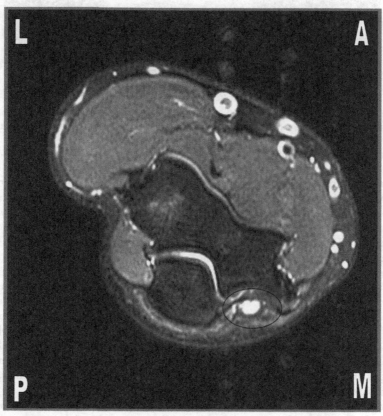

Figure 9.20 • Axial T2-weighted MR imaging of the elbow with fat suppression, demonstrating high signal intensity in the region of the ulnar nerve, which would ordinarily be of intermediate signal, in a case of ulnar neuropathy (oval).

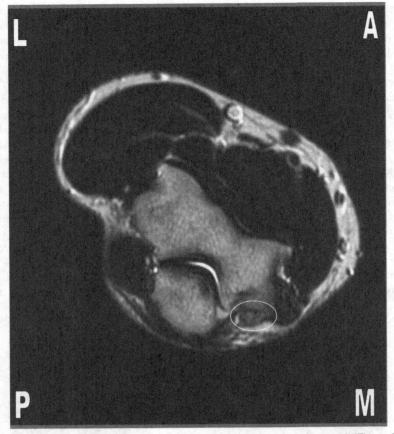

Figure 9.21 • Axial T1-weighted MR imaging of the elbow in the same patient illustrated in Figure 9.20 demonstrating thickening, heterogeneous signal intensity and irregularity of the ulnar nerve (oval) due to ulnar neuropathy.

can be responsible: developmental causes associated with an accessory muscle like the anconeus epitrochlearis[72,157,158] or an aberrant triceps insertion[159]; a shallow cubital tunnel[160]; post-traumatic causes associated with malunion or non-union of fractures[53,161]; muscle hypertrophy[162]; repeated valgus stress injuries[48,148]; and medial epicondylitis.[26,163] The clinical presentation can vary with the degree of entrapment from mild paraesthesia to severe deformation and muscle atrophy.[156]

The symptoms will manifest in the fifth digit and the medial aspect of the fourth digit, along the ulnar nerve distribution ... exactly the same symptoms as you may have experienced if you have every hit your 'funny bone'. It is important to elicit the presence of any ulnar nerve signs and symptoms proximal to the wrist, such as paraesthesia or weakness in the flexor carpi ulnaris muscle, as this can differentiate between 'Tunnel of Guyon' syndrome and more proximal entrapment of the nerve.[156,164]

Radial neuropathy is not as frequently seen as ulnar nerve entrapment.[28,54] Depending on the compression site, it may present clinically with either sensory and motor dysfunction or a motor deficit alone (posterior interosseous nerve syndrome). There will be findings of denervation in the muscles supplied by the radial nerve and sensory disturbances in the dorsal and radial aspects of the wrist and hand.[156,164] If the entrapment occurs distally, in the arcade of Frohse, there will only be muscular problems, as the radial nerve has by that time divided into a main sensory branch and the posterior interosseous branch, which supplies the supinator muscle and all the extensor muscles of the forearm with the exception of the extensor carpi radialis longus, which is supplied by the radial nerve before its bifurcation.[68,75,164]

In the general population, the median nerve is most often entrapped in the carpal tunnel of the wrist.[88] It may, however, be compressed in the elbow region,

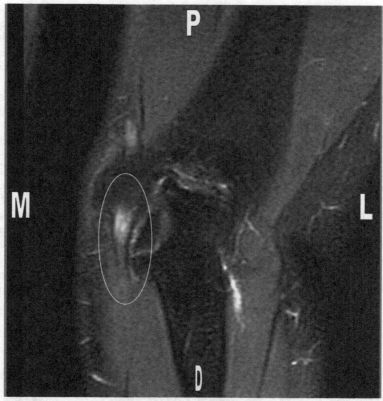

Figure 9.22 • Coronal T2-weighted MR imaging of the elbow in the same patient illustrated in Figures 9.20 and 9.21, with fat suppression, demonstrating high (bright) signal in the ulnar nerve with associated thickening (oval) due to ulnar neuropathy. P = proximal, D = distal.

most commonly in athletes.[54,55] This occurs at the level of the pronator muscle and is termed **pronator syndrome**. It is also possible for the anterior interosseous branch only to be affected.[165] The median nerve gives off this major branch after passing between the two origins of the pronator teres, approximately 5 cm inferior to the lateral epicondyle. The anterior interosseous nerve is a strictly motor branch supplying the pronator quadratus, the flexor pollicis longus and the radial half of the flexor digitorum profundus.[74,75]

Anterior interosseous nerve syndrome is demonstrated clinically as weakness of the thumb and index finger in conjunction with a complaint of proximal forearm pain. Patients with pronator syndrome generally experience an aching pain in the anterior portion of the proximal forearm and intermittent paraesthesia. Weakness or frank sensory loss is unusual.[156,164] Sources of entrapment leading to a pronator syndrome are multiple, including the ligament of Struthers,[55,84] muscle hypertrophy,[166] aberrant muscle origins,[167]

and soft tissue masses.[168] If there are concomitant findings in the median and radial nerve distribution, one should consider cervical radiculopathy or brachial plexitis as differential diagnoses.[164]

Bursitis

The olecranon and bicipitoradial bursae are not typically seen on MR imaging unless engorged with fluid. Patients will present with an antecubital mass or swelling at the posterior aspect of the elbow, depending on the affected bursa. Inflammatory conditions of the bursa can be imaged with MR and generally produce a high fluid signal intensity in the olecranon or bicipitoradial bursae on T2-weighted images and low signal intensity on T1-weighted images. The appearance of bicipitoradial bursitis, which can be insidious or present after athletic activity, is similar on MR imaging.[169,170]

MR is not necessary to manage bursitis in most cases; nonetheless, one must keep in mind that bursitis can be more than a reactive process at a site of high frictional stress. Inflammation of the olecranon bursa, for example, is classically seen after trauma, yet may also be present in inflammatory conditions such as rheumatoid arthritis and crystal deposition disorders such as gout.[171,172] Acute osteomyelitis in children and chronic osteomyelitis in adults is often associated with infectious bursitis. Performed usually only on cases that are refractory, MR imaging shows hyperintense marrow oedema on T1-weighted and T2-weighted images and cortical destruction.[173,174]

Articular conditions

Synovial folds or *plicae* represent a thickened fold of synovial tissue, situated at the lateral aspect of the radiocapitellar joint. They are also referred to as a *radiohumeral meniscus* or *labrum*.[175,176] Plicae are most commonly seen in the knee joint and are associated with chondromalacia on the adjacent articular surface.[177,178] The only plain film finding in the elbow may be sclerotic changes in the radial head and capitellum. As with their main differential diagnosis (loose bodies), they can be asymptomatic, or may cause 'snapping' of the elbow, locking and pain in the lateral aspect of the joint line.

Conditions typically associated with synovial articulations, such as inflammation, degeneration or proliferation, can affect the elbow and can be visualized with MR imaging (Figure 9.23A,B).

Rheumatoid arthritis (RA) is a common, systemic arthritic condition; involvement of the elbow joint is seen in 20% to 50% of rheumatoid patients.[144,179,180] The diagnosis is not usually dependent solely on imaging, but rather based on clinical criteria, which also include joint stiffness, presence of nodules and serological markers.[113,181] Nevertheless, elbow involvement may cause debilitating pain and joint

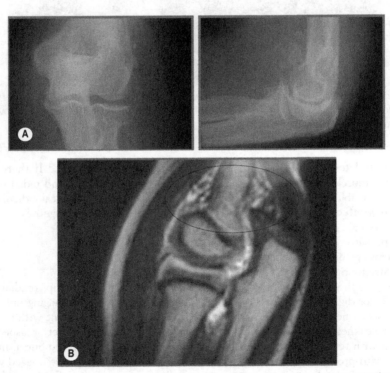

Figure 9.23 • (A) Anteroposterior and lateral conventional radiographs of the elbow demonstrating numerous intra-articular densities associated with a joint effusion. The likely diagnosis based on these findings is that of synovio-osteochondrometaplasia although there is a differential diagnosis depending on the clinical history, based on synovial-based lesions. (B) MR imaging of the elbow performed in the sagittal plane in the same patient, T1-weighted with intra-articular contrast, demonstrates a number of low signal intensity zones (oval) in the anterior and posterior aspect of the elbow joint associated with the articular distension, consistent with synovio-osteochondrometaplasia.

destruction in this condition, which begins as a proliferative synovitis and rapidly progresses to destruction of the articular cartilage and subchondral bone.[182] On plain film, this is demonstrated by a loss of joint space and bony erosions.[181] On MR images, thickening of the synovial membrane and associated pannus formation occurs and intra-articular fluid accumulates. An increased signal intensity from the oedematous synovium is seen, with hyperintense joint effusion. In a patient exhibiting clinical signs of rheumatoid arthritis, these are imaging signs that best confirm the diagnosis.[144]

Erosions, which exhibit decreased signal intensity, are radiologically visible and the pathognomonic nodules show as mixed signal intensity masses in the skin, synovium and tendons. Erosions in the cartilage and subchondral bone as well as any associated bursitis are also well visualized.[183] If intravascular contrast is used, the synovium will demonstrate enhancement, especially prominent on fat-saturation sequences. The destruction of both soft tissue structures and bone can lead to severe elbow instability. In late-stage RA, when the joint space is almost completely destroyed, MR may show a decrease in the synovitis.[183] Although other imaging modalities such as ultrasound may be used to follow the course of RA, MR imaging is able to evaluate better the subtle alterations to the bone as well as to the tendons that may not be detectable using ultrasound.

Osteoarthritis is seen less commonly in the elbow than in weight-bearing joints, and commonly there is a predisposing factor that has resulted in the degeneration of articular cartilage, such as trauma or arthropathy. Findings are typically evident on plain films.[181] MR imaging may be used to evaluate the integrity of the cartilage, identify focal defects or chondromalacia, and further qualify the findings seen on radiography. Osteoarthritis is a long-term complication of instability and impingement.[173,184]

Clinical pearls

- MR imaging of the elbow is useful in the clinical setting of acute trauma or chronic repetitive mechanical stress, both of which may result in pain and modification of the normal function of the elbow.
- MR imaging provides multiplanar, high-quality images with fine detail that can be very useful in the assessment of many elbow conditions, which are often not visible on plain film radiography and which are limited in their visualization using diagnostic ultrasound.
- MR imaging planes should include axial, sagittal and coronal slices with both T1- and T2-weighted sequences included in the study.
- MR imaging interpretation should commence with the fluid-sensitive sequences to determine regions of inflammation, fluid collection or bone oedema. These may assist in the localization and, later, the characterization of the elbow disorder.
- MR imaging may be helpful in assessing non-responsive patients suffering from overuse injuries such as epicondylitis.
- MR imaging can accurately determine the extent of tears or inflammatory changes in both ligaments and tendons, assisting in the prognosis and management of patients.
- During the MR imaging interpretation, pick an anatomical structure and follow it from its origin to insertion on all three planes.

References

1. Standring S, ed. Functional anatomy of the musculoskeletal system. In: *Gray's Anatomy: The Anatomical Basis of Clinical Practice*. 39th ed. Edinburgh: Elsevier; 2005.

2. Bates B, Hoekelman R. Interviewing and the health history. In: Bates B, ed. *A Guide to Physical Examination*. 3rd ed. Philadelphia: JB Lippincott; 1983:1–27.

3. Bates B. The musculoskeletal system. In: Bates B, ed. *A Guide to Physical Examination*. 3rd ed. Philadelphia: JB Lippincott; 1983:324–370.

4. Weinstein SM, Herring SA. Nerve problems and compartment syndromes in the hand, wrist, and forearm. *Clin Sports Med*. 1992;11(1):161–188.

5. Rojas IL, Provencher MT, Bhatia S, et al. Biceps activity during windmill softball pitching: injury implications and comparison with overhand throwing. *Am J Sports Med*. 2009;37(3):558–565.

6. Davidson PA, Pink M, Perry J, Jobe FW. Functional anatomy of the flexor pronator muscle group in relation to the medial collateral ligament of the elbow. *Am J Sports Med*. 1995;23(2):245–250.

7. Priest JD, Jones HH, Nagel DA. Elbow injuries in highly skilled tennis players. *J Sports Med*. 1974;2(3):139–149.

8. Priest JD. Tennis elbow. The syndrome and a study of average players. *Minn Med*. 1976;59(6):367–371.

9. Carroll R. Tennis elbow: incidence in local league players. *Br J Sports Med*. 1981;15(4):250–256.

10. Hang YS, Peng SM. An epidemiologic study of upper

extremity injury in tennis players with a particular reference to tennis elbow. *Taiwan Yi Xue Hui Za Zhi*. 1984;83(3):307–316.

11. Kitai E, Itay S, Ruder A, et al. An epidemiological study of lateral epicondylitis (tennis elbow) in amateur male players. *Ann Chir Main*. 1986;5(2):113–121.

12. Jacobson JA, Miller BS, Morag Y. Golf and racquet sports injuries. *Semin Musculoskelet Radiol*. 2005;9(4):346–359.

13. Hensley LD, Paup DC. A survey of badminton injuries. *Br J Sports Med*. 1979;13(4):156–160.

14. Jorgensen U, Winge S. Injuries in badminton. *Sports Med*. 1990;10(1):59–64.

15. Parziale JR, Mallon WJ. Golf injuries and rehabilitation. *Phys Med Rehabil Clin N Am*. 2006;17(3):589–607.

16. Plancher KD, Minnich JM. Sports-specific injuries. *Clin Sports Med*. 1996;15(2):207–218.

17. Wadsworth LT. When golf hurts: musculoskeletal problems common to golfers. *Curr Sports Med Rep*. 2007;6(6):362–365.

18. Wiesler ER, Lumsden B. Golf injuries of the upper extremity. *J Surg Orthop Adv*. 2005;14(1):1–7.

19. Loftice J, Fleisig GS, Zheng N, Andrews JR. Biomechanics of the elbow in sports. *Clin Sports Med*. 2004;23(4):519–530, vii–viii.

20. Verow P. Squash. *Practitioner*. 1989;233(1470):876, 878–879.

21. Cooney 3rd WP. Sports injuries to the upper extremity. How to recognize and deal with some common problems. *Postgrad Med*. 1984;76(4):45–50.

22. Meeuwisse WH, Sellmer R, Hagel BE. Rates and risks of injury during intercollegiate basketball. *Am J Sports Med*. 2003;31(3):379–385.

23. Heming M. Occupational injuries suffered by classical musicians through overuse. *Clinical Chiropractic*. 2004;7(2):55–66.

24. Klussmann A, Gebhardt H, Liebers F, Rieger MA. Musculoskeletal symptoms of the upper extremities and the neck: a cross-sectional study on prevalence and symptom-predicting factors at visual display terminal (VDT) workstations. *BMC Musculoskelet Disord*. 2008;9:96.

25. Eltayeb S, Staal JB, Kennes J, et al. Prevalence of complaints of arm, neck and shoulder among computer office workers and psychometric evaluation of a risk factor questionnaire. *BMC Musculoskelet Disord*. 2007;8:68.

26. Pascarelli EF, Hsu YP. Understanding work-related upper extremity disorders: clinical findings in 485 computer users, musicians, and others. *J Occup Rehabil*. 2001;11(1):1–21.

27. Silverstein B, Viikari-Juntura E, Kalat J. Use of a prevention index to identify industries at high risk for work-related musculoskeletal disorders of the neck, back, and upper extremity in Washington state, 1990–1998. *Am J Ind Med*. 2002;41(3):149–169.

28. Helliwell PS, Bennett RM, Littlejohn G, et al. Towards epidemiological criteria for soft-tissue disorders of the arm. *Occup Med (Lond)*. 2003;53(5):313–319.

29. Young MF. The physics of anatomy. In: *Essential Physics for Muscloskeletal Medicine*. Edinburgh: Elsevier; 2009.

30. Hindle A. Function of the upper limb. In: Trew M, Everett T, eds. *Human Movement: An Introductory Text*. 4th ed. Churchill Livingstone: Edinburgh; 2005:193–202.

31. Schwartz D, Reisdorff E. Fundamentals of skeletal radiology. In: *Emergency Radiology*. Colombus, OH: McGraw-Hill; 1999:L11–L26.

32. Rowe L, Yochum T. Radiographic positioning and normal anatomy. In: Yochum T, Rowe L, eds. *Essentials of Skeletal Radiology*. Baltimore: Williams and Wilkins; 1987:1–93.

33. Kijowski R, De Smet AA. The role of ultrasound in the evaluation of sports medicine injuries of the upper extremity. *Clin Sports Med*. 2006;25(3):569–590, viii.

34. Balint P, Sturrock RD. Musculoskeletal ultrasound imaging: a new diagnostic tool for the rheumatologist? *Br J Rheumatol*. 1997;36(11):1141–1142.

35. Kane D, Grassi W, Sturrock R, Balint PV. Musculoskeletal ultrasound—a state of the art review in rheumatology. Part 2: Clinical indications for musculoskeletal ultrasound in rheumatology. *Rheumatology (Oxford)*. 2004;43(7):829–838.

36. Yoon JS, Walker FO, Cartwright MS. Ultrasonographic swelling ratio in the diagnosis of ulnar neuropathy at the elbow. *Muscle Nerve*. 2008;38(4):1231–1235.

37. Yoon JS, Hong SJ, Kim BJ, et al. Ulnar nerve and cubital tunnel ultrasound in ulnar neuropathy at the elbow. *Arch Phys Med Rehabil*. 2008;89(5):887–889.

38. Yoon JS, Kim BJ, Kim SJ, et al. Ultrasonographic measurements in cubital tunnel syndrome. *Muscle Nerve*. 2007;36(6):853–855.

39. Wiesler ER, Chloros GD, Cartwright MS, et al. Ultrasound in the diagnosis of ulnar neuropathy at the cubital tunnel. *J Hand Surg [Am]*. 2006;31(7):1088–1093.

40. Okamoto M, Abe M, Shirai H, Ueda N. Diagnostic ultrasonography of the ulnar nerve in cubital tunnel syndrome. *J Hand Surg [Br]*. 2000;25(5):499–502.

41. Park GY, Lee SM, Lee MY. Diagnostic value of ultrasonography for clinical medial epicondylitis. *Arch Phys Med Rehabil*. 2008;89(4):738–742.

42. Tran N, Chow K. Ultrasonography of the elbow. *Semin Musculoskelet Radiol*. 2007;11(2):105–116.

43. Serafini G, Zadra N. Anaesthesia for MRI in the paediatric patient. *Curr Opin Anaesthesiol*. 2008;21(4):499–503.

44. Jaramillo D, Laor T. Pediatric musculoskeletal MRI: basic principles to optimize success. *Pediatr Radiol*. 2008;38(4):379–391.

45. Smidt N, Lewis M, van der Windt DA, et al. Lateral epicondylitis in general practice: course and prognostic indicators of outcome. *J Rheumatol*. 2006;33(10):2053–2059.

46. Bohndorf K, Kilcoyne RF. Traumatic injuries: imaging of peripheral musculoskeletal injuries. *Eur Radiol*. 2002;12(7):1605–1616.

47. Hoy G, Wood T, Phillips N, et al. When physiology becomes pathology: the role of magnetic resonance imaging in evaluating bone marrow oedema in the humerus in elite tennis players with an upper limb pain syndrome. *Br J Sports Med*. 2006;40(8):710–713.

48. Thornton R, Riley GM, Steinbach LS. Magnetic resonance imaging of sports injuries of the elbow. *Top Magn Reson Imaging.* 2003;14(1):69–86.

49. Fritz RC. MR imaging of osteochondral and articular lesions. *Magn Reson Imaging Clin N Am.* 1997;5(3):579–602.

50. Ercoli C, Boncan RB, Tallents RH, Macher DJ. Loose joint bodies of the temporomandibular joint: a case report. *Clin Orthod Res.* 1998;1(1):62–67.

51. Chan BK, Bell SN. Bilateral avascular necrosis of the humeral trochleae after chemotherapy. *J Bone Joint Surg Br.* 2000;82(5):670–672.

52. Cunningham PM. MR imaging of trauma: elbow and wrist. *Semin Musculoskelet Radiol.* 2006;10(4):284–292.

53. Bartels RH, Verbeek AL. Risk factors for ulnar nerve compression at the elbow: a case control study. *Acta Neurochir (Wien).* 2007;149(7):669–674. discussion 74.

54. Rich BC, McKay MP. The cubital tunnel syndrome: a case report and discussion. *J Emerg Med.* 2002;23(4):347–350.

55. Bencardino JT, Rosenberg ZS. Entrapment neuropathies of the shoulder and elbow in the athlete. *Clin Sports Med.* 2006;25(3):465–487, vi–vii.

56. Bilge T, Yalaman O, Bilge S, et al. Entrapment neuropathy of the median nerve at the level of the ligament of Struthers. *Neurosurgery.* 1990;27(5):787–789.

57. Rogers MR, Bergfield TG, Aulicino PL. The failed ulnar nerve transposition. Etiology and treatment. *Clin Orthop Relat Res.* 1991;(269):193–200.

58. Merolla G, Staffa G, Paladini P, et al. Endoscopic approach to cubital tunnel syndrome. *J Neurosurg Sci.* 2008;52(3):93–98.

59. Tanenbaum LN. Clinical 3T MR imaging: mastering the challenges. *Magn Reson Imaging Clin N Am.* 2006;14(1):1–15.

60. Wessely M, Hurtgen-Grace K, Grenier J-M. Elbow MRI. Part 1. Normal imaging appearance of the elbow. *Clinical Chiropractic.* 2006;9(4):198–205.

61. Teh J. Imaging of the elbow. *Imaging.* 2007;19:220–233.

62. Nuffield Orthopaedic Centre NHS Trust. MRI Protocols. Available from: www.noc.nhs.uk/SerARef/radiology/mriprotocols.htm; 2009; Accessed 28.02.09.

63. Wessely M, Grenier J-M. Elbow MRI. Part 2: The imaging of common disorders affecting the elbow region. *Clinical Chiropractic.* 2007;10(1):43–49.

64. Brunton LM, Anderson MW, Pannunzio ME, et al. Magnetic resonance imaging of the elbow: update on current techniques and indications. *J Hand Surg [Am].* 2006;31(6):1001–1011.

65. Fowler KA, Chung CB. Normal MR imaging anatomy of the elbow. *Magn Reson Imaging Clin N Am.* 2004;12(2):191–206, v.

66. Standring S, ed. *Gray's Anatomy - Pectoral girdle and upper limb: General organization and surface anatomy of the upper limb.* (Section 48). Edinburgh: Elsevier; 2009.

67. Green J, Silver P. Exploring the limbs. In: *An Introduction to Human Anatomy.* Oxford: Oxford University Press; 1981:27–51.

68. Standring S, ed. *Gray's Anatomy - Pectoral girdle and upper limb: Elbow.* (Section 51). Edinburgh: Elsevier; 2009.

69. Moore K. The upper limb. In: *Clinically Oriented Anatomy.* 2nd ed. Baltimore: Williams and Wilkins; 1985:626–793.

70. O'Driscoll S. Coronoid fracture classification. Available from: www.eorif.com/Elbowforearm/images; 2009; Accessed 09.03.09.

71. O'Hara JJ, Stone JH. Ulnar nerve compression at the elbow caused by a prominent medial head of the triceps and an anconeus epitrochlearis muscle. *J Hand Surg [Br].* 1996; 21(1):133–135.

72. Hsu RW, Chen CY, Shen WJ. Ulnar nerve palsy due to concomitant compression by the anconeus epitrochlearis muscle and a ganglion cyst. *Orthopedics.* 2004;27(2):227–228.

73. Kim YS, Yeh LR, Trudell D, Resnick D. MR imaging of the major nerves about the elbow: cadaveric study examining the effect of flexion and extension of the elbow and pronation and supination of the forearm. *Skeletal Radiol.* 1998; 27(8):419–426.

74. Green J, Silver P. The blood supply and nerve supply to the upper limb. In: *An Introduction to Human Anatomy.* Oxford: Oxford University Press; 1981:69–88.

75. Standring S, ed. *Gray's Anatomy - Pectoral girdle and upper limb: Forearm.* (Section 52). Edinburgh: Elsevier; 2009.

76. Green J, Silver P. The muscles and joints of the upper limb. In: *An Introduction to Human Anatomy.* Oxford: Oxford University Press; 1981:89–112.

77. Munshi M, Pretterklieber ML, Chung CB, et al. Anterior bundle of ulnar collateral ligament: evaluation of anatomic relationships by using MR imaging, MR arthrography, and gross anatomic and histologic analysis. *Radiology.* 2004;231(3):797–803.

78. Rowe L, Yochum T. Trauma. In: Yochum T, Rowe L, eds. *Essentials of Skeletal Radiology.* 2nd ed. Baltimore: Williams and Wilkins; 1996:653–794.

79. Lin F, Kohli N, Perlmutter S, et al. Muscle contribution to elbow joint valgus stability. *J Shoulder Elbow Surg.* 2007;16(6):795–802.

80. Lynch JR, Waitayawinyu T, Hanel DP, Trumble TE. Medial collateral ligament injury in the overhand-throwing athlete. *J Hand Surg [Am].* 2008;33(3):430–437.

81. Berg EE, DeHoll D. Radiography of the medial elbow ligaments. *J Shoulder Elbow Surg.* 1997;6(6):528–533.

82. Dunning CE, Zarzour ZD, Patterson SD, et al. Ligamentous stabilizers against posterolateral rotatory instability of the elbow. *J Bone Joint Surg Am.* 2001;83-A(12):1823–1828.

83. Dunning CE, Zarzour ZD, Patterson SD, et al. Muscle forces and pronation stabilize the lateral ligament deficient elbow. *Clin Orthop Relat Res.* 2001;(388):118–124.

84. Lee BP, Teo LH. Surgical reconstruction for posterolateral rotatory instability of the elbow. *J Shoulder Elbow Surg.* 2003;12(5):476–479.

85. Sener E, Takka S, Cila E. Supracondylar process syndrome. *Arch Orthop Trauma Surg.* 1998;117(6–7):418–419.

86. Lordan J, Rauh P, Spinner RJ. The clinical anatomy of the supracondylar spur and the ligament of Struthers. *Clin Anat.* 2005;18(7):548–551.

87. Siqueira MG, Martins RS. The controversial arcade of Struthers. *Surg Neurol.* 2005;64(suppl 1): S1:17–20, discussion S1:20–21.

88. Campbell WW, Landau ME. Controversial entrapment neuropathies. *Neurosurg Clin N Am.* 2008;19(4):597–608, vi–vii.

89. Gudmundsen TE, Ostensen H. Accessory ossicles in the elbow. *Acta Orthop Scand.* 1987;58(2): 130–132.

90. Obermann WR, Loose HW. The os supratrochleare dorsale: a normal variant that may cause symptoms. *AJR Am J Roentgenol.* 1983;141(1): 123–127.

91. Ishikawa H, Hirohota K, Kashiwagi D. A case report of patella cubiti. *Z Rheumatol.* 1976;35(11–12):407–411.

92. Kopuz C, Sancak B, Ozbenli S. On the incidence of third head of biceps brachii in Turkish neonates and adults. *Kaibogaku Zasshi.* 1999;74(3):301–305.

93. Standring S, ed. *Gray's Anatomy - Pectoral girdle and upper limb: Upper arm.* (Section 50). Edinburgh: Elsevier; 2009.

94. Macalister A. Additional observations on muscular anomalies in human anatomy (third series), with a catalogue of the principal muscular variations hitherto published. *Trans Roy Ir Acad Sci.* 1875;25:1–134.

95. Vollala VR, Nagabhooshana S, Bhat SM, et al. Multiple arterial, neural and muscular variations in upper limb of a single cadaver. *Rom J Morphol Embryol.* 2009;50(1): 129–135.

96. Kim KC, Rhee KJ, Shin HD. A long head of the biceps tendon confluent with the intra-articular rotator cuff: arthroscopic and MR arthrographic findings. *Arch Orthop Trauma Surg.* 2009;129(3):311–314.

97. Kim KC, Rhee KJ, Shin HD, Kim YM. Biceps long head tendon revisited: a case report of split tendon arising from single origin.

98. Schoenleber SJ, Spinner RJ. An unusual variant of the biceps brachii. *Clin Anat.* 2006;19(8):702–703.

99. Abu-Hijleh MF. Three-headed biceps brachii muscle associated with duplicated musculocutaneous nerve. *Clin Anat.* 2005;18(5): 376–379.

100. Jacoby SM, Herman MJ, Morrison WB, Osterman AL. Pediatric elbow trauma: an orthopaedic perspective on the importance of radiographic interpretation. *Semin Musculoskelet Radiol.* 2007;11(1):48–56.

101. De Boeck H. Radiology of the elbow in children. *Acta Orthop Belg.* 1996;62(suppl 1):34–40.

102. Ansah P, Vogt S, Ueblacker P, et al. Osteochondral transplantation to treat osteochondral lesions in the elbow. *J Bone Joint Surg Am.* 2007;89(10):2188–2194.

103. Takahara M, Mura N, Sasaki J, et al. Classification, treatment, and outcome of osteochondritis dissecans of the humeral capitellum. *Surgical technique. J Bone Joint Surg Am.* 2008;90(suppl 2 Pt 1):47–62.

104. Takahara M, Mura N, Sasaki J, et al. Classification, treatment, and outcome of osteochondritis dissecans of the humeral capitellum. *J Bone Joint Surg Am.* 2007;89(6):1205–1214.

105. Mitsunaga MM, Adishian DA, Bianco AJ Jr. Osteochondritis dissecans of the capitellum. *J Trauma.* 1982;22(1):53–55.

106. Klekamp J, Green NE, Mencio GA. Osteochondritis dissecans as a cause of developmental dislocation of the radial head. *Clin Orthop Relat Res.* 1997;(338):36–41.

107. Marshall KW, Marshall DL, Busch MT, Williams JP. Osteochondral lesions of the humeral trochlea in the young athlete. *Skeletal Radiol.* 2009; 38(5):479–491.

108. Kennedy J. What are osteochondral defects? Available from: http://www.osteochondraldefects.com; 2009; Accessed 02.03.09.

109. Rowe L, Yochum T. Hematological and vascular disorders. In: Yochum T, Rowe L, eds. *Essentials of Skeletal Radiology.* 2nd ed.

Arch Orthop Trauma Surg. 2008;128(5):495–498.

Baltimore: Williams and Wilkins; 1996:1243–1326.

110. Kijowski R, De Smet AA. Radiography of the elbow for evaluation of patients with osteochondritis dissecans of the capitellum. *Skeletal Radiol.* 2005;34(5):266–271.

111. Beers M, Berkow R. Avascular necrosis. In: *The Merck Manual.* 17th ed. Merck & Co: West Point, PA; 1999:453–454.

112. Peterson RK, Savoie 3rd FH, Field LD. Osteochondritis dissecans of the elbow. *Instr Course Lect.* 1999;48:393–398.

113. Helms C. Arthritis. In: *Fundamentals of Skeletal Radiology.* Philadelphia: Elsevier Saunders; 2005:113–140.

114. Ytrehus B, Carlson CS, Ekman S. Etiology and pathogenesis of osteochondrosis. *Vet Pathol.* 2007;44(4):429–448.

115. Kobayashi K, Burton KJ, Rodner C, et al. Lateral compression injuries in the pediatric elbow: Panner's disease and osteochondritis dissecans of the capitellum. *J Am Acad Orthop Surg.* 2004;12(4):246–254.

116. Kaeding CC, Whitehead R. Musculoskeletal injuries in adolescents. *Prim Care.* 1998;25(1):211–223.

117. Stoane JM, Poplausky MR, Haller JO, Berdon WE. Panner's disease: X-ray, MR imaging findings and review of the literature. *Comput Med Imaging Graph.* 1995;19(6):473–476.

118. Jawish R, Rigault P, Padovani JP, et al. Osteochondritis dissecans of the humeral capitellum in children. *Eur J Pediatr Surg.* 1993;3(2):97–100.

119. De Smet AA, Fisher DR, Graf BK, Lange RH. Osteochondritis dissecans of the knee: value of MR imaging in determining lesion stability and the presence of articular cartilage defects. *Am J Roentgenol.* 1990;155(3): 549–553.

120. De Smet AA, Fisher DR, Burnstein MI, et al. Value of MR imaging in staging osteochondral lesions of the talus (osteochondritis dissecans): results in 14 patients. *Am J Roentgenol.* 1990;154(3): 555–558.

121. Bradley JP, Petrie RS. Osteochondritis dissecans of the humeral capitellum. Diagnosis and treatment. *Clin Sports Med.* 2001;20(3):565–590.

122. Pena E, Calvo B, Martinez MA, Doblare M. Effect of the size and location of osteochondral defects in degenerative arthritis. A finite element simulation. *Comput Biol Med.* 2007;37(3):376–387.

123. Steinbach LS, Fritz RC, Tirman PF, Uffman M. Magnetic resonance imaging of the elbow. *Eur J Radiol.* 1997;25(3):223–241.

124. Beingessner DM, Dunning CE, Gordon KD, et al. The effect of radial head fracture size on elbow kinematics and stability. *J Orthop Res.* 2005;23(1):210–217.

125. Itamura J, Roidis N, Mirzayan R, et al. Radial head fractures: MRI evaluation of associated injuries. *J Shoulder Elbow Surg.* 2005;14(4):421–424.

126. Tejwani NC, Mehta H. Fractures of the radial head and neck: current concepts in management. *J Am Acad Orthop Surg.* 2007;15(7):380–387.

127. Loder RT. The demographics of equestrian-related injuries in the United States: injury patterns, orthopedic specific injuries, and avenues for injury prevention. *J Trauma.* 2008;65(2):447–460.

128. O'Dwyer H, O'Sullivan P, Fitzgerald D, et al. The fat pad sign following elbow trauma in adults: its usefulness and reliability in suspecting occult fracture. *J Comput Assist Tomogr.* 2004;28(4):562–565.

129. Gordon KD, Duck TR, King GJ, Johnson JA. Mechanical properties of subchondral cancellous bone of the radial head. *J Orthop Trauma.* 2003;17(4):285–289.

130. Landin LA, Danielsson LG. Elbow fractures in children. An epidemiological analysis of 589 cases. *Acta Orthop Scand.* 1986;57(4):309–312.

131. Mackenney PJ, McQueen MM, Elton R. Prediction of instability in distal radial fractures. *J Bone Joint Surg Am.* 2006;88(9):1944–1951.

132. Cohen MS. Fractures of the coronoid process. *Hand Clin.* 2004;20(4):443–453.

133. Zeiders GJ, Patel MK. Management of unstable elbows following complex fracture-dislocations—the "terrible triad" injury. *J Bone Joint Surg Am.* 2008;90(suppl 4):75–84.

134. Lindenhovius AL, Jupiter JB, Ring D. Comparison of acute versus subacute treatment of terrible triad injuries of the elbow. *J Hand Surg [Am].* 2008;33(6):920–926.

135. Loomer RL. Elbow injuries in athletes. *Can J Appl Sport Sci.* 1982;7(3):164–166.

136. McKee MD, Schemitsch EH, Sala MJ, O'Driscoll SW. The pathoanatomy of lateral ligamentous disruption in complex elbow instability. *J Shoulder Elbow Surg.* 2003;12(4):391–396.

137. Josefsson PO, Nilsson BE. Incidence of elbow dislocation. *Acta Orthop Scand.* 1986;57(6):537–538.

138. Macias CG, Wiebe R, Bothner J. History and radiographic findings associated with clinically suspected radial head subluxations. *Pediatr Emerg Care.* 2000;16(1):22–25.

139. Macias CG. Radial head subluxation. *Acad Emerg Med.* 2000;7(2):207–208.

140. Schunk JE. Radial head subluxation: epidemiology and treatment of 87 episodes. *Ann Emerg Med.* 1990;19(9):1019–1023.

141. Quan L, Marcuse EK. The epidemiology and treatment of radial head subluxation. *Am J Dis Child.* 1985;139(12):1194–1197.

142. Helms C. Trauma. In: *Fundamentals of Skeletal Radiology.* Philadelphia: Elsevier Saunders; 2005:78–112.

143. Kijowski R, Tuite M, Sanford M. Magnetic resonance imaging of the elbow. Part II: Abnormalities of the ligaments, tendons, and nerves. *Skeletal Radiol.* 2005;34(1):1–18.

144. Melloni P, Valls R. The use of MRI scanning for investigating soft-tissue abnormalities in the elbow. *Eur J Radiol.* 2005;54(2):303–313.

145. Kooima CL, Anderson K, Craig JV, et al. Evidence of subclinical medial collateral ligament injury and posteromedial impingement in professional baseball players. *Am J Sports Med.* 2004;32(7):1602–1606.

146. O'Holleran JD, Altchek DW. The thrower's elbow: arthroscopic treatment of valgus extension overload syndrome. *HSS J.* 2006;2(1):83–93.

147. McKee MD, Schemitsch EH, Sala MJ, O'Driscoll SW. The pathoanatomy of lateral ligamentous disruption in complex elbow instability. *J Shoulder Elbow Surg.* 2003;12(4):391–396.

148. Richard MJ, Aldridge 3rd JM, Wiesler ER, Ruch DS. Traumatic valgus instability of the elbow: pathoanatomy and results of direct repair. *J Bone Joint Surg Am.* 2008;90(11):2416–2422.

149. Marti RK, Kerkhoffs GM, Maas M, Blankevoort L. Progressive surgical release of a posttraumatic stiff elbow. Technique and outcome after 2–18 years in 46 patients. *Acta Orthop Scand.* 2002;73(2):144–150.

150. Bauman JT, Sotereanos DG, Weiser RW. Complete rupture of the distal biceps tendon in a woman: case report. *J Hand Surg [Am].* 2006;31(5):798–800.

151. Ramsey ML. Distal biceps tendon injuries: diagnosis and management. *J Am Acad Orthop Surg.* 1999;7(3):199–207.

152. Durr HR, Stabler A, Pfahler M, et al. Partial rupture of the distal biceps tendon. *Clin Orthop Relat Res.* 2000;(374):195–200.

153. Martin CE, Schweitzer ME. MR imaging of epicondylitis. *Skeletal Radiol.* 1998;27(3):133–138.

154. Savnik A, Jensen B, Norregaard J, et al. Magnetic resonance imaging in the evaluation of treatment response of lateral epicondylitis of the elbow. *Eur Radiol.* 2004;14(6):964–969.

155. Eustace S, Johnston C, O'Neill P, O'Byrne J. The elbow. In: *Sports Injuries: Examination, Imaging and Management.* Edinburgh: Elsevier Churchill Livingstone; 2007:333–356.

156. Bannister R. Disorders of the nerve roots and peripheral nerves. In: *Brain and Bannister's Clinical Neurology.* 7th ed. Oxford: Oxford University Press; 1992:420–458.

157. Boero S, Sénès F, Catena N. Pediatric cubital tunnel syndrome by anconeus epitrochlearis: a case report. *J Shoulder Elbow Surg.* 2009;18(2):e21–e23.

158. Dahners LE, Wood FM. Anconeus epitrochlearis, a rare cause of cubital tunnel syndrome: a case report. *J Hand Surg [Am].* 1984;9(4):579–580.

159. Matsuura S, Kojima T, Kinoshita Y. Cubital tunnel syndrome caused by abnormal insertion of triceps brachii muscle. *J Hand Surg [Br].* 1994;19(1):38–39.

160. Abe M, Ishizu T, Shirai H, et al. Tardy ulnar nerve palsy caused by cubitus varus deformity. *J Hand Surg [Am].* 1995;20(1):5–9.

161. Barrios C, Ganoza C, de Pablos J, Canadell J. Posttraumatic ulnar neuropathy versus non-traumatic cubital tunnel syndrome: clinical features and response to surgery. *Acta Neurochir (Wien).* 1991; 110(1–2):44–48.

162. Matsuzaki A. Membranous tissue under the flexor carpi ulnaris muscle as a cause of cubital tunnel syndrome. *Hand Surg.* 2001;6(2):191–197.

163. Grana W. Medial epicondylitis and cubital tunnel syndrome in the throwing athlete. *Clin Sports Med.* 2001;20(3):541–548.

164. Lindsay K, Bone I, Callander R. Localised neurological disease and its management. In: *Neurology and Neurosurgery Illustrated.* Edinburgh: Elsevier; 1991: 213–466.

165. Bridgeman C, Naidu S, Kothari MJ. Clinical and electrophysiological presentation of pronator syndrome. *Electromyogr Clin Neurophysiol.* 2007;47(2):89–92.

166. Ng AB, Borhan J, Ashton HR, et al. Radial nerve palsy in an elite bodybuilder. *Br J Sports Med.* 2003;37(2):185–186.

167. Paraskevas G, Natsis K, Ioannidis O, et al. Accessory muscles in the lower part of the anterior compartment of the arm that may entrap neurovascular elements. *Clin Anat.* 2008;21(3): 246–251.

168. Fitzgerald A, Anderson W, Hooper G. Posterior interosseous nerve palsy due to parosteal lipoma. *J Hand Surg [Br].* 2002;27(6): 535–537.

169. Siemons W, Kegels L, Van Oyen J, et al. Bicipitoradial bursitis. *JBR-BTR.* 2007;90(5):456.

170. Blankstein A, Ganel A, Givon U, et al. Ultrasonographic findings in patients with olecranon bursitis. *Ultraschall Med.* 2006;27(6): 568–571.

171. Watrous BG, Ho Jr G. Elbow pain. *Prim Care.* 1988;15(4):725–735.

172. Jin W, Lee JH, Yang DM, et al. Olecranon bursitis communicating with an olecranon cyst in rheumatoid arthritis. *J Ultrasound Med.* 2007;26(6):857–861.

173. Schweitzer M, Morrison WB. Arthropathies and inflammatory conditions of the elbow. *Magn Reson Imaging Clin N Am.* 1997;5(3):603–617.

174. Llinas L, Olenginski TP, Bush D, et al. Osteomyelitis resulting from chronic filamentous fungus olecranon bursitis. *J Clin Rheumatol.* 2005;11(5): 280–282.

175. Ruch DS, Papadonikolakis A, Campolattaro RM. The posterolateral plica: a cause of refractory lateral elbow pain. *J Shoulder Elbow Surg.* 2006;15(3):367–370.

176. Steinert AF, Goebel S, Rucker A, Barthel T. Snapping elbow caused by hypertrophic synovial plica in the radiohumeral joint: a report of three cases and review of literature. *Arch Orthop Trauma Surg.* 2010 Mar;130(3):347–351.

177. Farkas C, Gaspar L, Jonas Z. The pathological plica in the knee. *Acta Chir Hung.* 1997;36(1–4):83–85.

178. Boles CA, Butler J, Lee JA, et al. Magnetic resonance characteristics of medial plica of the knee: correlation with arthroscopic resection. *J Comput Assist Tomogr.* 2004;28(3):397–401.

179. Lehtinen JT, Kaarela K, Ikavalko M, et al. Incidence of elbow involvement in rheumatoid arthritis. A 15 year endpoint study. *J Rheumatol.* 2001;28(1):70–74.

180. Ehrlich GE. Incidence of elbow involvement in rheumatoid arthritis. *J Rheumatol.* 2001;28(7): 1739.

181. Rowe L, Yochum T. Arthritic disorders. In: Yochum T, Rowe L, eds. *Essentials of Skeletal Radiology.* 2nd ed. Baltimore: Williams and Wilkins; 1996: 795–974.

182. Beers M, Berkow R. Diffuse connective tissue disease. In: *The Merck Manual.* 17th ed. Merck & Co: West Point, PA; 1999: 416–445.

183. Guermazi A, Taouli B, Lynch JA, Peterfy CG. Imaging of bone erosion in rheumatoid arthritis. *Semin Musculoskelet Radiol.* 2004;8(4):269–285.

184. Kato H, Hirayama T, Minami A, et al. Cubital tunnel syndrome associated with medial elbow ganglia and osteoarthritis of the elbow. *J Bone Joint Surg Am.* 2002;84-A(8):1413–1419.

The wrist and hand

Michelle A. Wessely   Julie-Marthe Grenier   Martin Young

Introduction

The clinical evaluation of the wrist and hand regularly results in the use of diagnostic imaging to determine the origin of the patient's pain or complaint. Commonly, radiographs are taken to assess the osseous structures in particular; however, due to the complexity of the wrist and hand, coupled with the importance of this region in the ability to perform activities of daily living (ADLs), it is often vital that the soft tissue components can be scrutinized to achieve an accurate diagnosis.

In the past, further imaging has consisted of computed tomography (CT) and, in more recent times, ultrasound; however, the detail afforded by magnetic resonance (MR) imaging in determining the anatomical relationships of structures such as the fibrocartilage complex and the ligaments and tendons, which confer the function and stability to the wrist, and hand, has increasingly resulted in MR imaging being adopted to evaluate the detail of this region of the body.

History and examination

Much of what has already been written about the history-taking for the shoulder and elbow also holds true for the wrist and hand: it is part of a kinematic chain and clinical thinking must be directed to the other components of that chain, which may be responsible both for disrupting distal biomechanics and perpetuating symptoms and for referring proximal pathology.[1] It is also necessary to be alert for 'double crush' mechanisms of neural entrapment: the nerves that pass through the wrist are also subject to entrapment in the elbow, arm and thoracic outlet, which can refer pain or be comorbid with local entrapment.[2]

More than any other area, it is essential to enquire about the patient's side of handedness, occupation and activities of daily living. Even in the face of an obvious precipitating cause, factors such as repetitive activity, computer use, writing and ergonomics can profoundly affect both management and prognosis.

Examination of the wrist and hand, perhaps unsurprisingly, reflects that of the ankle and foot, with emphasis on observation; active and passive ranges of motion; neurological assessment; digital palpation; and muscle testing. There is, again, a paucity of meaningful special orthopaedic tests; the one exception to this is *Finkelstein's test* for stenosing tenosynovitis of the tendons of extensor pollicis brevis and abductor pollicis longus.[3] This test involves the patient opposing their thumb so that it lies across the palm, then grasping it with the fingers so that it lies within a clenched fist. The examiner then forcibly adducts the thumb to recreate the patient's symptoms. The examination should also include evaluation of the elbow, shoulder, thoracic outlet and cervical spine.[4]

The presence of obvious and persistent neurological signs and symptoms would, in the first instance, be likely to precipitate referral for nerve conduction studies; otherwise, diagnostic imaging is the next step for the inconclusive examination or unresponsive patient.[5,6]

Clinical indications

MR imaging of the wrist and hand is performed in a variety of clinical scenarios. For example, in the case of trauma-induced wrist pain, MR imaging of the

DOI: 10.1016/B978-0-443-06726-6.00010-X

wrist is useful to determine damage to the soft tissues, such as the scapholunate ligament and triangular fibro-cartilage complex, both crucial in maintaining the stability and, therefore, function of the wrist. The same is true of the hand, which is often comorbid with the wrist, and where lesions commonly affect the extensor and flexor mechanisms, both in cases of trauma and non-traumatic deformities.

MR imaging allows visualization of the anatomical structures that enables assessment of the anatomical and functional relationships of the area. In addition to the tissues that may be affected directly by trauma, complications may be also evaluated – such as the development of avascular necrosis, which commonly affects the scaphoid as a complication of fractures. This condition may be studied with great sensitivity using MR imaging and at an earlier stage than with radiography and this may, in some circumstances, alter the clinical prognosis and management of the patient. MR imaging is also useful in assessing the status of the median nerve, and for evaluating the presence of fibrosis, or scar tissue, that may be impeding full recovery for the patient with carpal tunnel syndrome.

Protocols

MR imaging of the wrist and hand may be performed with the patient supine or prone. The prone position is usually reserved for larger patients, where the wrist and hand are placed over the head of the patient, in the 'Superman' position. A surface coil will invariably be applied to the patient's wrist or hand to improve the signal-to-noise ratio and maximize the quality of the image.

The MR imaging study will normally consist of all three imaging planes: coronal, axial and sagittal, which are normally planned from the axial scout view. T1-weighted and T2-weighted sequences are usually performed in one or more imaging planes, with a slice thickness of 1 to 3 mm being adopted. However, depending on the clinical indication for MR imaging of the wrist and hand, particular sequences or even planes may be selected. In the wrist, the imaging study includes the distal radius and ulna up to the bases of the metacarpal bones. In the hand, the imaging study will normally include the distal carpal row to just beyond the distal aspects of the fingers.[7]

For either area, contrast may be added, depending on the nature of the clinical situation being investigated. The contrast may be added via the intravenous route, to attempt to differentiate a soft tissue mass or active inflammation[8] or, in some institutions, injected directly in to the joint to perform MR arthrography[9]; however, due to the inherent contrast from the fluid in the wrist, these procedures are not usually necessary. Some institutions have advocated imaging with varying positions of the wrist, placing the patient in pronation and supination in order to further study the ligamentous relationships in these positions[10]; however, this has not been adopted as standard protocol in most imaging institutions.

Normal and abnormal imaging appearances of the wrist and hand

Perhaps it is because of the wealth of structures contained in a very limited space that it is, unlike in all of the previous chapters, easier to consider normal and abnormal pathology together on a topic-by-topic basis: it is useful to develop a standard order in which to evaluate these structures so as to be methodical for each imaging study that is presented to the practitioner.

Osseous structures

The coronal imaging study will provide information regarding a number of areas, including the overall gross alignment (Figure 10.01, Box 10.01). On these images, the convex head of the ulna and the articular surface of the distal radius should be at the same level; any variance from this can indicate abnormal stresses being placed on the wrist, and is associated with a number of syndromes (Table 10.01).[11–15]

It is also essential to determine that all the carpal bones are present in the proximal and distal carpal rows (Figure 10.01). Carpal coalition is a condition whereby incomplete segmentation has occurred, resulting in two or more of the carpal bones appearing fused; most commonly, the lunate and triquetrum or the capitate and hamate,[16–18] although any adjacent bones may seemingly be involved.[19–25] The distal carpals may also be congenitally fused with the metacarpals, the most common coalition being between the second metacarpal and trapezoid.[26] Accessory ossicles may be present, which represent a normal variation, usually without clinical consequence to either the patient or

Figure 10.01 • Coronal T1-weighted MR imaging of the wrist demonstrating the proximal and distal carpal rows in detail. Note the alignment of the carpal bones in both carpal rows as well as the homogeneous signal intensity in this patient where the bony structures are normal. In addition, the triangular fibrocartilaginous complex is seen as a low signal region just proximal to the lunate and triquetrum (oval).

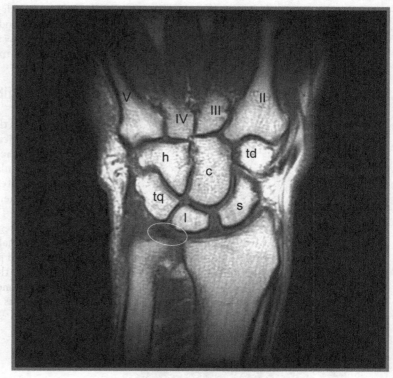

Box 10.01

Key to anatomical structures in annotated figures

c   Capitate
h   Hamate
l   Lunate
p   Pisiform
s   Scaphoid
td Trapezoid
tm Trapezium
tq Triquetrum
*   Hook of the hamate
#   Triangular fibrocartilage complex
I, II, III, IV, V – metacarpals
1. Interosseous muscles
2. Dorsal intercarpal ligament
3. Extensor retinaculum
4. Abductor pollicis longus tendon
5. Extensor pollicis brevis tendon
6. Extensor carpi radialis brevis tendon
7. Extensor carpi radialis longus tendon
8. Extensor carpi ulnaris tendon

9. Extensor pollicis longus
10. Extensor digitorum & indicis tendons
11. Extensor digiti minimi
12. Flexor carpi ulnaris tendon
13. Flexor digitorum superficialis
14. Flexor digitorum profundus
15. Flexor pollicus longus
16. Flexor carpi radialis
17. Radial artery
18. Ulnar artery and nerve
19. Median nerve
20. Thenar muscles
21. Flexor & abductor digiti minimi
22. Flexor retinaculum
23. Extensor digitorum and tendon
24. Flexor tendons of the digits
25. Dorsal digital vein
26. Palmar digital artery
27. Radial collateral ligament

Table 10.01 Syndromes associated with distal radioulnar misalignment

Ulna proximal to radius > 2 mm	Radius proximal to ulna > 2 mm
Avascular necrosis of the lunate (Kienböck's disease) or scaphoid	Impaction between ulna and lunate
Epiphyseal injury	Triangular fibrocartilage complex tear
Rett syndrome	Distal radial growth-plate injury (most commonly associated with child gymnasts)
Chondromalacia of the ulnar head	
Scapholunate disassociations	

physician; one exception to this is the presence of an *os styloideum*, a common bony protuberance located on the dorsal surface of the base of the second and third metacarpals, which may be associated with degenerative changes, bursitis or ganglia.[26,27]

In patients with a history of trauma, ossification may occur in and around tendons, resulting in the appearance of osseous lesions about the wrist and hand, a form of myositis ossificans (Figure 10.02).[28]

Triangular fibrocartilage complex

Familiarity with the soft tissue structures of the wrist and hand is particularly important, owing to their role in maintaining the stability of the wrist. In the coronal plane, the triangular fibrocartilage complex (TFCC) is well demonstrated with its contributing structures, including the meniscus and ulnar collateral ligament (Figure 10.01). The TFCC is a biconcave structure located in the region of the wrist between the ulna and the proximal carpal row, with attachments to the ulnar styloid process by bands of tissue and similarly attached to the radius (Figure 10.03). It stabilizes the ulnocarpal and radioulnar joints, facilitates complex movements at the wrist and distributes loads

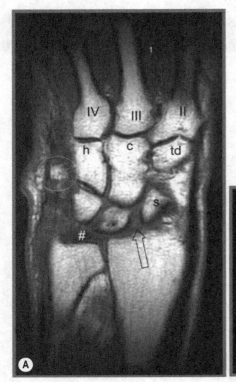
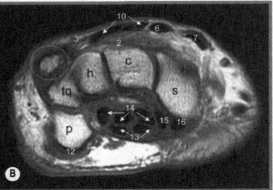

Figure 10.02 • MR imaging of the wrist in the coronal (A) and axial (B) planes using T1-weighted sequences. The circles outline a region of increased signal intensity corresponding to bony marrow, owing to the presence of ossification within the extensor carpi ulnaris tendon from a previous trauma. Also of note is the apparent widening of the scapholunate joint distance (arrow), although this may be normal and needs to be verified on the surrounding slices.

Continued

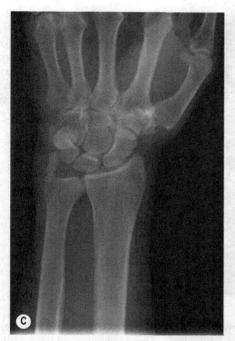

Figure 10.02—cont'd • A follow-up radiograph (C) demonstrates the large regions of increased density located just distal to the ulnar styloid process, most likely due to the previous injury to this region, forming myositis ossificans around the extensor carpi ulnaris.

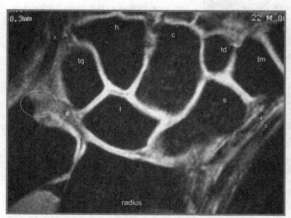

Figure 10.03 • MR imaging of the wrist in the coronal plane, three-dimensional volume acquisition using a gradient echo sequence in a 22-year-old male with pain in and about the wrist. This imaging study demonstrates the triangular fibrocartilage complex in exquisite detail, with visualization of the meniscus homologue, which then has fibres that continue to insert onto the ulnar styloid process (oval). Disruption anywhere along this region may result in instability to the wrist.

from the carpus to the ulna.[29,30] Between the TFCC and the radius is a region of intermediate signal on MR images, which represents hyaline cartilage.

Tendons

The tendons of the wrist can be best evaluated in the axial plane; in the hand, the sagittal plane is, initially, the primary plane for diagnostic information. The normal appearance of a tendon in the wrist and hand is that of a low signal intensity structure that is both linear and continuous. About the wrist, the tendons are divided into compartments for both anatomical and imaging description. The two main regions for the tendons of the wrist are the extensor and flexor groups (Figure 10.04). The median nerve lies amongst the flexor tendons as they travel through the wrist and may be involved in the development of symptoms and signs of carpal tunnel syndrome (Figure 10.05).[31] The extensor tendons run along the dorsal aspect of the wrist towards the hand and may cross over each other, leading to friction syndromes. These tendons may vary in their shape, with the extensor carpi radialis brevis appearing rather elongated in the axial plane (Figure 10.06). The tendons are normally surrounded by a small degree of fluid, which can accumulate in conditions such as tenosynovitis. This can be caused by direct trauma or by systemic disorders that promote a generalized inflammatory process, such as rheumatoid arthritis (Figure 10.07) and are often accompanied by osseous involvement such as erosions.

Nerves

Median nerve

Neural structures can be assessed well with MR imaging. When a patient presents with symptoms and signs of carpal tunnel syndrome, differentiation from proximal neuropathies can be challenging and the MR image may be useful to determine the presence and extent of any local irritation to the median nerve.[32] The median nerve should normally be of a slightly grey or higher signal intensity as compared with the surrounding tendons in the carpal tunnel of normal dimension.[31] In the proximal carpal tunnel, the nerve is slightly flatter than the surrounding tube-like flexor tendons. As it travels more distally through the carpal tunnel, it becomes even flatter in shape.

Carpal tunnel syndrome may arise due to a number of conditions, but is primarily considered a

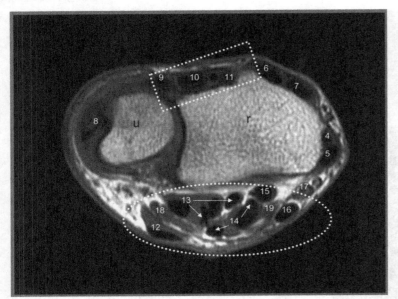

Figure 10.04 • Axial T1-weighted MR image of the wrist demonstrating the relationship between the bony structures of the distal radius and ulna with the compartmentalized tendons. Note the extensor group (rectangle) and the flexor compartment (oval).

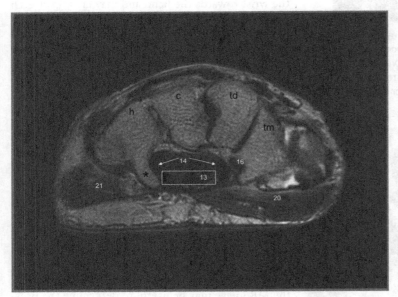

Figure 10.05 • Axial T2-weighted MR image of the wrist at the level of the hook of the hamate [*]. The tendons within the carpal tunnel, small oval regions of low signal intensity, are noted; the superficial volar-placed tendons are those of flexor digitorum superficialis. Those deeper and more posterior represent the tendons of flexor digitorum profundus.

compressive neuropathy.[33] Such compression may occur due to a simple local lesion, such as a ganglion within the carpal tunnel, or from a tenosynovitis of the flexor tendons, causing a decrease in the space that the median nerve occupies within the tunnel.[34–36] Relevant imaging findings from carpal tunnel syndrome may therefore include the presence of tenosynovitis of the flexor tendons, which will appear as areas of increased signal intensity about the tendons on the T2-weighted sequences. The addition of intravenous contrast may enhance a T1 sequence. The nerve may demonstrate an increase in its size and signal intensity on the fluid-sensitive sequences (Figure 10.08). MR imaging is not used routinely in the primary diagnosis of carpal tunnel syndrome,[6] but is best employed to determine the cause of symptoms and signs in persistent cases or to evaluate scar tissue formation following surgery, which can itself be a cause of median nerve irritation (Figure 10.09).[37,38]

Figure 10.06 • Axial T1-weighted MR imaging of the wrist at the level of the hook of the hamate demonstrating the tendons about the wrist, in particular those of the carpal tunnel (oval). In addition, along the dorsum over the wrist, regions of low signal intensity overlying the carpal bones represent the tendons of the extensors, including that of extensor carpi radialis brevis.

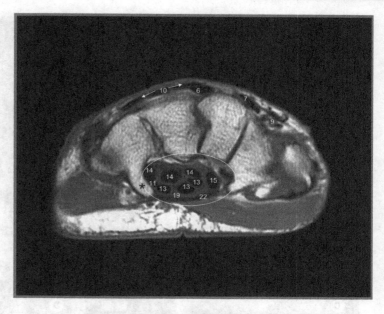

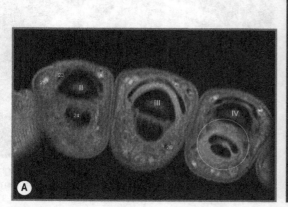

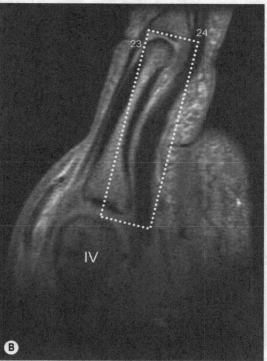

Figure 10.07 • Axial, T1-weighted, fat-saturated sequence of the fourth finger (**A**), where the tendons are noted as low signal intensity structures. In this patient, whereas the flexor tendons of the second and third digits are of normal signal intensity and size, the flexor tendons about the fourth digit are larger than normal and a moderate amount of soft tissue swelling is noted around this region. A similar region is seen about the extensor tendons of the third finger. This patient has rheumatoid arthritis, which may result in a synovitis, as well as rupture of tendons. In the sagittal plane, the T1-weighted fat-saturated image (**B**) shows thickening of the flexor tendon (rectangle) due to a synovitis stimulated by rheumatoid arthritis.

Continued

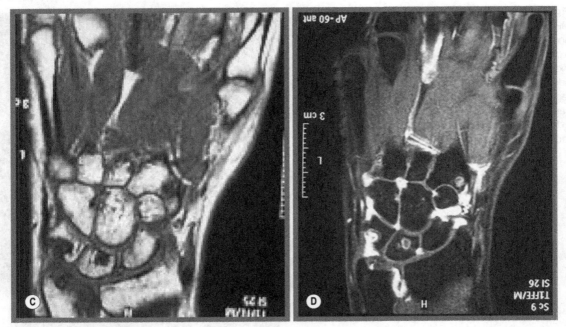

Figure 10.07—cont'd • Figure (C) shows a T1-weighted, coronal plane image of a 20-year-old female patient with a diagnosis of rheumatoid arthritis and demonstrates multiple, low signal lesions affecting the carpus. On the fluid-sensitive STIR sequence (D), these lesions, particularly obvious in the lunate, are of high signal and fairly well demarcated.

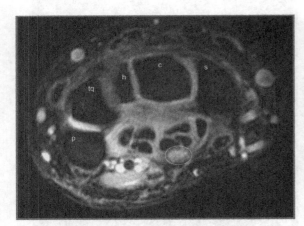

Figure 10.08 • T2-weighted, fat-saturation MR imaging of the proximal carpal row in the axial plane, in which the region of the carpal tunnel is diffusely high-signal, particularly around the tendons. Also of note is the high signal intensity and deformation of the median nerve situated within the carpal tunnel (oval). These findings are consistent with carpal tunnel syndrome.

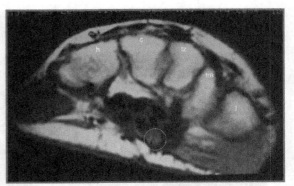

Figure 10.09 • Axial T1-weighted MR imaging of the right wrist of a 41-year-old female who had refractory symptoms following carpal tunnel surgery. The imaging was performed before the second intervention to determine the presence and extent of any scar tissue and to confirm the cause of her continuing symptoms. Thickening and fibrosis is noted about the median nerve (circle) and retraction of the tendons within the carpal tunnel in the volar direction is also seen.

Because of the potential complications of surgical intervention, conservative care is recommended; steroid injections and splinting can often be effective and both manual therapy and acupuncture have shown some benefit to patients.[39–42]

Ulnar nerve

The ulnar nerve may be compressed in the *tunnel of Guyon*, which lies between the pisiform and hamate and under their interconnecting ligament. Common causes of compression include ganglia, trauma and the presence of accessory muscles, all of which can be easily identified on MR imaging.[43] The site of compression needs to be differentiated from cubital tunnel syndrome (Chapter 9), which will affect the extensor carpi ulnaris in addition to distally innervated structures; however, it is also possible to differentiate between compression of the deep and superficial branches (Box 10.02).

Ligaments

Game-keeper's thumb is an avulsion injury of the base of the proximal phalanx, commonly related to a forced abduction movement in sports such

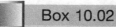

Box 10.02

Deep and superficial terminal branches of the ulnar nerve
Superficial terminal branch

Palmaris brevis
Medial palmar skin

Deep terminal branch

The three short muscles of the fifth digit
Third and fourth lumbricals
Adductor pollicis
Interossei
Flexor pollicis brevis

as skiing or from the recoil of a gun (hence the eponymic name) whereby the ulnar collateral ligament is disrupted along with a small fragment of bone from its insertion into the proximal phalanx. This ligament is important for conferring stability to the thumb, and, although basic imaging may be used to demonstrate the bony lesion, MR imaging depicts the bony and soft tissue injury with exquisite detail, which is important in the prognosis and most appropriate clinical management of the patient (Figure 10.10).

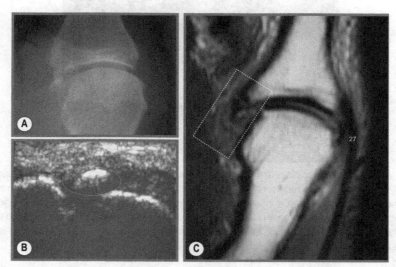

Figure 10.10 • Imaging of a patient with severe pain and limitation in the range of movement of the thumb following injury. The plain film radiograph (**A**) demonstrates a small, bony fragment at the base of the proximal phalanx. Ultrasound of the same region (**B**) again demonstrates the presence of a region of echo due to the bony fragment (oval); however, MR imaging of the first digit in the coronal plane using a T1-weighted sequence (**C**) demonstrates not only the bony fragment but also the disruption to the ligamentous complex (rectangle) surrounding this lesion, which is clinically much more significant and which often requires surgical intervention to repair and restore the normal biomechanics to the thumb.

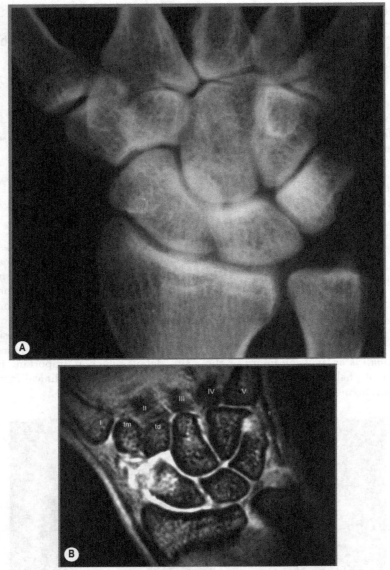

Figure 10.11 • (A) Posteroanterior plain film radiograph of a patient describing wrist pain focused over the anatomical snuff-box. There was a recent history of a fall onto the outstretched hand; these films were taken a few days after the incident. No evidence of a fracture is noted in the carpal bones. (B) MR image of the wrist of the same patient. In this image, a coronal plane, STIR sequence, a large area of increased signal intensity is noted in the distal aspect of the scaphoid due to the presence of a fracture; the exact location is difficult to confirm on this single slice.

MR imaging may also be used to determine the presence of radiographically occult fractures (Figure 10.11). The scaphoid is the most commonly fractured bone in the wrist, and, if initial radiographs are negative, options may consist of immobilizing the patient and re-radiographing 10 days later, or, if such facilities exist, performing MR imaging to determine the presence of any fracture and also to follow the development of potential complications such as avascular necrosis. This condition can also develop spontaneously in the paediatric lunate (Kienböck's disease) (Figure 10.12).[44,45]

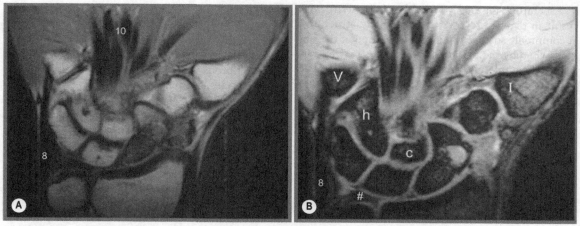

Figure 10.12 • MR imaging of the wrist in a patient with a recent history of trauma complaining of pain in the region of the anatomical snuff-box. The T1-weighted sequence (A) clearly demonstrates a region of low signal intensity in the proximal pole of the scaphoid bone. A linear region of low signal intensity is also noted in the waist of the scaphoid. On the T2-weighted sequence (B), a region of increased signal intensity is seen in the distal pole of the scaphoid as well as an area of cortical disruption along the lateral aspect of the scaphoid, owing to the presence of a fracture. The MR imaging confirms the presence of a fracture with the development of avascular necrosis of the proximal pole, a complication of the trauma.

Falls on the outstretched hand (FOOSH) may also affect the ligaments about the wrist, which need to be scrutinized, particularly on the coronal sequence. The ligaments, such as the scapholunate ligament, should be seen as a linear low-signal continuous structure connecting the scaphoid and lunate. In the case of disruption of the ligament, a slightly increased distance may be noted between the scaphoid and lunate (normal range is 2 to 4 mm) as well as disruption of the linear signal, which appears discontinuous or irregular (Figure 10.13).[43,45]

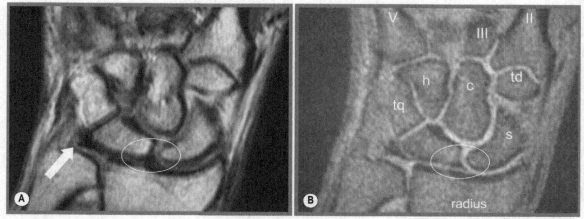

Figure 10.13 • Coronal, T1-weighted (A) and T2-weighted (B) MR imaging of a post-traumatic wrist. The patient complained of pain and a sensation of clicking about the lateral aspect of their wrist. The T1-weighted imaging demonstrates a lack of continuity of the scapholunate ligament (ovals) with a possible retraction of the insertion of the triangular fibrocartilage complex insertion onto the ulnar styloid process (arrow). On the T2-weighted sequence, again the discontinuity is noted between the scaphoid and lunate where there should normally be a linear low signal intensity representing the ligament. This finding is due to a tear of the scapholunate ligament, which may cause instability in the wrist.

Lacerating injuries to the hand or wrist may result in damage to soft tissue or bony structures. A commonly sustained injury is laceration of the fingers, whereby the tendons of the fingers may be partially or completely ruptured (Figure 10.14). The patient usually presents with a history of acute trauma, commonly involving a sharp utensil, with clinical deformity of the finger and the inability to perform flexion or extension. Whereas ultrasound may be useful to determine the extent of injury, it is highly operator-dependent.[46] MR imaging will provide superior information with respect to both bony and soft tissue damage, providing important information regarding the clinical diagnosis and management of the patient.

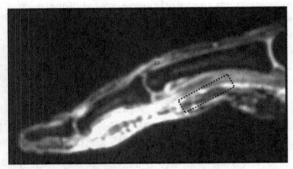

Figure 10.14 • Sagittal T2-weighted sequence in a patient who had been attacked with a knife and who, shortly after the incident, noted that she was unable to move her finger normally. After the physical examination, MR imaging was ordered. This shows that there is discontinuity of the flexor digitorum profundus tendon, which has been lacerated and retracted to the level of the proximal interphalangeal articulation (rectangle). This lesion will require surgical intervention in order to repair the extent of retraction so as to restore the mechanics of the digit.

Tumours

The majority of neoplasms in the wrist and hand are benign; the most common cause of such growths are ganglia, fibrous-walled masses attached to ligaments, joint capsules and tendon sheaths. More commonly found in females, they only become painful when pressing against adjacent structures; their cause appears to relate to chronic irritation.[47] MR imaging will reveal ganglia as low intensity structures on T1-weighted imaging; on T2-weighted imaging, the signal intensity is higher though generally diffuse with characteristic thin, low signal lines representing septa that subdivide the internal architecture of the ganglion. The most common differential is the presence of accessory, anomalous muscles, most commonly *extensor digitorum manus brevis*, found on the dorsum of the wrist medial to the tendon of extensor indices. The characteristic location helps to differentiate it from a ganglion.[29,43]

The second commonest soft tissue mass about the wrist is the giant cell tumour of the tendon sheath; a localized form of pigmented villonodular synovitis, characteristically noted on the volar digital surfaces; their differentiation is further helped by their appearance as low signal intensity structures on both T1- and T2-weighted images.[43]

Arthritis and infection

Infectious and arthritic processes commonly affect the hand and wrist and MR imaging allows for superb contrast of soft tissue and bone marrow changes, showing in exquisite detail changes that remain occult on other imaging modalities. These typical changes have been well detailed in the previous chapters.

References

1. Young MF. The physics of anatomy. In: *Essential Physics for Musculoskeletal Medicine*. Edinburgh: Elsevier; 2009.
2. Pierre-Jerome C, Bekkelund SI. Magnetic resonance assessment of the double-crush phenomenon in patients with carpal tunnel syndrome: a bilateral quantitative study. *Scand J Plast Reconstr Surg Hand Surg.* 2003;37(1): 46–53.
3. Kutsumi K, Amadio PC, Zhao C, et al. Finkelstein's test: a biomechanical analysis. *J Hand Surg Am.* 2005;30(1):130–135.
4. Bates B. The musculoskeletal system. In: Bates B, ed. *A Guide to Physical Examination.* 3rd ed. Philadelphia: JB Lippincott; 1983:324–370.
5. Keith MW, Masear V, Amadio PC, et al. Treatment of carpal tunnel syndrome. *J Am Acad Orthop Surg.* 2009;17(6):397–405.
6. Keith MW, Masear V, Chung K, et al. Diagnosis of carpal tunnel syndrome. *J Am Acad Orthop Surg.* 2009; 17(6):389–396.
7. Kaplan P, Helms C, Dussault R, Anderson M. *Musculoskeletal MRI*. Philadelphia: WB Saunders; 2001.

8. Eshed I, Althoff CE, Schink T, et al. Low-field MRI for assessing synovitis in patients with rheumatoid arthritis. Impact of Gd-DTPA dose on synovitis scoring. Scand J Rheumatol. 2006;35(4):277–282.

9. Theumann NH, Etechami G, Duvoisin B, et al. Association between extrinsic and intrinsic carpal ligament injuries at MR arthrography and carpal instability at radiography: initial observations. Radiology. 2006;238(3):950–957.

10. Pfirrmann CW, Theumann NH, Chung CB, et al. What happens to the triangular fibrocartilage complex during pronation and supination of the forearm? Analysis of its morphology and diagnostic assessment with MR arthrography. Skeletal Radiol. 2001;30(12): 677–685.

11. Singh A, Singh OP. A rare injury of distal radial and ulnar epiphysis. J Indian Med Assoc. 2007;105(8): 466, 468.

12. Glasson EJ, Bower C, Thomson MR, et al. Diagnosis of Rett syndrome: can a radiograph help? Dev Med Child Neurol. 1998;40(11): 737–742.

13. Darrow Jr JC, Linscheid RL, Dobyns JH, et al. Distal ulnar recession for disorders of the distal radioulnar joint. J Hand Surg Am. 1985;10(4):482–491.

14. DiFiori JP, Puffer JC, Aish B, Dorey F. Wrist pain, distal radial physeal injury, and ulnar variance in young gymnasts: does a relationship exist? Am J Sports Med. 2002;30(6): 879–885.

15. Caine D, Howe W, Ross W, Bergman G. Does repetitive physical loading inhibit radial growth in female gymnasts? Clin J Sport Med. 1997;7(4):302–308.

16. Mellado JM, Calmet J, Domenech S, Sauri A. Clinically significant skeletal variations of the shoulder and the wrist: role of MR imaging. Eur Radiol. 2003;13(7): 1735–1743.

17. Marburger R, Burgess RC. Symptomatic lunate-triquetral coalition. J South Orthop Assoc. 1995;4(4):307–310.

18. Delaney TJ, Eswar S. Carpal coalitions. J Hand Surg Am. 1992; 17(1):28–31.

19. Terrence JJJ. Congenital fusion of the trapezium and trapezoid. Rom J Morphol Embryol. 2008; 49(3):417–419.

20. Silverman AT, Shin SS, Paksima N. Asymptomatic pisiform-hamate coalition: a case report. Am J Orthop. 2007;36(6):E88–E90.

21. Louaste J, Amhajji L, Rachid K. [Pisiform-hamate synostosis with ulnar neuropathy. Case report]. Chir Main. 2007;26(3):170–172.

22. Kawamura K, Yajima H, Takakura Y. Pisiform and hamate coalition: case report and review of literature. Hand Surg. 2005;10(1):101–104.

23. Boya H, Ozcan O, Arac S, Tandogan R. Incomplete scapholunate and trapeziotrapezoid coalitions with an accessory carpal bone. J Orthop Sci. 2005;10(1): 99–102.

24. Ingram C, Hall RF, Gonzalez M. Congenital fusion of the scaphoid, trapezium, trapezoid and capitate. J Hand Surg Br. 1997;22(2): 167–168.

25. Oner FC, de Vries HR. Isolated capitatolunate coalition: a case report. J Bone Joint Surg Br. 1994;76(5):845–856.

26. Alemohammad AM, Nakamura K, El-Sheneway M, Viegas SF. Incidence of carpal boss and osseous coalition: an anatomic study. J Hand Surg Am. 2009;34(1):1–6.

27. Hazlett JW. The third metacarpal boss. Int Orthop. 1992;16(4):369–371.

28. Berquist T. MRI of the Musculoskeletal System. 4th ed. Philadelphia: Lippincott Williams and Wilkins; 2000.

29. Standring S, ed. Gray's Anatomy – Pectoral girdle and upper limb: Wrist and hand (Section 53). Edinburgh: Elsevier; 2009.

30. Moore K. The upper limb. In: Clinically Oriented Anatomy. 2nd ed. Baltimore: Williams and Wilkins; 1985:626–793.

31. Bower JA, Stanisz GJ, Keir PJ. An MRI evaluation of carpal tunnel dimensions in healthy wrists: Implications for carpal tunnel syndrome. Clin Biomech (Bristol, Avon). 2006;21(8):816–825.

32. Kim S, Choi JY, Huh YM, et al. Role of magnetic resonance imaging in entrapment and compressive neuropathy – what, where, and how

to see the peripheral nerves on the musculoskeletal magnetic resonance image: part 1. Overview and lower extremity. Eur Radiol. 2007; 17(1):139–149.

33. Lindsay K, Bone I, Callander R. Localised neurological disease and its management. In: Neurology and Neurosurgery Illustrated. Edinburgh: Elsevier; 1991:213–466.

34. Crowley B, Gschwind CR, Storey C. Selective motor neuropathy of the median nerve caused by a ganglion in the carpal tunnel. J Hand Surg Br. 1998;23(5):611–612.

35. Nourissat G, Fournier E, Werther JR, et al. Acute carpal tunnel syndrome secondary to pyogenic tenosynovitis. J Hand Surg Br. 2006;31(6):687–688.

36. Rashid M, Sarwar SU, Haq EU, et al. Tuberculous tenosynovitis: a cause of carpal tunnel syndrome. J Pak Med Assoc. 2006;56(3):116–118.

37. Stutz NM, Gohritz A, Novotny A, et al. Clinical and electrophysiological comparison of different methods of soft tissue coverage of the median nerve in recurrent carpal tunnel syndrome. Neurosurgery. 2008; 62(3 suppl 1): 194–199 discussion 199–200.

38. Stutz N, Gohritz A, van Schoonhoven J, Lanz U. Revision surgery after carpal tunnel release— analysis of the pathology in 200 cases during a 2 year period. J Hand Surg Br. 2006;31(1):68–71.

39. Napadow V, Kettner N, Liu J, et al. Hypothalamus and amygdala response to acupuncture stimuli in carpal tunnel syndrome. Pain. 2007;130(3):254–266.

40. Napadow V, Liu J, Li M, et al. Somatosensory cortical plasticity in carpal tunnel syndrome treated by acupuncture. Hum Brain Mapp. 2007;28(3):159–171.

41. Burke J, Buchberger DJ, Carey-Loghmani MT, et al. A pilot study comparing two manual therapy interventions for carpal tunnel syndrome. J Manipulative Physiol Ther. 2007;30(1):50–61.

42. Claes F, Verhagen WI, Meulstee J. Current practice in the use of nerve conduction studies in carpal tunnel syndrome by surgeons in The Netherlands. J Hand Surg Eur Vol. 2007;32(6):663–667.

43. Helms C, Major N, Anderson MW, et al. Wrist and hand. In: *Musculoskeletal MRI*. 2nd ed. Philadelphia: Elsevier Saunders; 2009:244–272.

44. Memarsadeghi M, Breitenseher MJ, Schaefer-Prokop C, et al. Occult scaphoid fractures: comparison of multidetector CT and MR imaging—initial experience. *Radiology*. 2006; 240(1):169–176.

45. Rowe L, Yochum T, eds. *Essentials of Skeletal Radiology*. 2nd ed. Baltimore: Williams and Wilkins; 2004.

46. Rasmussen OS. Sonography of tendons. *Scand J Med Sci Sports*. 2000;10(6):360–364.

47. Bogumill GP, Sullivan DJ, Baker GI. Tumors of the hand. *Clin Orthop Relat Res*. 1975;(108): 214–222.

The temporomandibular articulation

Michelle A. Wessely   Martin Young

Introduction

The temporomandibular articulation (TMA) is formed between the ovoid mandibular condyle and its complementary elliptical articulating surface on the glenoid fossa of the temporal bone (Figure 11.01).[1,2] Although a true synovial joint, it eludes traditional classification and different authors will place it in different groups.

Many simpler texts will term it a hinge joint (ginglymus)[3]; however, this overlooks the gliding phase of movement, typical of arthrodial joints – for this reason, some authors classify the joint in a unique category, terming it *ginglymoarthrodial*.[4] Although this describes the joint from a functional standpoint, structurally it is more commonly classified as a *bicondylar joint*; that is an ellipsoidal (or condylar) joint – one in which an ovoid head of one bone moves in an elliptical cavity of another (permitting all movements except axial rotation) with the additional feature of a meniscus between the articular surfaces. This feature also defines it as a *complex* joint.[5–7]

Regardless of the semantics over the joint's classification (it is most probably easiest to regard it as unique; there is no directly comparable joint), the important thing for the clinician to understand is that it is composed of a series of complicated, interrelated osseous and soft tissue structures, each of which may be implicated in clinical syndromes. As such, the joint can be responsible for a significant level of morbidity with local symptoms including pain, restriction, stiffness, crepitus and clicking.[8] It can also be responsible for referred pain syndromes and is an often overlooked cause of headache[9–11]; facial pain[12,13]; vertigo, tinnitus and ear symptoms[14–18]; and interrelated dysfunction elsewhere in the stomatognathic system (the dentition, mandible, cranium, spine and pelvis).[19–21]

The osseous structures centre around the articulating surfaces and the adjacent coronoid process; the soft tissue elements include the articular disc and its various attachments, a multitude of delicate ligaments, muscular insertion points and synovial and capsular components.[2,3] There is considerable dispute about the contribution of these various elements to the symptoms of temporomandibular disorder (TMD),[8] and diagnosis always needs to be carefully correlated with history and clinical findings; however, magnetic resonance (MR) imaging offers the clinician the chance to evaluate the articular disc in great detail. It is essential, therefore, to be able to differentiate the well-documented physiological, age-related changes from pathological conditions, which include internal derangement, tears, abnormal displacement (with or without reduction), dislocation and perforation. These, in turn, must be differentiated from internal signal abnormalities.[22]

History and examination

Because of the sequelae to and comorbidity with TMD, it is important to elicit a basic dental history from all patients. This should cover several key points (Box 11.01).[23,24] As with any clinical history, it is also necessary to undertake a systems review and to explore psychological history, which is particularly pertinent in chronic cases.[24,25]

DOI: 10.1016/B978-0-443-06726-6.00011-1

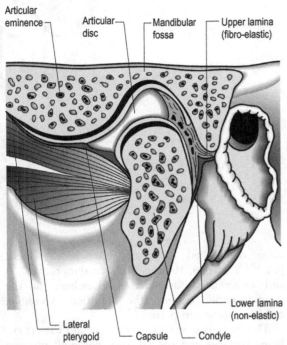

Articular
eminence — Articular — Mandibular — Upper lamina
disc — fossa — (fibro-elastic)

Lower lamina
(non-elastic)

Lateral
pterygoid — Capsule — Condyle

Figure 11.01 • The temporomandibular articulation is formed between the ovoid mandibular condyle and its complementary elliptical articulating surface on the glenoid fossa of the temporal bone.

Box 11.01

The key points in eliciting a basic dental history from patients with temporomandibular disorder

- Location of pain
- Onset and progression of symptoms
- Characteristics of pain
  - Quality
  - Intensity
  - Radiation and referral
  - Variation
  - Associated symptoms
- Aggravating and relieving factors
- Past dental interventions

Owing to the interrelated complexity of head and face pain disorders, it is necessary to evaluate non-masticatory structures in order to properly establish a differential diagnosis. This screening should comprise examination of the eyes, ears, cervical spine and cranial nerves.[26–28]

The examination of the temporomandibular joint should cover the muscles of mastication, the joint itself and the teeth.[24] Whereas this last is more properly the province of the dentist or orthodontist, it is perfectly simple for any competent clinician to note the absence or significant decay of teeth, excessive wear or obvious malocclusion – all of which can be primary causative factors in TMD[29–33] – and, if necessary, refer for an expert opinion and reconstructional or orthodontic intervention.

The examination of myofascial structures should start with observation of facial symmetry and evidence of muscle atrophy. Digital palpation should then be used to elicit the presence of myofascial trigger points in the muscles of mastication – temporalis, masseter and the medial and lateral pterygoids – plus associated muscles, including the digastric, suprahyoid, sternocleidomastoid and the intrinsic and extrinsic muscles of the cervical spine.[34]

Because the pterygoids can be hard to palpate, functional manipulation can be used to assess these muscles. This is accomplished by contracting the muscles by clenching, both against the opposing teeth and a separator, and by protruding against resistance and then stretching by passive and active opening of the mouth. An increase in pain is regarded as a positive finding, although this needs to be carefully differentiated from intracapsular pain and restriction (Table 11.01).[24,35]

When evaluating temporomandibular gait, any lateral deviation on opening and closing should be noted, as well as the smoothness of transition from swing to glide phases. Trismus (popping, clicking or grating sounds from within the joint) can often be felt more easily than heard if the fingers are placed lightly over the joints during gait; alternatively, a stethoscope may be used. When the mouth is fully open, the maximum interincisal distance should be between 53 and 58 mm in an adult, equivalent to the width of the middle three fingers.[36–39]

Differential diagnosis

Temporomandibular disorders need to be differentiated from other facial pain syndromes, including: osseous disease; dental conditions; salivary and lymphatic disorders; neuropathic pain and headache; and miscellaneous conditions such as atypical facial pain.[40] This is usually easy to achieve by competent history-taking and examination without recourse to diagnostic imaging.[8]

Table 11.01 Outcomes for and interpretation of functional manipulation of the jaw

Activity	Medial pterygoid	Inferior lateral pterygoid	Superior lateral pterygoid	Intracapsular disorder
Clenching on teeth	Increased pain	Increased pain	Increased pain	Increased pain
Clenching on separator (unilaterally)	Increased pain	No pain	Increased pain	No pain
Opening widely	Increased pain	Slightly increased pain	No pain	Increased pain
Protruding against resistance	Slightly increased pain	Increased pain	No pain	Increased pain
Protruding against resistance with unilateral separator	Slightly increased pain	Increased pain	Slightly increased pain (if clenching)	No pain

Box 11.02

Classification of temporomandibular disorders

I. Disorders of the muscles of mastication
II. Disorders of the temporomandibular joint
  A. Derangement of the condyle-disc complex
  B. Structural incompatibility of the articular surface
  C. Inflammatory disorders
III. Chronic mandibular hypomobility
IV. Congenital/developmental growth disorders

The different aetiologies of TMD also need to be differentiated, as the underlying cause will obviously affect both management and prognosis. The classification of TMD is detailed in Box 11.02; diagnostic imaging is of particular use in differentiating types II and IV TMD.[8]

Clinical indications for diagnostic imaging

Temporomandibular disorders can be classified as extra-articular or intra-articular, or can of course be a combination of both. Extra-articular causes of TMD are usually muscular in origin and are a common clinical entity presenting to a wide variety of primary healthcare practitioners. Aetiological factors include bruxism, often exacerbated by stress or anxiety, trauma, and occlusal disruption.[41]

The intra-articular causes of temporomandibular disorders, also known as arthrogenous TMD, are most commonly attributed to abnormalities affecting the meniscus: displacement, either temporary or

chronic, degenerative joint disease, inflammatory disorders such as rheumatoid arthritis, infection or, rarely, tumour processes.[8,42,43] Discal pathology is where MR imaging may be most useful, to determine the resting position of the meniscus and assess its movement during temporomandibular gait.[44] Some meniscal dysfunction is also related to myopathology; for example, anterior disc displacement in the closed position, which reduces with opening, has been linked with a lateral pterygoid spasm, evidence of which may be detectable with MR imaging.[45,46]

In former years, imaging of the TMA consisted of routine radiography, including the panoramic views which can provide some information regarding the shape, size and general state of the mandibular condyles (Figure 11.02); conventional tomography was

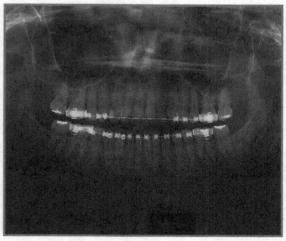

Figure 11.02 • Panoramic digital imaging of the mandible illustrating the typical appearance of this image.

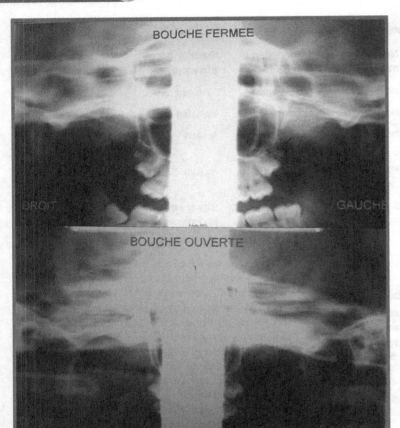

BOUCHE FERMEE

DROIT   GAUCHE

BOUCHE OUVERTE

Figure 11.03 • Conventional tomography of open mouth (*bouche ouverte*) and closed mouth (*bouche fermée*) to demonstrate the typical appearance of this type of imaging.

also used to assess the open and closed mouth (Figure 11.03).[47] High-resolution ultrasound may also be sensitive enough to detect gross internal derangement affecting the TM joint.[48–50] Although computed tomography (CT) has also provided detail regarding the bony parameters of the TMA, MR imaging excels in the evaluation of the soft tissue components of the TMA, so often the origin of the patient's complaint.[49,51,52] Current knowledge of TMA pathologies has largely relied on both the clinical presentations of a range of conditions as well as the use of basic, invasive and not always helpful imaging modalities. With the advent of MR imaging, the understanding of the osseous component of articulations has been furthered and the soft tissues in and about the articulation have also moved firmly into the spotlight.[22,47,49]

The distinct advantage of MR imaging and MR arthrography is that they allow for the excellent visualization of both bony and soft tissue anatomy using a technique that is only minimally invasive (Figures 11.04, 11.05). The advancement of the technology of imaging has led to significant improvement in the understanding of the complex nature of the anatomy and hence the pathology encountered in the TMA.[53–55]

Protocol

MR imaging of the TMA requires that the patient be lying supine, with a 3-inch (7.5-cm) surface coil attached to both articulations. It is common for both TMAs to be imaged during the same study, even if only one side is symptomatic. Images are collected in the closed-mouth position and then, with the use of a splint, the patient is imaged with the mouth open. If contrast is to be added, this will be performed after the initial MR imaging sequences.

Normally, the patient is imaged in the axial plane to determine the orientation of the anterior condyles. From this, the sagittal oblique sequences are planned, with the slices perpendicular to this line, in both the closed- and then the open-mouth

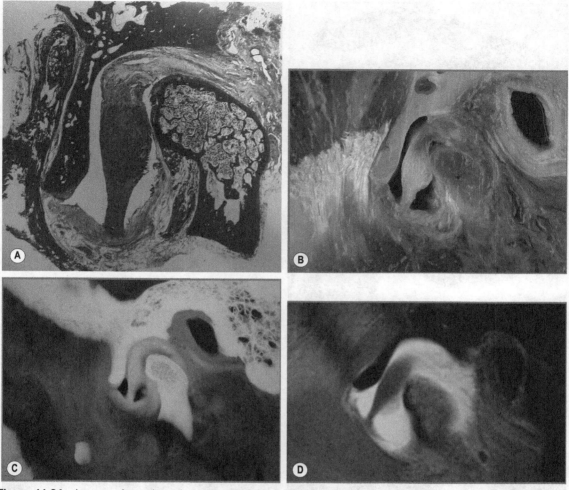

Figure 11.04 • Images of a male cadaver jaw. (A) Sagittal oblique slice through the temporomandibular articulation/joint (TMA) demonstrating the gross histological/anatomical appearance of the meniscus with its direct relationship with the articular capsule anteriorly. (B) Sagittal oblique 2–3-mm slice through the specimen to demonstrate the anatomical appearance at ×1 magnification, allowing the reader to correlate (A) with this, the appearance of the meniscus and its relationship with the TMA. (C) Sagittal oblique slice Faxitron (radiograph) of the same specimen demonstrating the relationship of the internal articular components with the rest of the TMA. (D) MR arthrogram performed in the sagittal oblique plane demonstrating the correlation of the preceding imaging with cross-sectional imaging of the TMA, noting in particular the meniscus and its relationship with the articular capsule.

position (Figures 11.06, 11.07), noting in particular the location of the meniscus in both positions. Coronal oblique images may also be performed and are planned off the initial axial sequence along the long axis of the condyles. Both T1-weighted and T2-weighted images may be performed, in both the closed- and open-mouth positions, depending on the preference of the imaging centre and based on the type of MR machine.[56–58]

Normal imaging anatomy

Osseous structures

Normally, on the sagittal image, the condyles should be oval in shape and covered by a thin layer of cortical bone (Figure 11.08), which on the MR image will appear with low signal intensity. The signal

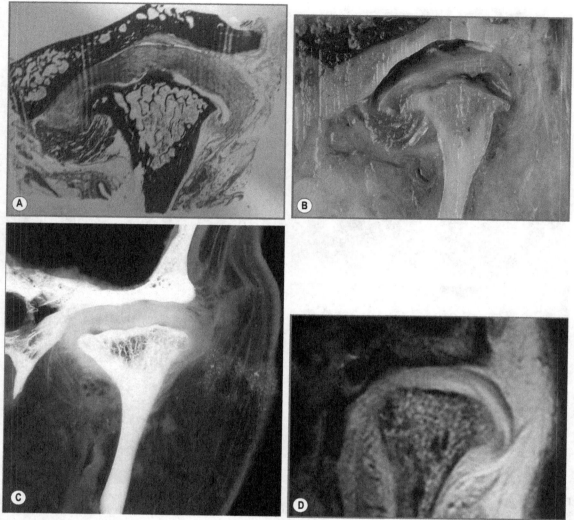

Figure 11.05 • Images of the same male cadaver as Figure 11.04. (A) Coronal slice through the right TMA at a microscopic level (right is lateral). Note the irregularities of the mandibular condyle, which represents a normal variation of the condylar surface, not usually appreciated on plain radiographs but which can be appreciated on special imaging. (B) The same specimen seen with the naked eye, allowing appreciation of the relationship between the previous image and the gross anatomy. (C) Faxitron image (radiograph) performed in the AP view demonstrating the relationship between the meniscus, mandibular condyle and the glenoid fossa of the temporal bone. (D) MR T1-weighted arthrogram showing how the meniscus is draped over the mandibular condyle, which is somewhat irregular.

intensity should be homogeneous and, on the fluid-sensitive sequences, should be intermediate to low signal. On the T1-weighted sequence, the signal intensity should be brighter than on T2-weighting and be the same as that in the remaining normal bone marrow visualized elsewhere on the image (Figure 11.09).

Articular disc

The articular disc is a lozenge or elongated oval shape and has a superior and inferior surface. The superior surface is concavo-convex from anterior to posterior to conform to the contours of the articular fossa and condyle. The inferior surface is moulded to the

Figure 11.06 • Sagittal oblique, T1-weighted MR image of a normal temporomandibular articulation (TMA) in the closed-mouth position. Note the relationship of the mandibular condyle to the external auditory meatus (star), which can assist with image orientation when reading the image. In this stance, both the anterior and posterior aspects of the meniscus are draped over the TMA (oval).

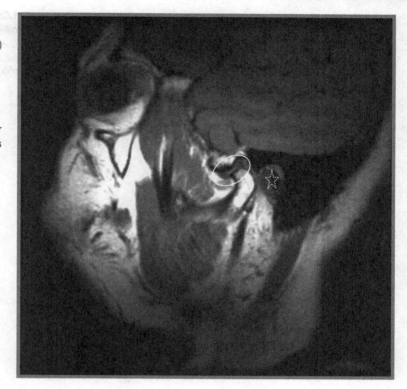

Figure 11.07 • Sagittal oblique, T1-weighted image of a normal temporomandibular articulation in the open-mouth position. Note the altered position of the mandibular condyle with respect to the glenoid fossa of the temporal bone (Figure 11.02). Anterior translation of the mandibular condyle has occurred, with an alteration of the relationship with the meniscus (oval).

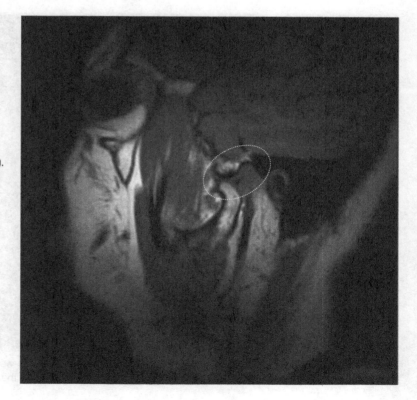

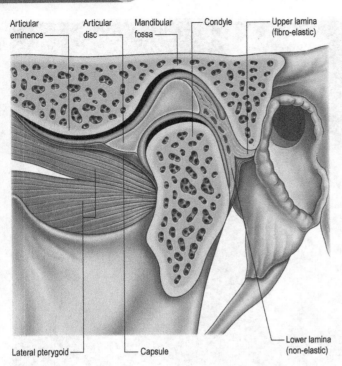

Articular eminence — Articular disc — Mandibular fossa — Condyle — Upper lamina (fibro-elastic)

Lateral pterygoid — Capsule — Lower lamina (non-elastic)

Figure 11.08 • A sagittal section of the temporomandibular joint demonstrating the location, shape and relations of the articular disc. Reproduced, with permission, from Gray's Anatomy 39e, Standring S, ed, (Elsevier, 2005)

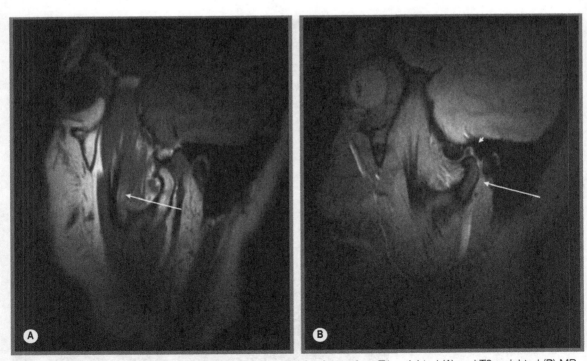

Figure 11.09 • Normal appearance of the mandibular condyles (arrows) on T1-weighted (A) and T2-weighted (B) MR images. The meniscus is outlined by fluid and is visible immediately superior to the condyle (arrowhead in B).

condyle of the mandible and is, therefore, concave (Figure 11.08).[1,59] The disc completely divides the TMA into two distinct compartments – superior and inferior, both of which are usually compressed – and, ordinarily, there is no interconnection; however, in the older population there can be a significant degree of degeneration in the region of the disc. This may result in partial or complete perforation of the disc, thus allowing communication between the superior and inferior joint spaces.[2,60,61]

The disc is attached both to the fibrous capsule and to the lateral pterygoid muscle anteriorly. There are extensions that pass medial and laterally, which head towards and insert into the mandibular condyle. The posterior portion of the disc divides into superior and inferior portions, or *lamellae*. The upper, or superior, lamella inserts into the posterior margin of the mandibular fossa and is composed of fibroelastic tissue. The lower, or inferior, lamella is attached to the posterior condyle but is not elastic and is composed of white fibres.[53]

The thickest portion of the disc is just posterior to the central portion at a position that corresponds with the deepest part of the mandibular fossa. The disc has been further divided into various parts according to the anatomical appearance – anterior extension, anterior band, intermediate zone, posterior band and the bilaminar zone (upper and lower lamellae).[1]

Morphological evaluation of the superior and inferior surface of the disc reveals some distinct differences in the nature of pathological changes. The inferior surface is by far the more commonly affected in patients, though without discal symptoms, suggesting that there may be no correlation between the presence or absence of disc derangement and the degree of change to disc morphology. Although the exact function and related biomechanical properties of the disc have not been fully determined clearly, the highly ordered crimped nature of the collagen indicates its viscoelastic ability to be loaded, and to become stiffer with time.[62,63] There is also a change in the properties of the collagen of the disc with time; it becomes stiffer.[63] This loss of proteoglycans and increased water content probably makes the disc more susceptible to mechanical stresses and increases the risk of disc disruption.

On the microscopic level, fibres extend from anterior to posterior and also in the vertical direction. The chief component of the disc is the glycosaminoglycan chondroitin sulphate. There is a direct relationship between the disc morphology with respect to its length and degree of displacement.

As the degree of displacement increases, so the convexity of the posterior slope of the articular eminence decreases. As the disc displacement increases, so do the inferior, superior and posterior joint spaces.[64]

The meniscus of the TMA is visible in all planes on MR imaging: sagittal oblique, axial and coronal oblique. The appearance of a normal meniscus is that of a biconcave structure of low signal intensity covering the mandibular condyle (Figures 11.04, 11.05). The signal intensity within the meniscus is usually homogeneous, although this depends somewhat on the age of the patient; in the older patient, small alterations in intrameniscal signal intensity may be considered normal.

In the sagittal oblique plane, the meniscus should be directly superior to the mandibular condyle in the closed-mouth position. On the T2-weighted (fluid-sensitive) sequences, the meniscus is outlined by the fluid located in the superior and inferior compartments; this is particularly pronounced on the sagittal oblique slices (Figure 11.09). There is neither means to quantify the volume of fluid that is considered normal or abnormal nor agreement as to what defines these terms; indeed, some authors consider that any fluid noted on the fluid-sensitive sequences should be considered evidence of a joint effusion. The assessment is, therefore, largely down to the experience of the individual radiologist.[30,65–69]

The meniscus is attached posteriorly to the articular capsule. The posterior meniscal attachment may be anatomically divided into three sections: from anterior to posterior, the temporal posterior attachment, the intermediate posterior attachment and the condylar posterior attachment. This last cannot be seen on MR imaging due to the current lack of resolution; however, the first two regions can be identified.[70,71] The attachment is best identified on the sagittal oblique view, where a small band or line of low signal intensity is noted to connect the posterior part of the meniscus to the articular capsule. This can be noted in the closed-mouth and then also in the open-mouth position (Figure 11.10): it should be visible in both positions and demonstrate complete continuity with the meniscus. More specifically, the temporal posterior attachment should be visible in the closed-mouth position as a structure of low signal intensity located posterior to the mandibular condyle. It should be a thin, slightly curved region of tissue. In the open-mouth position, the temporal posterior attachment becomes more arched and is usually noted in the

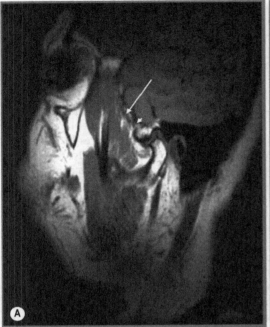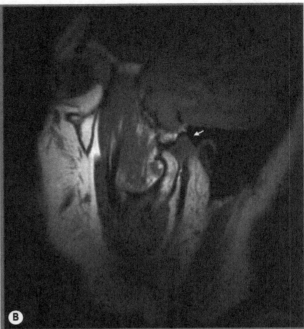

Figure 11.10 • Sagittal T1-weighted MR image of the normal temporomandibular articulation (TMA) performed in the closed-mouth (A) and open-mouth (B) positions. The attachment between the meniscus and the posterior articular capsule can be seen as a thin band of low signal intensity, which should be continuous with the posterior disc (arrow). The superior, temporal attachment, located immediately posterior to the mandibular condyle, is slightly curved but becomes notably more curved when the mouth is open (arrowhead).

normal patient, placed more superiorly, towards the glenoid fossa.

Although the anterior attachment of the meniscus may be visualized, this may not be a constant feature. When seen, the attachment is noted as a low linear signal intensity connecting the thicker meniscus with the articular capsule.

Using MR imaging and this knowledge of normal discal anatomy, the disc can be assessed for disorders involving its displacement, which may reduce in the open-mouth position, remain unreduced in the open-mouth position or be displaced and/or perforated, the latter of which is the more clinically severe.[72] Symptoms related to disc dysfunction may include pain, tenderness and/or noise over the articulation, limited ability to open the mouth, earache and headache.[8]

Muscles (Figures 11.11–11.16)

Of the muscles of mastication, the lateral pterygoid muscle has received the most attention, is the most intimately related to the TMA and has been

implicated as an aetiological factor in disc pathology[46,70,73]; however, the medial pterygoid, masseter and temporalis muscles can also be aetiological factors and are frequently comorbid in TMD.

Lateral pterygoid

The *lateral pterygoid* muscle is divided into two heads: the upper or *superior head* and the lower or *inferior head* (Figures 11.11, 11.13). The superior head originates from the sphenoid bone and the infratemporal surface and crest of the greater wing of the sphenoid bone. The inferior head originates from the lateral surface of the lateral pterygoid plate. The buccal nerve and the maxillary artery pass between the two heads, both of which extend posteriorly to insert into the pterygoid fovea, inferior to the condyloid process of the mandible and into the articular capsule of the TM joint. Some controversy exists as to whether there is also an insertion into the meniscus; although this is often touted as established fact,[1,2,4,74,75] actual cadaveric studies show that there is usually only an attachment to

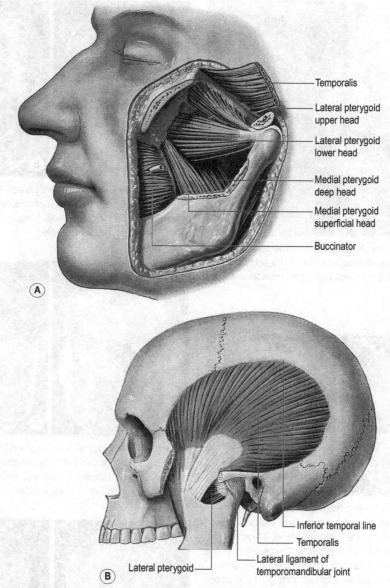

Temporalis

Lateral pterygoid
upper head

Lateral pterygoid
lower head

Medial pterygoid
deep head

Medial pterygoid
superficial head

Buccinator

(A)

Inferior temporal line

Temporalis

Lateral ligament of
temporomandibular joint

Lateral pterygoid

(B)

Figure 11.11 • The muscles of mastication: (A) the pterygoids; (B) the temporalis. (The masseter, which originates on the deep and inferior surfaces of the zygomatic arch and inserts onto the ramus and coronoid process of the mandible, has been removed.) Reproduced, with permission, from Gray's Anatomy 39e, Standring S, ed, (Elsevier, 2005)

the capsule, which, in turn, has connection to the disc.[70,76,77]

The action of the two discrete elements of the lateral pterygoid muscle is complex and has only recently been fully appreciated. When the muscles contract bilaterally, the condyle is pulled anteriorly and inferiorly, assisting the digastric and geniohyoid muscles in opening the jaw. If only one lateral pterygoid contracts, the jaw rotates about a vertical axis passing roughly through the opposite condyle and is pulled contralaterally. This action, together with that of the medial pterygoid (see below), provides most of the medially directed force used when grinding food between teeth of the same side.

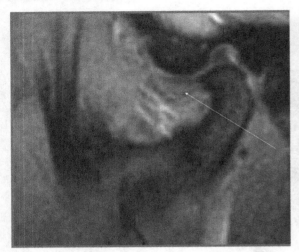

Figure 11.12 • Sagittal oblique, T2-weighted MR imaging of the TMA in the closed-mouth position in a symptomatic patient. A portion of the lateral pterygoid muscle can be noted (arrow).

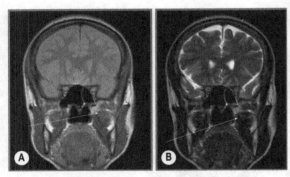

Figure 11.13 • MR imaging through the TMA, which here formed part of an MR imaging study of the brain. Both images are performed in the coronal plane, T1-weighted (A) and T2-weighted (B) demonstrating the position of the lateral pterygoid muscle (arrow), noting the upper and lower portions of the muscle, corresponding to the upper and lower head. In this patient, the muscle is homogeneous with no evidence of atrophy or asymmetry.

The superior head is inactive during jaw opening and most active when the jaws are clenched, although most of the power generated is due to contraction of masseter and temporalis. The latter muscle also acts to potentially pull the condyle posteriorly, and the action is prevented by the simultaneous contraction of the superior head of lateral pterygoid.[1,4]

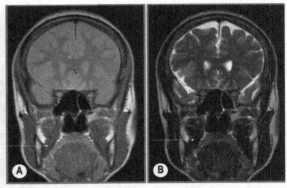

Figure 11.14 • Coronal, T1-weighted (A) and T2-weighted (B) MR imaging of the TMA demonstrating the position of the medial pterygoid muscle (arrow), located just inferior to the lateral pterygoid muscle.

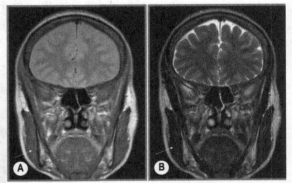

Figure 11.15 • Coronal, T1-weighted (A) and T2-weighted (B) MR imaging of the TMA demonstrating the position of the masseter (arrow), where it is possible to appreciate the superficial nature of this muscle.

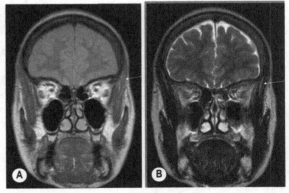

Figure 11.16 • Coronal, T1-weighted (A) and T2-weighted (B) MR imaging of the TMA demonstrating the position of the temporalis muscle (arrow), a much more diminutive muscle as compared with the masseter (Figure 11.15).

Medial pterygoid

As with the lateral pterygoid, its medial counterpart has two heads (Figures 11.11, 11.14). The *deep medial pterygoid* forms the major part of the muscle and arises from the medial surface of the lateral pterygoid plate of the sphenoid, deep to the lower lateral head of lateral pterygoid. The smaller, *superficial medial pterygoid* arises from the pyramidal process of the palatine bone and the maxillary tuberosity. The insertion of both heads is the medial, posteroinferior surface of the ramus and angle of the mandible.[1,4] The muscles act to elevate and protrude the mandible. When acting independently, they pull the chin to the opposite side; used alternately, they can therefore produce a grinding motion.[2]

Masseter

The masseter muscle comprises three layers, the fibres of which blend anteriorly. The largest of these layers is the *superficial masseter*, which arises from the maxillary process of the zygoma and the anterior two-thirds of the inferior border of the zygomatic arch. Its fibres pass posteriorly and inferiorly, to insert into the angle and lower posterior half of the lateral surface of the mandibular ramus. The *middle masseter* arises from the anteromedial two-thirds and posteroinferior one-third of the zygomatic arch, inserting into the central part of the ramus of the mandible. The *deep masseter* arises from the deep surface of the zygomatic arch and inserts into the upper part of the mandibular ramus and its coronoid process (Figure 11.15).[1] There is still debate as to whether fibres of masseter are attached to the anterolateral part of the articular disc of the temporomandibular joint; however, cadaveric studies suggest that the actual attachment is to an area of pseudodiscal material termed the premeniscal lamina.[78,79]

Temporalis

The largest masticatory muscle arises from the temporal fossa and the deep surface of the temporal fascia. Its fibres converge and descend into a tendon that attaches to the medial surface, apex, anterior and posterior borders of the coronoid process and to the anterior border of the mandibular ramus. Fibres of temporalis may occasionally have attachment to the articular disc (Figures 11.12, 11.16).[70,78,79]

Ligaments

The ligamentous capsule of the TMA extends superiorly from the articular tubercle of the temporal bone anteriorly to the region of the squamotympanic fissure posteriorly. In between these two extremes, the capsule has fibres that conform to the contour of the mandibular fossa. Inferiorly, the capsule descends to the level of the neck of the mandible. In the closed-mouth position, the superior portion of the capsule is loose, in contrast to the inferior portion, which is taut.[1,75]

The articular capsule should be visible on the sagittal oblique view, particularly the fluid-sensitive sequences or those where contrast has been added. The capsule is usually noted as a thin, linear structure extending anteriorly and posteriorly. The anterior attachment of the meniscus has a direct insertion into the anterior capsule, which may be visible. However, just because the direct attachment site is not visualized, does not necessarily mean that there is a disruption; it may instead be due to the orientation of the MR slice not corresponding to the capsule anatomy. Similarly, the posterior attachment is usually, but not always, seen connecting with the articular capsule.

Apart from the joint capsule, the ligaments of the TMA are small and rarely injured in isolation. The most frequent cause of ligamentous injury in this joint is dislocation, which can often be associated with a fracture of the mandible.[80,81] There are three ligaments to note (Figure 11.11):

The *sphenomandibular ligament* lies medial to the joint capsule, with which it can sometimes blend. It is a flat, thin band that descends from the spine of the sphenoid, widening as it reaches the lingula of the mandibular foramen. Some fibres traverse the medial end of the petrotympanic fissure and attach to the anterior malleolar process.[82,83]

The (lateral) *temporomandibular ligament* is a broad ligament that arises from the zygomatic process of the temporal bone and extends inferiorly and posteriorly to attach to the lateral surface and posterior border of the neck of the condyle.[84,85]

The *stylomandibular ligament* is a thickened band of deep cervical fascia stretching from the apex and anterior surface of the styloid process of the temporal bone to the angle and posterior border of the mandible. Its function as a ligament has been debated and it can offer little in the way of biomechanical support to the joint; however, it has been postulated that it has a proprioceptive role, and injury to the ligament can cause considerable pain and dysfunction: Ernest syndrome.[1,86,87]

Normal variants and diagnostic pitfalls

Osseous variants

There is an interesting difference between the male and female adolescent population with respect to the contour of the articular surface of the TMA. Statistically significant differences in joint space and contour of the eminence-loading surface have been noted with a normal disc position. In addition, when an anterior disc position in the closed mouth was noted, a noticeable difference in the anatomy of the surrounding bone relationships was also seen; perhaps this goes part of the way to explain the slightly higher prevalence of TMA dysfunction in females.[88]

Muscular variants

There can be considerable variation in the muscles of mastication and these can be detected on MR imaging. This appears to be most clinically significant in the lateral pterygoid muscle, where two types of insertion have been described. In type 1, the superior head of the lateral pterygoid muscle appears to be attached to the meniscus and the inferior head of the lateral pterygoid muscle to the condyle. In type 2, fibres of the lateral pterygoid muscle appear to be attached to both disc and capsule whilst those of the inferior head again attach to the condyle. It has been postulated that, in type 1, the meniscus may be able to displace more easily, which in turn leads to dysfunction in the lateral pterygoid muscle, resulting in muscle atrophy. Equally, hypertonicity of this muscle in type 1 patients may predispose to meniscal displacement.[46]

Pathological conditions

Meniscus

The most common mechanical lesion to affect the TMA is that of discal derangement and this structure needs to be fully examined in the closed- and then open-mouth position, with the possible addition of contrast as deemed necessary.[89,90]

The meniscus can frequently develop a tear within it, often as part of the degenerative process in the older patient, and this may be symptomatic. The easiest way of detecting such a lesion is by assessing the signal intensity of the meniscus on the fluid-sensitive sequences. Normally, the meniscus should be a low signal intensity structure with attachments anteriorly and posteriorly.[42,91]

In a degenerative meniscal tear, a small collection of bright or high signal areas will be located within the body of the meniscus. With meniscal tears that are associated with trauma, in addition to these areas of high signal, joint effusion may be noted. This may act as a natural capsule dilator, accentuating the appearance of the meniscal tear and making it easier to identify. In a traumatic meniscal lesion, associated findings may occur in the attachment of the meniscus to the anterior and, more commonly, the posterior attachments to the articular capsule, which need to be assessed. Although the attachments may not be visible along the whole of their length, a close evaluation on all the slices needs to be performed in order to ensure that the meniscus is intact.[92]

Following the assessment of the signal intensity of the meniscus, the positional relationship needs to be evaluated with respect to the mandibular condyle and articular eminence, or glenoid fossa. Although MR techniques have even been developed to assess the TMA during small incremental degrees of opening, the normal protocol is to assess the patient with the mouth closed, establishing the position of the meniscus, and then having the mouth opened in a secured position to assess for any positional change in the meniscus, which should remain associated with the mandibular condyle, although some slight superior migration is regarded as normal.[93,94]

Most frequently, meniscal displacement occurs anteriorly; this is best assessed on the sagittal images. However, the meniscus can displace medially or laterally, and, in these cases, the coronal or axial images will offer the best visualization.[95,96]

Regardless of the direction of translation of the disc, meniscal displacement can occur in two ways. Either the displacement will occur with meniscal reduction during opening or closing, or the meniscus will remain displaced; what is referred to as non-reducing displacement (Figures 11.17, 11.18). The latter condition is the more challenging to manage and, in general, is associated with a higher level of symptomatology. Whilst assessing the position of the meniscus, it is also useful to look for evidence of degenerative joint disease of the TMA; there is an association between the presence of meniscal displacement and the presence of degenerative joint disease.[93,97,98]

Figure 11.17 • Sagittal oblique, T1-weighted MR images of a 21-year-old female suffering pain in both TMAs. In the closed-mouth position (A), note the anteriorly located position of the meniscus, which is entirely draped anterior to the mandibular condyle (oval) owing to dislocation of the meniscus. In the open-mouth position (B), the meniscus (oval) appears to have reduced.

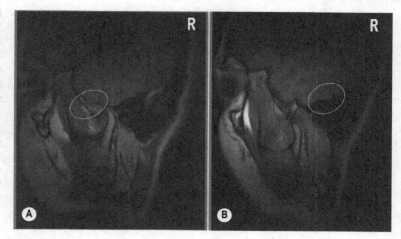

Figure 11.18 • Sagittal oblique, T1-weighted MR images of a 40-year-old female with right jaw pain. In the closed-mouth position (A), the meniscus is completely dislocated anteriorly. In the open-mouth position (B), the meniscus does regain some engagement with the mandibular condyle, representing a degree of recapture; however, this is markedly less than in Figure 11.17B.

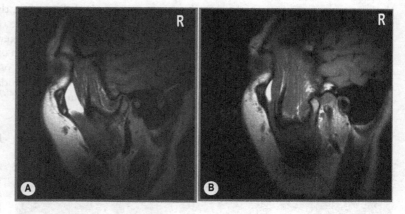

Articular conditions

The mandibular condyles can be affected by various disorders, causing a change in their morphology or the signal intensity therefrom (Figure 11.12). In certain conditions, such as juvenile chronic arthritis, there is an underdevelopment of the mandibular condyles during skeletal growth, which results in bilateral hypoplasia. In other patients, the hypoplasia can be unilateral, resulting from clinical situations such as direct trauma to the TMA (Figure 11.19). Mandibular hypoplasia will be noted on both routine and special imaging as an underdevelopment of the mandibular condyle; the challenge for the clinician is to correlate the findings to the patient's presentation and history to determine whether it is congenital, developmental or acquired. Associated internal derangements, particularly meniscal lesions, may be found with mandibular hypoplasia, presumably because of the altered biomechanical stress placed upon the articulation.[99–101]

The signal intensity of the mandibular condyle may be altered due to either an articular disorder, leading to the development of abnormality in the subchondral bone, or disorders affecting the bony marrow. Articular disorders affecting the mandibular condyle include degenerative joint disease, rheumatoid arthritis and less common conditions such as gout and calcium pyrophosphate crystal deposition disease (CPPD).[98] The synovial membrane that covers the majority of the TMA may also be affected by local processes (including infection and degenerative joint disease) or by systemic synovial-based processes, including rheumatoid arthritis, tuberculosis, gout and pigmented villonodular synovitis.[63,102]

Degenerative joint disease (DJD) will manifest as irregularity of the articular surface, with thinning of the articular cartilage, osteophyte formation, and

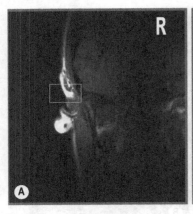
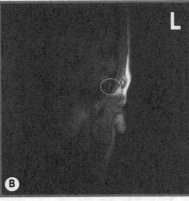

Figure 11.19 • Coronal oblique, T1-weighted MR images of the TMAs in the closed-mouth position. This 24-year-old female patient was complaining of pain in the left TMA. Note the appearance of the normal right mandibular condyle (A), which, in this plane, is smooth and round, with no evidence of irregularity or deformity (rectangle). By contrast, in the left joint (B), the mandibular condyle is irregular and hypoplastic, both images being of the same size proportionally.

subchondral cysts. Although routine radiography can be used to evaluate the TMA for DJD, if internal derangements are suspected, special imaging may be more appropriate. Degenerative changes to the articular surfaces of the TMA are found most often in the lateral third of the joint. Remodelling occurs where there is an alteration of the normal articular contours of the joint and is commonly seen as thinning of the cartilage, possibly as a physiological response to the biomechanical stresses placed upon it. If a contrast study has been performed during the MR imaging, the articular cartilage may be visible and demonstrate this thinning, which can be variable in extent. Degenerative changes are associated with perforation of the disc as well as more classical signs, including osteophyte formation, subchondral cysts and denudation of the articular cartilage (Figure 11.20).[60,97]

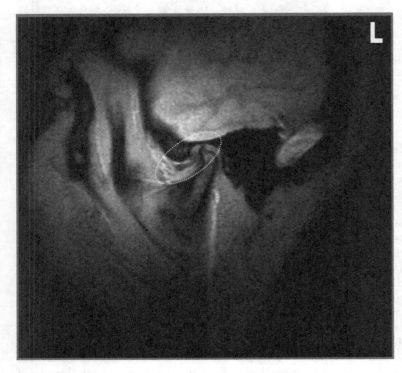

Figure 11.20 • Sagittal oblique, T1-weighted MR image in the closed-mouth position. This 24-year-old female patient had pain in the left articulation. There are two prominent findings with relation to the TMA. There is a loss of the normal round smooth surface of the mandibular condyle, suggesting abnormality. This appearance may be the result of previous trauma or other causes, including an articular-based condition such as rheumatoid arthritis, which may alter the growth and appearance of the mandibular condyle depending at what age the condition arose. The second finding is, again, displacement of the meniscus anteriorly in the closed-mouth position, due to a dislocation (oval encompasses both observations). In this image, it is even possible to determine the anterior insertions of the meniscus in the articular capsule by noting two small thread-like low signal intensity structures leading off anteriorly from the meniscus.

In rheumatoid arthritis, marginal erosions may be seen, with thinning of the articular cartilage particularly prominent. In addition, secondary DJD findings will need to be assessed and synovial effusion may also be detectable. With the use of intravenous gadolinium, active synovitis may be detectable. Internal derangements of the TMA are often associated with rheumatoid arthritis and will be visible on MR imaging.[103,104]

The bony marrow of the mandibular condyle may be affected by osseous pathology. Avascular necrosis of the mandible is a phenomenon that has a well-documented association with medications used to treat osteoporosis; this makes evaluation of the mandibular condyle a particularly important target for clinicians with patients who are being managed with such pharmacological interventions. Patients may complain of discomfort about the TMA, with limitation in the normal range of movement and pain during particular movements that solicit the articulation; the physical examination may also suggest abnormality of the joint. Routine radiography may be able to detect avascular necrosis; however, the sensitivity and specificity of MR imaging in the detection of avascular necrosis,

particularly at an early stage, is well documented.[105,106] Avascular necrosis of the mandibular condyle is shown as a region of high signal on the fluid-sensitive sequences, in a somewhat heterogeneous appearance in the subchondral bone, which may extend to the neck of the mandible. On the T1-weighted image, irregular heterogeneous regions of low signal will be noticed interspersed in the subchondral bone. Associated lesions of the menisci may be noted.[100,107,108]

Clinical pearls

- Patients are imaged in both the closed- and then open-mouth position, allowing for the assessment of disc displacement.
- Often both TMAs are imaged, providing useful comparative information and often revealing clinically silent abnormalities.
- MR imaging allows evaluation of the other soft tissues, which are an often overlooked source of pain, as well as the meniscus.

References

1. Standring S, ed. In: *Gray's Anatomy – Infratemporal region and temporomandibular joint*. (Section 30). Edinburgh: Elsevier; 2009.

2. Moore K. The head. In: *Clinically Oriented Anatomy*. 2nd ed. Baltimore: Williams and Wilkins; 1985:794–982.

3. Green J, Silver P. The scalp and face. In: *An Introduction to Human Anatomy*. Oxford: Oxford University Press; L294–L308, 1981.

4. Okeson J. Functional anatomy and biomechanics of the masticatory system. In: *Management of Temporomandibular Disorders and Occlusion*. 6th ed. St Louis: Elsevier Mosby; 2008:2–24.

5. Young MF. The physics of anatomy. In: *Essential Physics for Musculoskeletal Medicine*. Edinburgh: Elsevier; 2009.

6. Koenigsberg R, ed. *Churchill's Illustrated Medical Dictionary*. New York: Churchill Livingstone; 1989.

7. Standring S, ed. Functional anatomy of the musculoskeletal system. In: *Gray's Anatomy: The Anatomical Basis of Clinical Practice*. 39th ed. Edinburgh: Elsevier; 2005.

8. Okeson J. Signs and symptoms of temporomandibular disorders. In: *Management of Temporomandibular Disorders and Occlusion*. 6th ed. St Louis: Elsevier Mosby; 2008: 164–215.

9. Taub D, Stiles A, Tucke AG. Hemicrania continua presenting as temporomandibular joint pain. *Oral Surg Oral Med Oral Pathol Oral Radiol Endod*. 2008;105(2): e35–e37.

10. Mongini F. Temporomandibular disorders and tension-type headache. *Curr Pain Headache Rep*. 2007;11(6):465–470.

11. Lupoli TA, Lockey RF. Temporomandibular dysfunction: an often overlooked cause of chronic headaches. *Ann Allergy Asthma Immunol*. 2007;99(4): 314–318.

12. Isong U, Gansky SA, Plesh O. Temporomandibular joint and muscle disorder-type pain in U.S. adults: the National Health Interview Survey. *J Orofac Pain*. 2008;22(4):317–322.

13. Janal MN, Raphael KG, Nayak S, Klausner J. Prevalence of myofascial temporomandibular disorder in US community women. *J Oral Rehabil*. 2008;35(11):801–809.

14. Bjorne A. Assessment of temporomandibular and cervical spine disorders in tinnitus patients. *Prog Brain Res*. 2007;166:215–219.

15. Bjorne A, Agerberg G. Reduction in sick leave and costs to society of patients with Meniere's disease after treatment of temporomandibular and cervical spine disorders: a controlled six-year cost-benefit study. *Cranio*. 2003;21(2):136–143.

16. Bjorne A, Agerberg G. Symptom relief after treatment of temporomandibular and cervical spine disorders in patients with Meniere's disease: a three-year

follow-up. *Cranio.* 2003;21(1): 50–60.

17. Wright EF. Otologic symptom improvement through TMD therapy. *Quintessence Int.* 2007;38(9):e564–e571.

18. Tuz HH, Onder EM, Kisnisci RS. Prevalence of otologic complaints in patients with temporomandibular disorder. *Am J Orthod Dentofacial Orthop.* 2003;123(6):620–623.

19. Howat J. *Chiropractic: Anatomy and Physiology of Sacro Occipital Technique.* Oxford: Cranial Communication Systems; 1999.

20. Chaitow L, Commeaux Z. *Cranial Manipulation.* Edinburgh: Elsevier; 2005.

21. Alcantara J, Plaugher G, Klemp DD, Salem C. Chiropractic care of a patient with temporomandibular disorder and atlas subluxation. *J Manipulative Physiol Ther.* 2002; 25(1):63–70.

22. Wessely M, Young MF. Magnetic resonance imaging of the temporomandibular joint. *Clinical Chiropractic.* 2008;11(1):37–44.

23. Bates B. The musculoskeletal system. In: Bates B, ed. *A Guide to Physical Examination.* 3rd ed. Philadelphia: JB Lippincott; 1983: 324–370.

24. Okeson J. History and examination for temporomandibular disorders. In: *Management of Temporo-mandibular Disorders and Occlusion.* 6th ed. St Louis: Elsevier Mosby; 2008:216–285.

25. Yatani H, Studts J, Cordova M, et al. Comparison of sleep quality and clinical and psychologic characteristics in patients with temporomandibular disorders. *J Orofac Pain.* 2002; 16(3): 221–228.

26. Drum RK, Fornadley JA, Schnapf DJ. Malignant lesions presenting as symptoms of craniomandibular dysfunction. *J Orofac Pain.* 1993;7(3): 294–299.

27. Yoon SZ, Lee SI, Choi SU, et al. A case of facial myofascial pain syndrome presenting as trigeminal neuralgia. *Oral Surg Oral Med Oral Pathol Oral Radiol Endod.* 2009; 107(3):e29–e31.

28. Foreman PA. Chronic orofacial pain: a clinical challenge. *N Z Dent J.* 2008;104(2):44–48.

29. Kanehira H, Agariguchi A, Kato H, et al. Association between stress and temporomandibular disorder. *Nihon Hotetsu Shika Gakkai Zasshi.* 2008;52(3):375–380.

30. Costa AL, D'Abreu A, Cendes F. Temporomandibular joint internal derangement: association with headache, joint effusion, bruxism, and joint pain. *J Contemp Dent Pract.* 2008;9(6):9–16.

31. Huang GJ, Drangsholt MT, Rue TC, et al. Age and third molar extraction as risk factors for temporomandibular disorder. *J Dent Res.* 2008;87(3): 283–287.

32. Huang GJ, Rue TC. Third-molar extraction as a risk factor for temporomandibular disorder. *J Am Dent Assoc.* 2006;137(11): 1547–1554.

33. Mackie A, Lyons K. The role of occlusion in temporomandibular disorders—a review of the literature. *N Z Dent J.* 2008;104(2):54–59.

34. Travell J, Simons D. *Myofascial Pain and Dysfunction.* Baltimore: Williams and Wilkins; 1992.

35. Thomas CA, Okeson JP. Evaluation of lateral pterygoid muscle symptoms using a common palpation technique and a method of functional manipulation. *Cranio.* 1987;5(2):125–129.

36. Agerberg G. Maximal mandibular movements in teen-agers. *Acta Morphol Neerl Scand.* 1974;12(2): 79–102.

37. Agerberg G, Osterberg T. Maximal mandibular movements and symptoms of mandibular dysfunction in 70-year old men and women. *Sven Tandlak Tidskr.* 1974;67(3):147–163.

38. Agerberg G. Maximal mandibular movements in young men and women. *Sven Tandlak Tidskr.* 1974;67(2):81–100.

39. Agerberg G. Maximal mandibular movements in children. *Acta Odontol Scand.* 1974;32(3): 147–159.

40. Suarez P, Clark G. Oral conditions of 1,049 patients referred to a university-based oral medicine and orofacial pain center. *Spec Care Dentist.* 2007;27(5):191–195.

41. Okeson J. Etiology of functional disturbances in the masticatory system. In: *Management of*

Temporomandibular Disorders and Occlusion. 6th ed. St Louis: Elsevier Mosby; 2008:130–163.

42. El-Essawy MT, Al-Nakshabandi NA, Al-Boukai AA. Magnetic resonance imaging evaluation of temporomandibular joint derangement in symptomatic and asymptomatic patients. *Saudi Med J.* 2008;29(10):1448–1452.

43. Jirman R, Fricova M, Horak Z, et al. Analyses of the temporomandibular disc. *Prague Med Rep.* 2007;108(4): 368–379.

44. Okeson J. Diagnosis of temporomandibular disorders. In: *Management of Temporomandibular Disorders and Occlusion.* 6th ed. St Louis: Elsevier Mosby; 2008: 285–332.

45. Bakke M, Moller E, Werdelin LM, et al. Treatment of severe temporomandibular joint clicking with botulinum toxin in the lateral pterygoid muscle in two cases of anterior disc displacement. *Oral Surg Oral Med Oral Pathol Oral Radiol Endod.* 2005;100(6): 693–700.

46. Taskaya-Yilmaz N, Ceylan G, Incesu L, Muglali M. A possible etiology of the internal derangement of the temporomandibular joint based on the MRI observations of the lateral pterygoid muscle. *Surg Radiol Anat.* 2005;27(1): 19–24.

47. Lewis EL, Dolwick MF, Abramowicz S, Reeder SL. Contemporary imaging of the temporomandibular joint. *Dent Clin North Am.* 2008;52(4): 875–890, viii.

48. Pereira LJ, Gaviao MB, Bonjardim LR, Castelo PM. Ultrasound and tomographic evaluation of temporomandibular joints in adolescents with and without signs and symptoms of temporomandibular disorders: a pilot study. *Dentomaxillofac Radiol.* 2007;36(7):402–408.

49. Tvrdy P. Methods of imaging in the diagnosis of temporomandibular joint disorders. *Biomed Pap Med Fac Univ Palacky Olomouc Czech Repub.* 2007;151(1):133–136.

50. Vilanova JC, Barcelo J, Puig J, et al. Diagnostic imaging: magnetic resonance imaging, computed tomography, and ultrasound. *Semin*

Ultrasound CT MR. 2007;28(3): 184–191.

51. Gonzalez YM, Greene CS, Mohl ND. Technological devices in the diagnosis of temporomandibular disorders. *Oral Maxillofac Surg Clin North Am.* 2008;20(2):211–220, vi.

52. Hussain AM, Packota G, Major PW, Flores-Mir C. Role of different imaging modalities in assessment of temporomandibular joint erosions and osteophytes: a systematic review. *Dentomaxillofac Radiol.* 2008;37(2):63–71.

53. Murakami K, Nishida M, Bessho K, et al. MRI evidence of high signal intensity and temporomandibular arthralgia and relating pain. Does the high signal correlate to the pain? *Br J Oral Maxillofac Surg* 1996;34(3): 220–224.

54. Westesson PL, Brooks SL. Temporomandibular joint: relationship between MR evidence of effusion and the presence of pain and disk displacement. *Am J Roentgenol.* 1992;159(3): 559–563.

55. Haley DP, Schiffman EL, Lindgren BR, et al. The relationship between clinical and MRI findings in patients with unilateral temporomandibular joint pain. *J Am Dent Assoc.* 2001;132(4): 476–481.

56. Kaplan P, Helms C, Dussault R, Anderson M. Temporomandibular joint. In: *Musculoskeletal MRI.* Philadelphia: WB Saunders; 2001: 169–173.

57. Taskaya-Yilmaz N, Ogutcen-Toller M. Magnetic resonance imaging evaluation of temporomandibular joint disc deformities in relation to type of disc displacement. *J Oral Maxillofac Surg.* 2001;59(8):860–865, discussion 5–6.

58. Gynther GW, Holmlund AB, Reinholt FP, Lindblad S. Temporomandibular joint involvement in generalized osteoarthritis and rheumatoid arthritis: a clinical, arthroscopic, histologic, and immunohisto-chemical study. *Int J Oral Maxillofac Surg.* 1997;26(1):10–16.

59. Joseph J. Locomotor system: temporomandibular joint. In: Hamilton W, ed. *Textbook of Human Anatomy.* 2nd ed. London: MacMillan; 1976:82–83.

60. Stratmann U, Schaarschmidt K, Santamaria P. Morphometric investigation of condylar cartilage and disc thickness in the human temporomandibular joint: significance for the definition of osteoarthrotic changes. *J Oral Pathol Med.* 1996;25(5):200–205.

61. Akerman S, Kopp S, Rohlin M. Histological changes in temporomandibular joints from elderly individuals. An autopsy study. *Acta Odontol Scand.* 1986;44(4):231–239.

62. Berkovitz BK. Crimping of collagen in the intra-articular disc of the temporomandibular joint: a comparative study. *J Oral Rehabil.* 2000;27(7):608–613.

63. Berkovitz BK. Collagen crimping in the intra-articular disc and articular surfaces of the human temporomandibular joint. *Arch Oral Biol.* 2000;45(9):749–756.

64. Smith HJ, Larheim TA, Aspestrand F. Rheumatic and nonrheumatic disease in the temporomandibular joint: gadolinium-enhanced MR imaging. *Radiology.* 1992;185(1):229–234.

65. Lee SH, Yoon HJ. MRI findings of patients with temporomandibular joint internal derangement: before and after performance of arthrocentesis and stabilization splint. *J Oral Maxillofac Surg.* 2009;67(2):314–317.

66. Emshoff R, Rudisch A. Temporomandibular joint internal derangement and osteoarthrosis: are effusion and bone marrow edema prognostic indicators for arthrocentesis and hydraulic distention? *J Oral Maxillofac Surg.* 2007;65(1):66–73.

67. Emshoff R, Brandlmaier I, Gerhard S, et al. Magnetic resonance imaging predictors of temporomandibular joint pain. *J Am Dent Assoc.* 2003;134(6):705–714.

68. Emshoff R, Brandimaier I, Bertram S, Rudisch A. Magnetic resonance imaging findings of osteoarthrosis and effusion in patients with unilateral temporomandibular joint pain. *Int J Oral Maxillofac Surg.* 2002;31(6): 598–602.

69. Rudisch A, Innerhofer K, Bertram S, Emshoff R. Magnetic resonance imaging findings of internal derangement and effusion in patients with unilateral temporomandibular joint pain. *Oral Surg Oral Med Oral Pathol Oral Radiol Endod.* 2001; 92(5):566–571.

70. Christo JE, Bennett S, Wilkinson TM, Townsend GC. Discal attachments of the human temporomandibular joint. *Aust Dent J.* 2005;50(3):152–160.

71. Sindelar BJ, Herring SW. Soft tissue mechanics of the temporomandibular joint. *Cells Tissues Organs.* 2005; 180(1):36–43.

72. Suenaga S, Ogura T, Matsuda T, Noikura T. Severity of synovium and bone marrow abnormalities of the temporomandibular joint in early rheumatoid arthritis: role of gadolinium-enhanced fat-suppressed T1-weighted spin echo MRI. *J Comput Assist Tomogr.* 2000;24(3): 461–465.

73. Usui A, Akita K, Yamaguchi K. An anatomic study of the divisions of the lateral pterygoid muscle based on the findings of the origins and insertions. *Surg Radiol Anat.* 2008;30(4):327–333.

74. Joseph J. Locomotor system: muscles of the head. In: Hamilton W, ed. *Textbook of Human Anatomy.* 2nd ed. London: MacMillan; 1976:154–158.

75. Palastanga N, Field D, Soames R. Head and brain. In: *Anatomy and Human Movement: Structure and Function.* 5th ed. Edinburgh: Elsevier Butterworth Heinemann; 2006:635–694.

76. Heylings DJ, Nielsen IL, McNeill C. Lateral pterygoid muscle and the temporomandibular disc. *J Orofac Pain.* 1995;9(1):9–16.

77. Zhang L, Sun L, Ma X. [A macroscopic and microscopic study of the relationship between the superior lateral pterygoid muscle and the disc of the temporomandibular joint]. *Zhonghua Kou Qiang Yi Xue Za Zhi.* 1998;33(5):267–269.

78. Le Toux G, Duval JM, Darnault P. The human temporo-mandibular joint: current anatomic and physiologic status. *Surg Radiol Anat.* 1989;11(4):283–288.

79. Merida Velasco JR, Rodriguez Vazquez JF, Jimenez Collado J. The relationships between the temporomandibular joint disc and related masticatory muscles in

humans. *J Oral Maxillofac Surg.* 1993;51(4):390–395, discussion 5–6.

80. Schwartz AJ. Dislocation of the mandible: a case report. *AANA J.* 2000;68(6):507–513.

81. Umstadt HE, Ellers M, Muller HH, Austermann KH. Functional reconstruction of the TM joint in cases of severely displaced fractures and fracture dislocation. *J Craniomaxillofac Surg.* 2000; 28(2):97–105.

82. Sencimen M, Yalcin B, Dogan N, et al. Anatomical and functional aspects of ligaments between the malleus and the temporomandibular joint. *Int J Oral Maxillofac Surg.* 2008;37(10):943–947.

83. Shiozaki H, Abe S, Tsumori N, et al. Macroscopic anatomy of the sphenomandibular ligament related to the inferior alveolar nerve block. *Cranio.* 2007;25(3):160–165.

84. Alomar X, Medrano J, Cabratosa J, et al. Anatomy of the temporomandibular joint. *Semin Ultrasound CT MR.* 2007;28(3): 170–183.

85. Tomas X, Pomes J, Berenguer J, et al. Temporomandibular joint soft-tissue pathology, II: Nondisc abnormalities. *Semin Ultrasound CT MR.* 2007; 28(3):205–212.

86. Brown CR. Ernest syndrome: insertion tendinosis of the stylomandibular ligament. *Pract Periodontics Aesthet Dent.* 1996; 8(8):762.

87. Shankland WE 2nd. Ernest syndrome as a consequence of stylomandibular ligament injury: a report of 68 patients. *J Prosthet Dent.* 1987;57(4):501–506.

88. Major PW, Kinniburgh RD, Nebbe B, et al. Tomographic assessment of temporomandibular joint osseous articular surface contour and spatial relationships associated with disc displacement and disc length. *Am J Orthod Dentofacial Orthop.* 2002;121(2):152–161.

89. Helms C, Major N, Anderson MW, et al. The temporomandibular joint.

In: *Musculoskeletal MRI.* 2nd ed. Philadelphia: Elsevier Saunders; 2009:172–176.

90. Ribeiro RF, Tallents RH, Katzberg RW, et al. The prevalence of disc displacement in symptomatic and asymptomatic volunteers aged 6 to 25 years. *J Orofac Pain.* 1997;11(1):37–47.

91. Katzberg RW, Westesson PL, Tallents RH, Drake CM. Anatomic disorders of the temporomandibular joint disc in asymptomatic subjects. *J Oral Maxillofac Surg.* 1996; 54(2):147–153, discussion 53–55.

92. Tomas X, Pomes J, Berenguer J, et al. MR imaging of temporomandibular joint dysfunction: a pictorial review. *Radiographics.* 2006;26(3):765–781.

93. Burnett KR, Davis CL, Read J. Dynamic display of the temporomandibular joint meniscus by using "fast-scan" MR imaging. *Am J Roentgenol.* 1987;149(5): 959–962.

94. Okeson J. Mechanics of mandibular movement. In: *Management of Temporomandibular Disorders and Occlusion.* 6th ed. St Louis: Elsevier Mosby; 2008:81–94.

95. Nebbe B, Major PW. Prevalence of TMA disc displacement in a pre-orthodontic adolescent sample. *Angle Orthod.* 2000;70(6):454–463.

96. Milano V, Desiate A, Bellino R, Garofalo T. Magnetic resonance imaging of temporomandibular disorders: classification, prevalence and interpretation of disc displacement and deformation. *Dentomaxillofac Radiol.* 2000; 29(6):352–361.

97. Kondoh T, Westesson PL, Takahashi T, Seto K. Prevalence of morphological changes in the surfaces of the temporomandibular joint disc associated with internal derangement. *J Oral Maxillofac Surg.* 1998;56(3):339–343, discussion 43–44.

98. Beers M, Berkow R. Temporomandibular disorders. In: *The Merck Manual.* 17th ed. Merck & Co: West Point, PA; 1999:772–776.

99. Pirttiniemi P, Peltomaki T, Muller L, Luder HU. Abnormal mandibular growth and the condylar cartilage. *Eur J Orthod.* 2009;31(1):1–11.

100. Larheim TA. Role of magnetic resonance imaging in the clinical diagnosis of the temporomandibular joint. *Cells Tissues Organs.* 2005; 180(1):6–21.

101. Singh DJ, Bartlett SP. Congenital mandibular hypoplasia: analysis and classification. *J Craniofac Surg.* 2005;16(2):291–300.

102. Larheim TA, Katzberg RW, Westesson PL, et al. MR evidence of temporomandibular joint fluid and condyle marrow alterations: occurrence in asymptomatic volunteers and symptomatic patients. *Int J Oral Maxillofac Surg.* 2001;30(2):113–117.

103. Scutellari PN, Orzincolo C. Rheumatoid arthritis: sequences. *Eur J Radiol.* 1998;27(suppl 1): S31–S38.

104. Ozcan I, Ozcan KM, Keskin D, et al. Temporomandibular joint involvement in rheumatoid arthritis: correlation of clinical, laboratory and magnetic resonance imaging findings. *B-ENT.* 2008; 4(1):19–24.

105. Kaplan P, Helms C, Dussault R, Anderson M. *Musculoskeletal MRI.* Philadelphia: WB Saunders; 2001.

106. Rowe L, Yochum T. Hematological and vascular disorders. In: Yochum T, Rowe L, eds. *Essentials of Skeletal Radiology.* 2nd ed. Baltimore: Williams and Wilkins; 1996:1243–1326.

107. Fu KY, Li YW, Zhang ZK, Ma XC. Osteonecrosis of the mandibular condyle as a precursor to osteoarthrosis: a case report. *Oral Surg Oral Med Oral Pathol Oral Radiol Endod.* 2009;107(1): e34–e38.

108. Campos PS, Freitas CE, Pena N, et al. Osteochondritis dissecans of the temporomandibular joint. *Dentomaxillofac Radiol.* 2005;34(3):193–197.

Index

Osseous structure *see* Bone(s)
Os supratrochleare, elbow, 193
Osteoarthritis, elbow, 207
Osteoblastoma, cervical spine
    neoplasms, 28–29
Osteochondral defects, foot and ankle,
    138–139, 139*f*
Osteochondral trauma, knee, 116, 117*f*
Osteochondritis dissecans, elbow, 194
Osteochondrosis, elbow, 194–195,
    195*f*
Osteoid osteoma, cervical spine
    neoplasms, 28–29
Osteomyelitis
    cervical spine, 29
    elbow, 206
    foot and ankle, 144
Osteophytes, lumbar spine vertebrae,
    71, 72
Osteoporosis, hip and pelvis, 98
Os trigonum syndrome, 128, 136

P

Paediatric considerations, foot and
    ankle, 136–138
Pain diagrams, hip and pelvis
    examination, 81
Palmaris longus muscle, 191
Panic attacks, as contraindication, 63
Pannus, cervical spine degenerative
    disease, 24–25
Paraspinal muscles, lumbar spine, 64
'Parson's knee,' knee examination, 102*t*
Partial tendon tears
    elbow tendons, 200–201
    rotator cuff disease, 164*f*, 165, 166*f*,
        168–169
Patella *see* Knee
Patella cubiti, elbow, 193
Patellar tracking syndrome, 102
Patient questions, 6
Patrick/FABER test, 82
Pellegrini–Stieda disease, 198–199
Pelvis *see* Hip and pelvis
Peroneus brevis tendon, 133, 133*f*
    diseases/disorders, 143
Peroneus longus tendon, 133, 133*f*
    diseases/disorders, 143
Peroneus tertius tendon, 134
Pes planus deformity, 141
Phase coherence, 2
Piedallu test, 82*t*
'Pitcher's elbow,' 202

Plantar fasciitis, foot and ankle,
    145–146, 145*f*
Polymyalgia rheumatica, shoulder pain
    vs., 150*t*
Popliteal bursa, knee, 110–111
Positioning
    rotator cuff disease, 168
    shoulder, 151–152
    wrist and hand, 213–214
Posterior cruciate ligament, 108, 110*f*
    injuries, 120, 122*f*
Posterior glenohumeral instability,
    173–174
Posterior impingement syndrome,
    136
Posterior internal impingement
    syndromes, 162
Posterior interosseous nerve, 188
Posterior labral tears, glenohumeral
    instability, 174
Posterior labrocapsular periosteal sleeve
    lesion (POLPSA), 174
Posterior longitudinal ligament (PLL),
    16
Posterior talofibular (PTAF) ligament,
    134
    diseases/disorders, 141
Posterior tendons, foot and ankle, 132
Posterior tibiofibular (PTIF) ligament,
    136
    diseases/disorders, 141
Posterosuperior labral absence,
    shoulder, 154
Postsurgical spine, lumbar spine,
    74–77
Pregnancy
    as contraindication, 63
    gadolinium contrast agents, 63–64
Pronator (median nerve) syndrome,
    elbow, 188, 202–203
Pronator teres muscle, 191
Prostate carcinoma, cervical spine
    metastases, 29
Proton density (PD) images
    contrast, 5
    shoulder, 151
Provocative tests, shoulder, 149–150
Proximal femur, 87, 90*f*
Psoas muscle, 64
Psoriatic arthritis, cervical spine, 25
Pulses, knee examination, 101–102
Pulse sequences, 5–6
    inversion recovery (IR), 6
    spin echo (SE), 5–6

Q

Quadriceps angle (Q-angle), knee
    examination, 102, 103*f*

R

Radial collateral ligament, 182*f*, 192
    trauma, 200, 200*f*
Radial fissures, lumbar spine disc
    disease, 69
Radial nerve, 188
    brachioradialis muscle, 188
    entrapment, 203
    neuropathy, 204
    supinator muscle, 188
Radial tunnel syndrome, 202–203
Radiculopathy, cervical disc herniation,
    11–12
Radiographic latent period, foot and
    ankle infections, 143–144
Radiography
    elbow, 182
    shoulder, 151
Radiohumeral meniscus (labrum),
    elbow, 206
Radius
    elbow dislocations, 197
    head fractures, 196–197
Referral forms, 6–7, 7*f*
Relaxation time, tissues, 3
Repeated strains, foot and ankle, 141
Repetition time (TR), contrast, 3, 3*f*
Requests (for magnetic resonance
    imaging), 77
Rheumatoid arthritis
    cervical spine, 25
    elbow, 206–207
    temporomandibular articulation,
        243
    wrist and hand, 217, 219*f*
Rotator cuff disease, 160, 161–169
    impingement syndromes, 161–165
        acromioclavicular joint osteophytes,
            161, 161*f*
        anterior internal impingement, 162,
            164*f*
        extrinsic impingement, 165
        glenohumeral instability, 161–162
        Hawkins test, 162, 163*f*
        intrinsic cuff degeneration, 162
        muscle hypertrophy, 162
        Neer test, 162, 163*f*
        os acromiale, 161, 161*f*

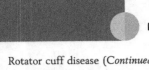

Printed in the United States
By Bookmasters